Dr Paula Baillie-Hamilton is a London-university-trained medical doctor and has previously worked in the following fields: cardiology, gastroenterology, rheumatology, paediatrics, emergency medicine, psychiatry, obstetrics and gynaecology, endocrinology, oncology, general medicine and general surgery. She also holds an academic doctorate for her research into the effects of toxic chemicals on human health at Christ Church, Oxford University.

She is now a Visiting Fellow in Occupational and Environmental Health at Stirling University. She is also a full member of the British Society for Allergy, Environmental and Nutritional Medicine and is one of the country's foremost experts on toxic chemicals and their harmful effects on our health, and has published full papers in international academic journals in this field.

Her first book, *The Detox Diet* (UK) (also known as *The Body Restoration Plan*) was published in the UK in April 2002. The book has also been translated into Dutch and German and to date over 250,000 copies are in print. She now writes for UK newspapers and magazines and the US-based magazine *Phenomena* about modern day health issues.

This book is dedicated to my dearly beloved husband Mike and wonderful children Angus, Bruce, Lucy and Rory ...

As well as to you and your children

Stop the 21st Century Killing You

Toxic chemicals have invaded our lives.
Fight back!
Eliminate toxins, tackle illness,
get healthy and live longer

DR PAULA BAILLIE-HAMILTON

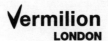

Vermilion
LONDON

3 5 7 9 10 8 6 4 2

First published in the United Kingdom in 2005 by Vermilion,
an imprint of Ebury Publishing
Random House UK Ltd.
Random House
20 Vauxhall Bridge Road
London SW1V 2SA

Random House Australia (Pty) Limited
20 Alfred Street, Milsons Point, Sydney,
New South Wales 2061, Australia

Random House New Zealand Limited
18 Poland Road, Glenfield,
Auckland 10, New Zealand

Random House (Pty) Limited
Endulini, 5A Jubilee Road, Parktown 2193, South Africa

Random House UK Limited Reg. No. 954009
www.randomhouse.co.uk

Papers used by Vermilion are natural, recyclable products
made from wood grown in sustainable forests.

A CIP catalogue record is available for this book from the British Library.

ISBN: 0091894670

Designed and typeset by seagulls

Printed and bound in Great Britain by
Mackays of Chatham plc, Chatham, Kent

Contents

Acknowledgements

It is a fact universally acknowledged that it is impossible to write a book without the support of others. So I would like to take this opportunity to thank all those who have played a pivotal role in the creation and production of this book.

The biggest thanks goes to my publisher Eileen Campbell who, with a flick of her magic wand, turned an idea into reality. I am also exceedingly indebted to Amanda Hemmings for her fantastic editorial advice and creative skills and everyone at Random House who has helped in the production of this book, in particular Julia Kellaway, who has co-ordinated the editing for this book in a highly professional and exemplary manner, Richard Emerson and Imogen Fortes. On the subject of editors, I would also like to thank my sister Julia for her extremely constructive editorial advice and for all her excellent help and support every step of the way.

Others I would particularly like to thank are my literary agent Robert Kirby and his very able assistant Catherine Cameron, my father John Hickman and mother Pat Hickman for looking after my children often at short notice so I could complete this book.

Lastly I would like to acknowledge Professor Kim Jobst and all the other people I have not mentioned who have played a role in supporting me personally or professionally in achieving my goals. Thank you all!

Author Note

Neither the publisher nor the author is engaged in rendering professional advice or services to the individual reader. The ideas, procedures and suggestions contained in this book are not intended as a substitute for consulting your physician. All matters regarding health require medical supervision. Neither the author nor the publisher shall be liable or responsible for any loss, injury or damage allegedly arising from any information or suggestion in this book.

Neither the publisher nor the author is responsible for specific health or allergy needs that may require medical supervision. While the author has made every effort to provide accurate telephone numbers and Internet addresses at the time of publication, neither the publisher nor the author assumes any responsibility for errors or for changes that occur after publication.

Introduction

Thank you for buying *Stop the 21st Century Killing You*. I hope this book will be of great benefit to you. It is packed with vitally important information and tips to help you to survive the twenty-first century in the best of health. It has been designed to increase your knowledge of the many factors underlying and triggering diseases, which to date conventional medicine has not adequately recognised or catered for. It will also present you with a whole host of proven ways in which alternative and complementary medical treatments could vastly improve your health.

This is the second book that I have written in this field. I have loved every minute of the extensive time and effort that has gone into researching and writing it. Over the years, I have discovered that the problems caused by the twenty-first century, such as increased pollution, changed lifestyles and poorer nutrition, appear to have played a major part in the numerous health epidemics that we are seeing today. The good news is that far from being an insoluble problem, there are many proven and effective ways in which the situation can be turned around, thus raising current levels of health to a new, higher plane.

This book uses the detox approach throughout. This means that, rather than just tackling disease symptoms, it also sets out to target the actual known causes of disease. It does this by providing you, the reader, with the often little publicised facts about how certain chemicals can actually damage your health, which diseases they trigger and how to rid them from your body.

One of my favourite occupations is talking to the people whose lives have been revolutionised by using these complementary methods. By understanding more about the origins of their disorders, they have been able to seek out the most effective cures for their own unique situations. In many instances, the results have been quite breathtaking.

To give you an example, several months after my first book *The Detox Diet* was published in the UK, I received a letter from a reader. Rather than summarising it, I would like to print the letter just as she wrote it to me.

'I am 59 years old and for the last 12 years I have had very poor health. Originally I was diagnosed with ME [myalgic encephalomyelitis] but last year, after contacting a specialist doctor, on investigating my medical history, and the events leading up to my physical collapse, she diagnosed organophosphate poisoning.

'When I read the article publicising your book I thought that, although it was written for people without serious organophosphate problems, it might help me. I obtained your book and have followed the advice closely, but without food restrictions. I am sure you will be pleased to hear that I am feeling normal, which is a condition I had thought I would never feel again.

'Now:

■ I sleep for eight hours per night;
■ I can stay up all day;
■ I have been able to walk around the shopping area without excruciating pain a few hours later;
■ I have begun to do my own housework;
■ I recently drove 120 miles without having to spend the next 48 hours in bed recovering;
■ Best of all I can make arrangements to go out knowing that I will be well enough to attend the event;
■ I used to sleep with a TENS [painkilling] machine strapped to my legs to dull the pain, and have only used it twice since I began your regime;
■ I am also losing weight and inches, but I am trying not to lose too much too quickly, as at my age my skin is not elastic and I am trying to avoid saggy skin. I can't thank you enough for the effort you put in to gather the enormous amount of information necessary to make a coherent manual for a healthy life.'

From this and a great deal more feedback from others, I know that it is realistically possible to make a positive impact and help people to turn their lives around. The knowledge that there is no book currently available to help people deal with all the issues covered here is what has inspired and driven me to write *Stop the 21st Century Killing You.*

The aim of this book is to guide you through the modern-day health maze. Whether you currently have one of the 30 or so illnesses covered in this book or are looking to optimise your health, it will tell you what to look out for – as well as the major twenty-first century health hazards that should be avoided. It will also explain how you can make the most of your situation.

This is followed by a wealth of information in the appendices designed to help you turn these exciting concepts into reality. There you will find out more about the toxic chemicals that could be damaging your health so you can start to avoid them. It will also explore the many options open to you to reverse the situation by revealing the best sources of nutrients from both foods and supplements and outlining the 8 most popular herbals. More practical advice to help guide you on your path to wellbeing can be found by contacting one of the many health organisations mentioned in the Useful Contacts section (page 319).

Whatever your particular reasons for being interested in your health, I wish you all the best on your voyage towards discovering what really works for you. There are some truly amazing health benefits waiting to be discovered, and some of them could make all the difference to your future wellbeing. I wish you good health and a very long and happy life.

part one

21st Century Health

1

21st Century Diseases

Diseases once thought of as rare are now widespread. In the year 1900, less than 4 per cent of the UK population died of heart disease and cancer combined. In 2002, this figure had increased to an unprecedented 65 per cent.

Good health – a vanishing dream?

If you have picked up this book, the chances are that you either think you have a twenty-first century disease and are trying to improve your health – or you are well and wanting to stay that way. Either way, you will know that good health is becoming more and more of a rare commodity. There has been a dramatic change in the pattern of disease over the last century, mainly due to the fact that in the past many people died of diseases, such as measles, that are no longer regarded as fatal due to basic

Diabetes: an example of a classic 21st century disease

Since first described over 3,000 years ago by the ancient Egyptians, the formerly rare disease of diabetes has over the last few decades been transformed into a potentially disabling and life-threatening condition affecting huge numbers of people. Now, despite all the advances modern science has to offer, this explosion in numbers of people affected means that more people per head of population are dying of diabetes than in 1900 – and that's 22 years before the discovery of insulin!

With the World Health Organization (WHO) predicting that the number of people with diabetes worldwide is set to double to 300 million by the year 2025, and with a staggering one in ten UK citizens set to develop diabetes in his or her lifetime, the current situation appears to be in freefall. (See chemicals linked to diabetes, page 174.)

Typical 21st century illnesses

- Allergies (including hay fever)
- Arthritis and connective tissue disorders
- Asthma
- Attention Deficit Hyperactivity Disorder (ADHD)
- Autoimmune diseases
- Cancer
- Chemical sensitivities
- Chronic fatigue syndrome (CFS)
- Depression
- Diabetes
- Dyslexia
- Eczema
- Food intolerances

- Heart disease
- High cholesterol
- Hypertension
- Immune system suppression
- Infertility
- Inflammatory bowel disease (IBD)
- Irritable bowel syndrome (IBS)
- Low energy levels
- Memory loss
- Multiple sclerosis (MS)
- Obesity
- Parkinson's disease (PD)
- Stroke
- Thyroid disease

improvements in the standard of living. As a consequence, people are now living long enough to contract degenerative diseases. However, the current day disease pattern cannot be explained away by an ageing population alone, as the whole pattern of diseases we are now affected by seems to have dramatically changed.

People have started to get diseases at younger ages and the number of infants and children contracting catastrophic illnesses has never been higher. Furthermore, totally new illnesses such as chronic fatigue syndrome (CFS), autism and chemical sensitivities have not only emerged but are already affecting large swathes of the population. In certain instances, the pace of change has been so remarkable that the number of those affected by many of these diseases appears to have doubled every few decades.

Ironically, we have never been so health conscious – with ever increasing numbers of people cutting out excess fat, counting calories and working out at the gym. So, in light of the existing evidence, it is fair to say that there seems to be something about the twenty-first century that appears to be killing us.

What is behind this 21st century disease plague?

As you can imagine, I am not the first scientist to question what is going on as, to date, many billions of pounds have been spent in researching these diseases. However, most of this research tends to focus on finding disease treatments rather than looking for the underlying causes of these illnesses. This has resulted in an ever-increasing number of drugs coming on to the market designed to 'tweak' the system, lessen aggravating symptoms but in most cases not cure the disease itself. So while the health of the pharmaceutical industry has never been better, the health of the population has continued to plummet, and will continue to do so unless we go back to basics and improve our efforts in preventing people from becoming ill in the first place.

So what appears to be at the heart of twenty-first century disease?

Man-made chemicals and heavy metals: The heart of the problem appears to be that over the past 100 or so years, the quantity of toxic chemicals in our environment has been rising to levels that have never been higher in man's entire history. Every single creature on the face of this earth is now permanently contaminated with these chemicals. The problem is that the human body was never designed to protect itself against this form of chemical onslaught. Unfortunately for us, one of the main consequences of our comparative inability to break down these chemicals is a build-up of chemicals in the body. The greater the build-up of chemicals, the more pronounced their ability to disrupt the smooth running of the body's systems. The consequence of this constant 24/7 poisoning has, not surprisingly, been the development and triggering of an escalating number of diseases, such as diabetes, asthma and cancer.

Chemicals + humans = chemical-triggered diseases

So in view of the ever increasing levels of chemical pollution now present, many leading scientists have hypothesised that these chemicals are probably playing a significant role in bringing about the twenty-first century disease epidemics. Let's be totally clear about this: with chemical production continuing to rise to ever greater heights, no one now can count him- or herself safe.

Medical ignorance could be exacerbating the situation

Despite the growing numbers of press reports linking chemicals and disease and the increasingly urgent warnings from those scientists specialising in environmental medicine, the rest of the medical world appears to be deaf to these fears.

This wide-scale apathy originates in medical school, as few doctors are even taught about most modern-day chemicals. Fewer still know where these chemicals can be found, let alone understand the ways in which they could be poisoning us. As a

The childhood vaccination programme – a damaged generation

Most doctors give numerous vaccines unquestioningly to young babies in the name of health protection. While the concept of vaccination seems to make sense, the use of the following raft of hidden chemical 'additives', used to make a vaccine cheaper and extend its shelf life, appears to have corrupted this basically sound concept:

- Mercury – a heavy metal used in the disinfectant/preservative 'thimerosal', and known to cause brain injury, autism, attention deficit hyperactivity disorder (ADHD) and autoimmune diseases.
- Aluminium – a toxic metal additive used to promote antibody response, associated with Alzheimer's disease, brain damage, seizures and cancer.
- Formaldehyde – a preservative, nerve-damaging and cancer-causing agent.
- Ethylene glycol (antifreeze).
- Monosodium glutamate (MSG) – a breakdown product of protein and common flavour enhancer well known for poisoning brain cells.
- Sulphites – cause genetic damage in some animals.
- Neomycin – an antibiotic, also previously registered for use in US pesticides, and known to cause reproductive and developmental harm, such as birth defects, infertility, sterility and impairment of normal growth and development. (See Appendix C.)

result, during most medical consultations, the concept that chemicals could have contributed in some way to a patient's problem would not even register as a remote possibility.

Consequently, not only are patients losing out on a potential opportunity to reverse or minimise any chemically triggered problem, but some of the solutions, which include chemicals such as pesticides, may in their own right be adding to the overall problem (see From Auschwitz to Alzheimer's, page 124).

It gets worse, as one of medicine's most important and hallowed 'preventive' treatment programmes, childhood vaccination, appears to be responsible for adding to the problem by significantly increasing the overall chemical body burden of every vaccinated child. For instance, before mercury was withdrawn from childhood vaccines in the USA, between 1989 and 1999, children who received all the recommended vaccinations would have absorbed their lifetime's 'safe' level of mercury by the time they were six months old. This 'mistake' was so serious that it even prompted an adviser to the National Immunization Program – Dr Neal Halsey of John Hopkins University – at a hearing in Cambridge three years ago, to admit that he felt bad that he didn't pick it up. Unfortunately, in the UK, despite being removed from regular childhood vaccinations, mercury in the form of thimerosal is still present in many of the non-routine vaccines given to children. (See box, European countries ban amalgam dental fillings over safety fears, page 38.) Indeed, a US congressman is calling for criminal penalties for any government agency that knew about the dangers of thimerosal in vaccines and did nothing to protect American children. Congressman Dan Burton (Republican-Indiana) during a Congressional Hearing: 'You mean to tell me that since 1929, we've been using thimerosal and the only test that you know of is from 1929 and every one of those people had meningitis and they all died?' For nearly an hour Burton repeatedly asked the Food and Drug Administration (FDA) and Centers for Disease Control and Prevention (CDC) officials what they knew and when they knew it. (Thimerosal contains a related mercury compound called ethyl mercury. Mercury is a toxic metal that can cause immune, sensory, neurological, motor and behavioural dysfunctions.)

Despite the almost continual assurances that vaccines are safe, the fact remains that no study has ever looked at the potential risks of injecting young babies with current levels of these chemical additives.

However, when the former Chief Vaccine Control Officer at the US FDA, Dr J Anthony Morris, stated, 'There is a great deal of evidence to prove that immunisation of children does more harm than good', it makes you wonder why the practice of injecting babies with known brain-damaging, potentially lethal and, in most cases, many totally unnecessary chemicals in the name of health (and in the absence of any safety studies) has been allowed to continue virtually unchallenged. (For more information on vaccines, thimerosal and mercury see pages 38, 96, 113, 137–8, 155, 273–6 and Appendix C.)

The way forward

This profound level of ignorance and general apathy on the part of the majority of the medical profession with respect to the potential danger we all now face from chemicals is what prompted me – not only a medical doctor and academic, but also a housewife and mother of four – to write this book. I, and a growing number of other highly qualified scientists who have made the effort to take an impartial look at what is going on, have been able to glimpse a world as yet unseen to the great majority of the medical profession.

Despite the situation appearing (it has to be said) pretty dire, knowing what is causing the problem can open the door to ways to tackle it. So what I would like you to do is suspend any prejudices you might have, read this book, then make up your own mind.

So whether you are the mother of a child who has developed what appears to be vaccine-induced autism, or you are an adult who has just been diagnosed with asthma, read on. This book has been written for you and for everyone else who has fallen victim to one of the twenty-first century diseases or who wants to protect him- or herself from everything modern day life appears to be throwing at them.

2

21st Century Toxins

'*A report from the World Health Organization recently concluded that dental amalgam fillings were the main source of mercury exposure in the population. Absorption from dental amalgam fillings is up to 10 times the amount from fish and seafood.*'

WORLD HEALTH ORGANIZATION:
ENVIRONMENTAL HEALTH CRITERIA SERIES, 1991

A polluted world

The creation and widespread use of man-made substances in the late twentieth century has resulted in every region of the planet being contaminated with a cocktail of toxins. Whether you go to the North Pole or to the Sahara desert, you will find these health-damaging chemicals everywhere.

It would be a mistake to think that the only people at risk are those who are exposed to them at work, for in this polluted environment in which we all now live, every one of us is exposed on a daily basis to massive amounts of these chemicals. While few people deliberately set out to expose themselves to toxins, the simple act of eating contaminated foods or using 'treated' products could be putting you at risk – without you even realising it.

Please do not believe that, just because you can't see them, they are not there. After all, the many hundreds of billions of kilograms of these man-made chemicals that are produced every single year have to go somewhere! We end up eating these chemicals in our foods as pesticides, additives, pollutants and contaminants from food containers. We drink them in tap water, which contains chemicals leached from contaminated soils, environmental pollutants, and even chemicals added deliberately, such as fluoride. We absorb them through our skin from cosmetics, toiletries, treated wood, pesticide-sprayed plants, treated areas of public parks, golf courses, bath water and swimming pools. We even inhale them in air contaminated with solvents (see Solvents and VOCs in Glossary, page 285), car fumes, industrial waste and environmental pollutants.

As a result, each of us is now heavily contaminated with on average 300–500 industrial toxins, few of which have been properly tested for their harmful effects at low concentrations, in the short term, in the long term, individually and when combined with other toxins. The persistent cumulative nature of many of these chemicals, together with the fact that we are at the top of the food chain, means humans are one of the most polluted species on earth. Each year it becomes more and more apparent that the introduction of these highly toxic chemicals into our lives has set off a twenty-first century disease time bomb. So what are these chemicals, and why are they so effective at damaging our health?

The chemicals behind our health problems

The chemicals that appear to be causing all these health problems can basically be divided into two main groups:

- Toxic metals (see Appendix A.4)
- Man-made chemicals (see Appendix A)

Toxic metals include substances such as lead, cadmium and mercury and they have been around for as long as we have, since they are part of our natural world. The problem is that, owing to the explosive increase in manufacturing, we are now exposed to levels far higher than our bodies were ever designed to withstand. The coping mechanisms that our bodies have developed over thousands of years are increasingly becoming saturated and so unable to protect us. Therefore it's not surprising to learn that studies regularly reveal that people with higher levels of these metals in their bodies are at much greater risk of developing virtually all of the twenty-first century illnesses listed on page 8.

The health risk posed by synthetic chemicals arises from their similarity to naturally produced substances, which allows them to be assimilated into all the natural bodily systems essential to supporting animal life, in combination with their unnatural new synthetic properties. So while they can interfere with normal body functioning, many of these compounds cannot be broken down or 'switched off' after having completed their work, unlike the natural substances they mimic. Instead they can keep on falsely stimulating or disrupting our bodies 24 hours a day, seven days a week. This low-grade but constant damage they cause to many of the body's systems is one of the reasons why they appear to pose such a major long-term health problem.

Although most synthetic chemicals are actually derived from natural substances, usually crude oil or coal, these chemicals are definitely not natural since they are all manufactured in chemical laboratories using techniques developed within the last 100 years. These relatively recently created processes have produced many synthetic chemicals which possess a totally new set of properties and shapes compared to those found in nature that they are designed to emulate. These properties include increased stability, increased longevity, high toxicity and reduced biodegradability. These new qualities are the reasons why synthetic substances are so widely used, as in many cases they can offer clear advantages over natural materials.

Chemicals that are extremely stable are used as fire retardants or insulators. Chemicals that powerfully manipulate bodily functions are used as medicines for humans and animals, or as pesticides to kill insects and many other forms of life. Chemicals that possess strong colours are used as pigments or food colourings. Chemicals that add malleability are used to make plastics flexible. Consequently, synthetic chemicals are now commonly used as pesticides, plastics, solvents, dyes, medicines, industrial chemicals, rubber, food preservatives and many other products besides. As scientists keep finding more uses for these new types of chemicals, the quantities produced keep on rising.

The rise in synthetic chemical production

Synthetic chemicals are extremely big business. Production in the USA alone in 1994 was worth a staggering $101 billion. The graph shows the phenomenal increase in production of these substances throughout the twentieth century.

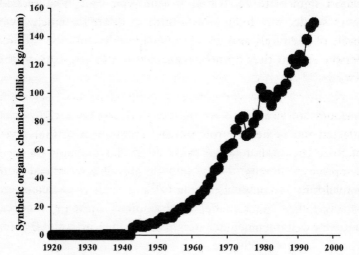

Graph showing the annual US production of synthetic chemicals over the twentieth century.[1]

However, these new properties appear to be at the heart of the problem as the toxicity we experience from such chemicals is due to the fact that our bodies are not designed to cope with synthetic chemicals. Over millions of years, our bodies have developed very sophisticated detoxification systems to rid themselves of most naturally produced toxins on a day-to-day basis. But these new synthetic compounds have structures totally alien to the normal toxins found in the environment. So while our waste-disposal system can manage to process some of these 'alien' chemicals, it is often completely unable to deal with others. Consequently, the ones that our system cannot shift tend to accumulate in the body, and studies show that, as with toxic metals, a high level of accumulated synthetic chemicals increases the risk of succumbing to all of the twenty-first century illnesses.

Chemical poisoning – immediate and long-term

So how exactly do toxic chemicals cause us physical harm? The toxic effects of chemicals can be divided into two main types of damage. The most obvious and best-documented way is direct poisoning by a relatively large quantity of chemicals – inducing almost immediate and often violent symptoms. The second, more subtle, way follows long-term exposure to much lower levels of chemicals and usually goes unnoticed by the affected person, so that they do not relate their health problems to this toxic build-up.

Not surprisingly, the quicker and more dramatic poisoning episodes are relatively easy to recognise, by both the person affected and by health professionals. This is because high levels of toxic chemicals tend to cause rapid and dramatic damage. Symptoms can range from mild flu-like illnesses through to convulsions, unconsciousness and death. Since these symptoms usually follow quickly after the poisoning incident, they are relatively well documented, and on the whole hard to ignore. On

New theory of chemically induced disease in the 21st century

Dr C S Miller, of the Department of Family Practice, University of Texas Health Science Center, at San Antonio, USA, believes that we are on the threshold of a new theory of disease – that it is triggered by toxic chemicals. She states, 'In the late 1800s, physicians observed that certain illnesses spread from sick, feverish individuals to those contacting them, paving the way for the germ theory of disease. The germ theory served as a crude but elegant formulation that explained dozens of seemingly unrelated illnesses affecting literally every organ system.

'Today we are witnessing another medical anomaly – a unique pattern of illness involving chemically exposed people who subsequently report multisystem symptoms and new-onset chemical and food intolerances. These intolerances may be the hallmark for a new disease process, just as fever is a hallmark for infection.'

She and others believe this new disease process might be the key to explain the emergence of a totally new type of chemically related disorders, such as Gulf War syndrome, chronic fatigue syndrome and attention deficit hyperactivity disorder.[2]

a wider scale, these high-dose poisoning episodes are a major problem accounting for a staggering three million cases of acute severe pesticide poisonings alone, including 220,000 fatalities worldwide every year.

Slow poisoning

These figures, considerable as they are, in all probability vastly underestimate the true damage that chemicals pose to our health. This is because, as yet, no one has found a way to record the number of people suffering from a whole range of chemically related illnesses triggered by much lower levels of chemical exposure. For instance, the exposure to low levels of cancer-inducing chemicals may not make people ill immediately, but could activate the development of cancer cells or cause other forms of damage that may only become apparent years, even decades, later. Because of the much longer time factors involved, the lower levels of chemicals involved and the massive quantity of toxic chemicals all around us, it is now far more difficult to draw a direct link between particular chemicals and the illnesses they cause. The other complication is that, since we all have a different genetic make-up and live in different environments, we may each react in a slightly different way to a given level and variety of chemicals.

One of the real problems preventing a fuller understanding of the health consequences of this long-term chemical damage stems from the relatively recent emergence of environmental medicine as a specialism, only a few decades ago, and the small number of trained specialists in this field. Because of the limited understanding and low profile of this subject, environmental medicine is one of the so-called 'Cinderella' medical specialisms. It does not attract major research budgets from pharmaceutical companies, in part because most treatments are based on chemical avoidance and nutritional supplements, none of which can be patented and sold at high prices. Also, very few health professionals learn about the subject during their training – I know that I certainly didn't when I was at medical school in the 1980s.

If the vast majority of healthcare professionals have very little

How great is your exposure to health damaging chemicals?

The more of these that apply to you, the greater your risk of developing a chemically triggered twenty-first century disease.

- Working with chemicals.
- Using pesticides around your house and garden (such as flyspray, weed-killer and flea powder).
- Using non-environmentally friendly cosmetics, toiletries and household cleaners.
- Exposure to chemicals in medicines (such as nit shampoo and mercury preservatives in vaccines).
- Eating mostly conventionally grown (non-organic) foods, especially the skins or outer leaves of fruit and vegetables.
- Eating too many processed foods, full of preservatives, colourings, flavourings and other additives.
- Eating contaminated seafood.
- Drinking unfiltered tap water.
- Drinking soft drinks from aluminium cans.
- Having mercury amalgam fillings in your teeth.
- Living in a major city (air pollution).

knowledge or awareness of the potential health risks involved from our exposure to chemicals, they won't be asking the right questions or looking for the relevant signs which would indicate chemical damage. And if you don't look for a problem, the chances are that you won't find it. So what can we do about protecting ourselves against these twenty-first century toxins?

Cutting down on toxins

The good news is that by making simple lifestyle changes, it is possible to significantly lower the level of these twenty-first century chemicals in the body. I will go into this area in much more detail in Chapter 4, but in brief, the main way this is achieved is via various proven and safe methods, based on nutritional supplements, which boost the body's natural ability to kick out toxins and act as an internal sponge, soaking up more persistent toxins so that they can be expelled from the body.

How contaminated is your seafood?

Where you source your seafood from can make all the difference to the level of chemicals it could contain. For example, one study carried out by scientists at Indiana University, published in *Science Magazine* in January 2004, revealed that the level of common seafood pollutants, such as 'cancer causing' toxins like PCBs, dioxins and organochlorines, varied greatly according to its origins. After a comprehensive testing programme of fish around the world, they found Scottish farmed salmon to contain the highest levels of all. Indeed, the levels were so high that, according to the Environmental Protection Agency (EPA) published guidelines, it was only safe to eat one portion of this fish every four months. In contrast, wild salmon from the Pacific, by the same guidelines, could be eaten up to eight times a month due to its lower level of chemicals. This staggering difference was thought to be mainly due to the more contaminated high-fat feed diet given to farmed fish.

While tackling your inner chemical load is very important, lowering your current and future exposure to toxins is just as vital. As well as speeding up your ability to detox, reducing your exposure to the most concentrated sources of chemicals will greatly help minimise your future chemical body burden.

It would be impractical to eliminate toxic chemicals completely from our everyday lives, but it is eminently possible to dramatically reduce the levels entering your body by prioritising – that is, avoiding the most concentrated forms of chemicals first. The key is to do *what* you can *when* you can. The good news is that we can all enjoy better health just by knowing the new rules – if you understand where the problem lies then you hold the key to the solution. A little effort focused in the right places will greatly assist you in achieving a healthier and more vibrant body and lifestyle, despite the proliferation of chemicals and other hazards. The next chapter sets out an easy-to-follow twenty-first century survival plan, which you can follow at your own pace. Even if you take up just one of these suggestions, it will make a difference.

3

21st Century Survival Plan
THE DETOX PROGRAMME

'Sugar substitutes cause worrying symptoms in many people, from memory loss to brain tumours. But despite US FDA approval as a 'safe' food additive, this was not always the case. Indeed, in 1991 the US National Institute of Health, a branch of the Department of Health and Human Services, published a bibliography – "Adverse effects of Aspartame" – listing no less than 167 reasons to avoid it.'

PAULA BAILLIE-HAMILTON, 'ARTIFICIAL SWEETENERS: FOOD ADDITIVES OR CHEMICAL WARFARE AGENTS?' *PHENOMENA* ISSUE 3 MAY/JUNE 2004

How to adapt to and survive 21st century life

We can all help ourselves to adapt to the environment we now live in. By learning a new set of easy-to-follow rules, we can make the changes necessary to give us the best chances possible to achieve and remain in good health. To be successful, you will have to pace yourself, since it will inevitably take time to absorb all this new information. Taking one small step at a time will enable you to focus your mind on one activity, and make real progress within a short time. Before you know it, you will have set in place most of the changes necessary to create a less polluted personal environment and lifestyle. While you don't have to follow the entire plan to achieve better health, the more that you are eventually able to incorporate into your daily life the better.

The three steps described below cover the entire plan. They are graded in order of how easy they are to achieve and their importance, starting with the easiest and most important.

Three steps to better health - at a glance

Step one
- Avoid most concentrated forms of chemicals, such as pesticides.
- Start taking nutritional supplements.

Step two
- Start buying more organic foods and wash and peel conventionally grown foods.
- Buy a water filter.
- Add more soluble fibre to your diet.

Step three
- Start taking regular exercise.
- Lower your exposure to toxins in other parts of your life.

Three steps to better health
STEP ONE:
By avoiding the use of most concentrated forms of chemicals you can go a very long way towards dramatically cutting your exposure to chemicals in everyday life. As pesticides, dental amalgam fillings and other forms of concentrated chemicals tend to contain the highest levels, tackling this area presents a pain-free way of significantly lowering your current and future exposure to toxic chemicals.

Regular vitamin and mineral supplements enable your body to process and remove much of its existing burden of toxins and help it to rid itself of the ones that you can't avoid ingesting in the future. For advice on the best supplements, see Chapter 4 and for good brands see Useful Companies, page 320.

STEP TWO:
The next step requires more effort and will be an ongoing process, as it will take time to change your shopping habits and

lifestyle accordingly. Be realistic about what you can achieve here. While it is very difficult to eat and drink 'clean' produce all the time, the greater the proportion of toxin-free produce in your diet, the better.

For most people, food is the most important way that chemicals enter the body. Chemicals in food originate from three main sources:

- Deliberately added chemicals. These include pesticides such as fungicides and insecticides; antibiotics; and additives such as colourings, preservatives, flavouring and artificial sweeteners. Conventional agriculture uses large amounts of pesticides to kill insects and weeds and to stop food spoiling. The foods containing the highest levels tend to be perishable items such as fresh fruit and vegetables, the majority of which contain one or more pesticides. Poultry and cattle farming use antibiotics as growth promoters. These chemicals end up in the meat you buy. Many food additives are also known to damage your health.
- Packaging contamination, i.e. food wrappers and takeaway food containers (see page 27).
- Environmental pollution. Some parts of the sea can be heavily polluted with heavy metals and persistent toxins such as organochlorines (see Appendix A, page 281). As a consequence, fish and other seafood can be contaminated. Environmental pollution levels tend to be highest in animal fat, particularly if the animal or fish is a predator (such as salmon) because organochlorines are highly fat-soluble and persistent chemicals and they accumulate up the food chain. So if, for example, a salmon eats a smaller fish that is contaminated with toxins, these toxins will be added to those already carried by the salmon.

Don't panic, go organic

One of the simplest ways of significantly reducing your dietary intake of chemicals is by buying organic foods (see Glossary, page 333). Organic foods are those grown under a system of agriculture that limits the addition of synthetic chemicals at all stages. The end result is that organic foods are not only less polluted but many studies have also found them to contain much higher levels of essential nutrients. You can easily tell if your food is organic as food sold as organic must, by law, possess a label that displays its organic certification number.

Fortunately, organic foods are becoming not only more widely available but more affordable too. For fruit and vegetables, which can contain some of the highest levels of pesticides if grown conventionally, organic is by far the best choice. Whilst organically reared salmon is by no means free from pollutants, its more natural diet means that it will tend to be less contaminated than the farmed alternative.

'Detoxing' conventionally grown foods

Whilst it would be good if we could all eat organically, for many, due to limited availability or budget, this is not an option. The good news is that in many cases you can dramatically cut the level of chemicals in conventionally grown fruit and vegetables by washing and peeling them to remove the surface chemicals. By reducing your intake of seafood (ensuring, of course, you are getting enough omega-3 oils in supplements) and cutting down on animal fats, as these tend to contain the highest levels of resistant toxic chemicals, you can dramatically cut your intake of chemicals. Even simple acts, such as removing visible fats from meats and fish and discarding the fat that comes off, can help detox those foods. Lastly, you should store food in glass, ceramic or other natural materials as this will prevent your foods getting yet another dose of chemicals leaching out from plastic or polystyrene storage containers.

How to read and trust labels

Processed foods in general tend to have lower levels of pesticides and, incidentally, nutrients as a consequence of a number of pesticide-lowering processes such as food preparation and cooking.

However, their higher levels of chemicals in the form of preservatives, colourings and flavourings – normally added post-processing – mean that they are far from being chemical free.

So, when you pick up a packet of food or drink, take a closer look at the label to make sure it has:

- no added synthetic colourings, flavourings or preservatives
- only natural sweeteners, as artificial sweeteners, such as aspartame, are known to have dozens of well-documented health damaging effects
- no hydrogenated or 'trans' fats as these can block your body's ability to absorb and use essential fatty acids.

In addition, make sure that the carton of fruit juice you buy is a fruit *juice* and is not described as a fruit *drink*, as these are more likely to contain potentially harmful additives. Cut down on your intake of animal fats, as these tend to contain the highest levels of persistent toxic chemicals, and substitute with vegetable oils.

The 'Dirty Dozen'

In my last book, *The Detox Diet*, using nationally published and publicly available data, I calculated which foods are likely to contain the highest levels of metabolism-blocking chemicals. At the number one spot, as you can see, eels are, according to my calculations, the most contaminated food, with the others following in descending order:

1. Eels (UK)
2. Fish oils (Canada)
3. Lamb (New Zealand)
4. Oranges (Spain)
5. Mint leaves (no country listed)
6. Cocoa butter (used in chocolate) (no country listed)
7. Dill (no country listed)
8. Salmon (farmed, UK)
9. Sugar snap peas (Kenya)
10. Geese (France)
11. Winter lettuce (UK)
12. Trout (farmed, UK)

Cleaning up your water

Tap water contains many chemicals that can enter the body either by mouth, or by being absorbed through the skin. Water can be contaminated with the former warfare gas chlorine, aluminium (deliberately added during processing), lead and plastics (from piping), and environmental pollutants (pesticides in agricultural areas). A sink-top or whole-house water filter will significantly lower the levels of chemicals in tap water. Bottled water also tends to be less polluted than tap water, particularly if stored in glass.

Soluble fibre

While the above will reduce your intake of chemicals, adding soluble fibre to your diet will help lower your existing toxic chemical load. You can take soluble fibre in the form of supplements such as pectin, psyllium seed husks or in foods such as peas, beans and other pulses. (See page 45 for details.)

STEP THREE:

Exercise is a great detoxifier. By increasing the level of exercise you do each week, you not only boost your ability to remove chemicals from your body, but also rebalance your natural levels of hormones and energise your metabolism (see page 57).

Lowering levels of environmental chemicals

There are numerous ways that chemicals can get into your body from your surroundings. In fact there are so many sources of chemicals, I will spend the rest of this chapter suggesting ways in which you can take control of the situation and detox all the major areas of your life. You will soon discover that there are many potential problem areas in your environment and it is simply not possible, or necessary, to do everything suggested at once. My advice to you is to start by lowering your exposure to the areas where you might find the chemicals that are closely connected to your health condition. Then it is simply a matter of doing as much as you can, as and when it suits you.

Areas ripe for detox

- Kitchen
- Laundry/utility room
- Bathroom
- Living room
- Bedroom
- Workroom/office
- Garden
- Shed/garage

Detoxing your home and environment

The level of chemicals we are being exposed to from our environment is at an all time high. Not only are we subjected to a barrage of chemicals from our food, we are also smothering ourselves with them every time we put on suntan lotion, face and body creams or the many other beauty products available to us all. We also breathe them in when we use a wide range of sprays and other chemical-filled products. We can even get a mouthful of highly toxic chemicals such as mercury – which, despite being banned in several other major European countries (see page 38), is still widely used by British dentists.

It is virtually impossible to cut chemicals out of your life permanently, but it is possible to slash the amount that gets through by paying a little attention to which products you use to clean your house, use in the garden, put on your face or place in your mouth. While it can take a bit of getting used to, any efforts you make in lowering your overall exposure to chemicals in your home and garden will be repaid in terms of better health and more energy.

I have started by flagging up the highest non-food sources of chemicals room by room, and have then progressed to other areas. Once you know where the highest concentrated sources of chemicals can be located, it will be possible to convert even the most polluted toxic home into a safe, relaxing, low-chemical oasis.

Kitchen clearout

Food preparation and storage: Even if your food is uncontaminated, there are many ways that chemicals can still sneak into it before it reaches your mouth, for example, from plastic or metal cooking containers and utensils and food coverings. The chemicals

Microwave warning

Despite the virtual omnipresence of microwave ovens, I would recommend that you avoid using them. My concern is largely based on a small-scale but high-quality study carried out by Dr Hans Hertel, a Swiss food scientist, who looked at the effect of microwaved food on humans. His conclusions were clear and alarming: microwave cooking altered the food's nutrients significantly enough that changes occurred in the participants' blood – changes that suggested deterioration. The changes included:

- Increased cholesterol levels.
- More leukocytes, or white blood cells (which can suggest poisoning).
- Production of radiolytic compounds (which are unknown in nature).
- Decreased red blood cell numbers and haemoglobin levels (which could indicate anaemia).

Dr Hertel and his team published these worrying results in 1992, but a Swiss trade organisation, the Swiss Association of Dealers for Electro-apparatuses for Households and Industry, had a gagging order issued, which prohibited Dr Hertel from declaring that microwaves were dangerous to health. The gagging order was removed in 1998, after a Swiss court ruled that the order violated his right to freedom of expression. Switzerland was ordered to pay Dr Hertel compensation as well.

in plastic are highly fat-soluble, so any fatty foods placed in direct contact with a plastic container will act like blotting paper and absorb many of the fat-soluble chemicals it contains. The longer the food is in contact and the higher the temperature, the greater the final level of food contamination will be. The same goes for aluminium cooking utensils and salty or acidic foods (such as fruit). For instance, fizzy acidic drinks in aluminium containers can have relatively high levels of metal contamination.

By replacing these with more natural alternatives, such as glass, wood, metal (stainless steel is fine) or clay-porcelain based containers, you can ensure that you will not get an extra mouthful of health-damaging chemicals.

Lastly, if using non-organically grown foods, wash and peel fruit and vegetables before cooking them or eating them raw. For vegetables you can't peel, such as broccoli, throw away any cooking water, as this tends to contain most of the pesticides.

Clear out your 'killing' corner: Virtually every kitchen has a 'killing corner', such as a cupboard or shelf that is filled to the brim with all manner of fly and cockroach sprays, insect-repellents, pets' flea powders and shampoos, along with a battery of other deadly synthetic chemicals. These should all be banished from your kitchen. But don't put them down the sink where they will poison the water supply – dispose of them responsibly. Take them to the appropriate place at your local authority's refuse site. Once you have achieved this, check out the following chemical-free ways of dealing with unwelcome visitors.

Food hygiene and alternative pest control: First things first. Always clear food away last thing at night to discourage potential pests from making your home theirs. To further discourage them, try spraying the room with a solution of essential citrus oils and water. Cockroaches can be eliminated by mixing equal parts of baking soda and powdered sugar. Spread this mixture where they congregate and repeat every one to two weeks until the pests have gone. To discourage ants you can use mint. Mix one cup of water with two teaspoons of essential oil of peppermint and spray the mixture wherever the ants come in – on windowsills, kitchen worktops and along skirting boards.

If your dog has fleas, rather than spraying the whole house with highly toxic chemicals, you could use a herbal shampoo, or spray your pet and then buy them a herbal flea-collar, which contains natural repellents such as pennyroyal or eucalyptus oils. There are even herbal flea powders to use on carpets and furnishings. They usually contain pyrethrum (a plant extract) or borax.

Indeed, there are so many natural remedies available for most insects and pests, I don't have the space to cover them all here. I suggest you check out your local health food shop or herbalist. Alternatively look on the Internet for suppliers.

De-chemical your laundry/utility room
The vast majority of domestic cleaning products contain an abundance of toxic chemicals, most of which could seriously impact upon your health. The best thing to do is to clear them

all out, and look for healthier alternatives. To be honest, despite the continuing media hype, cleaning a home doesn't need complex and expensive ingredients: white vinegar, baking soda, or borax diluted with water in liquid or paste form all make cheap and safe cleaning products. Vinegar and water is excellent for cleaning windows. Lemon juice will work wonders for washing dishes or cleaning your bathroom or sink areas.

If this approach doesn't appeal to you, you'll find plenty of alternative environmentally friendly cleaning solutions in your local health shop or supermarket. *Ecover* is one brand, which I tend to use for virtually all my cleaning needs, from washing powder to dishwasher tablets. If there are particular products you really can't find a replacement for, it's a good idea to seal them up in an airtight container such as a tin. This will significantly reduce the amount of vapour they release into the air, which would otherwise end up in your lungs.

And if you get someone in to clean the carpets, insist on them using steam cleaners. My brother-in-law suffered weeks of ill health after his carpet was recently 'cleaned' with lashings upon lashings of toxic chemicals. Better still, buy your own steamer. Not only can it clean carpets but it may also help remove existing chemicals on carpets. You could also use it to clean other household fabrics on sofas or curtains – though it would be advisable to check the fabric cleaning label first as some materials might not take kindly to steam.

Bathroom bliss

Although you may not realise it, many beauty and personal cleansing products are far from natural. In fact, most are stuffed with synthetic chemicals, such as pesticides, preservatives, plastics, fluoride and artificial scents. These are used to make their products smell nicer, feel and look better and to last longer. However, together they all add up to a massive load of poisonous chemicals, the vast majority of which we could all live quite happily without.

When trying to assess which ones are good and which are dubious, the usually extensive list of ingredients can make things very confusing. The easiest way forward is to adopt the phrase 'if in doubt, chuck it out!' The increasing demand for low-chemical beauty products has revolutionised the industry, resulting in more and more companies specialising in this area. Choose companies that sell natural, environmentally friendly, or best of all, organic products. Good ones are *Green People* and *Dr Hauschka*. These both have an extensive range of beauty and skin care products. The direct marketing companies known as *Neways* and *Nutrimetics* also offer a large range of high-quality natural products. Okay, it might take you a little time, effort and more money to find alternatives for your favourite products, but believe me, the rewards will most definitely be worthwhile.

There are also more and more companies selling fluoride-free toothpaste, although I have yet to see any fluoride-free varieties sold in supermarkets. My family's clear favourite is aloe vera/tea tree mint flavour toothpaste, a zingily minty mouth sensation made by the company *Kingfisher*. *Tom's of Maine* produce a great natural deodorant, which is also amazingly free of aluminium and other unwanted chemicals normally found in such products. I prefer their *unscented 'Nature's deodorant'*, although you may catch a mild whiff of coriander when you first put it on. It contains the rare combination – for a deodorant anyway – of being both highly effective and safe. But if you like scented versions these are also available.

Lastly, room fresheners tend to be full of synthetic chemicals, so if you do want your bathroom to have a pleasant whiff, try pouring tiny amounts of natural essential oils on a flower based potpourri.

Check out your medicine cabinet: The other main source of chemicals in your bathroom is likely to be your medicine cabinet. I am not talking about prescription drugs, as I am certainly not encouraging anyone who is ill to stop taking their medication. The products that I want to warn you about are the 'medicated' shampoos specifically designed for head infestations such as nits and head lice.

These may contain powerful insecticides, which are intended to be put directly on to the skin, where a proportion of the chemicals will then be absorbed straight into the body. Your doctor, pharmacist or alternative health-care specialist may be able to recommend alternatives, such as fine-tooth combing and natural remedies. These are just as effective as potentially highly toxic medicated formulae – if not more so, as increasing numbers of parasites have now developed a resistance to many chemical treatments.

Where chemicals tend to be found in a typical living room

Air your air: The largest amount of chemicals in the average room that are likely to enter your body tend to be in contaminated air. Thus, the simple and quickest way of getting rid of them is to open your windows. Make sure you open windows at

How green is your carpet?

Most woollen carpets are dyed with synthetic dyes, made from a wide range of chemicals. But the trouble really starts with the wool itself. To carry the heavily promoted Woolmark® label, wool has to be treated with pyrethroids, for example the Beyer chemical company's Eulan®, to a minimum concentration of 130 milligrams per kilogram. Pyrethroids act as nerve poisons, and their use in carpets has been banned in the USA for 15 years.

So 'pure wool' carpets are not usually very pure. The problem gets even worse if they have a 'latex' backing. In most cases this actually means synthetic latex. First of all, this is not bio-degradable, unlike natural latex, which means that most latex-backed carpets should only be disposed of as expensive chemical waste. Secondly, synthetic latex contains an unhealthy cocktail of anti-ageing chemicals. Thirdly, it contains vulcanisation agents that include styrene, a cancer-producing chemical. It is the styrene which gives new carpets their special smell. So what's the alternative? While you can buy organic carpet, it can involve a high cost and a potentially very long wait to get it. However, unlike virtually every other carpet on the market, it won't come with these unwanted chemical extras.

One final point that needs to be considered before buying a carpet is that all carpets collect a large quantity of household dust. As this dust acts as a sanctuary for toxic chemicals, having fewer carpets in your home means lower levels of floor-borne toxins for children, adults and pets to walk on and absorb into their skin.

the front and back of the house, as this will increase the flow of air. This is particularly important in new houses, as many of them are now hermetically sealed. Ventilating the house for just half an hour can make all the difference.

Even if you live in a city, indoor air still tends to be far more polluted than the air outside, so it is still a good idea to allow some ventilation. Of course, if you live next to a very busy road it would be wise to close the windows during peak-hour traffic. If the outside air is exceptionally polluted, consider investing in an air filter, which removes pollutants, many of which will contain chemicals from exhaust fumes.

Another way of reducing airborne chemicals is by filling your home with plants. It has been found that spider plants, Boston ferns, elephant-ear philodendron, English ivy and aloe vera are highly effective at absorbing solvents from the atmosphere.

Other sources of chemicals in a typical living room: The main types of chemicals contaminating a typical living room stem from the use of the following:

- Pesticides used in wood treated for dry rot, and all-wool carpets treated for moth-proofing.
- Plastic in household fittings and ornaments.
- Flame-retardants in many fabrics.
- Solvents in carpets, fibreboard, chipboard and paints.

As you can imagine, building materials or furnishings that incorporate these offenders may be potentially loaded with toxic chemicals. Because of this the average room can have many potential hot spots. In most cases, not much can be done. The expense would probably be too great and there are not enough viable alternatives. But there are some steps you can take. For example, try to source furnishings made from natural, untreated fabrics when replacing old furnishings and fittings.

If having a room renovated, ask your builder to use environmentally friendly products, such as those sold by the London-based company *Construction Resources* (see Appendix D).

As well as providing a fabulous source of information, these companies should help you to source low-chemical versions of virtually everything you will ever need. Better still, in many cases the environmentally friendly option is not more expensive and may actually be much cheaper.

Although it is impossible to offer advice on specific projects, there are a few general rules that apply across the board:

- Try to use fixings such as screws and nails that don't require adhesives.
- If you have to use an adhesive, then silicon rubber glue, latex, hide glue and water washable wood glue are less toxic than epoxy resins.
- The best sealants are made of pure silicone or linseed oil putty.
- When using wood, use solid untreated hard wood (from an environmentally responsible source), rather than chemically treated soft wood such as pine. Definitely avoid plywood, MDF (medium density fibreboard) or chipboard.
- Use wooden window frames rather than PVC fittings.
- Avoid products that are made of plastics and treated with fire-retardants if possible, using only products that are naturally fire-resistant.

Bedroom toxins – what's under your mattress?

The bedroom is a particularly important room, as most of us spend over one-third of our lives there. Consequently, if any room needs to be free of chemicals this should be the one. The easiest and most effective way of detoxing this room is simply to keep your window open at night – but just make sure you have a burglar latch to keep out other unwanted bodies.

Because of the current fire regulations, most mattresses are now treated with flame-retardants. While it is possible to buy an organic mattress, a simple step is to cover the mattress with a blanket in addition to the usual sheet. Choose pillows filled with natural fibres such as cotton, wool or feathers.

Your wardrobe tends to be the other major source of chemicals. Some will originate from clothes that contain plastics, such as synthetic leather or waterproof clothing. You can even be responsible for adding chemicals yourself if you dry-clean your clothes (because of the solvents used in the cleaning process), or if you use certain chemically treated mothballs to prevent insect damage.

In order to keep the chemical content of clothes and fabrics as low as possible, buy clothes and fabrics made of natural fibres and use natural substances such as lavender oils to prevent insect damage. If you consider yourself or any other wearer of an item of clothing to be at low risk from fire, avoid clothes treated with flame-retardant chemicals. If you dry-clean your clothes, hang them out to air in a well-ventilated place for a few days before putting them back in your wardrobe. Better still, find a dry-cleaner who uses steam instead of solvents.

What's in your workroom/office?

Those working with chemicals tend to get their greatest overall levels of chemicals from their work environment. Chemicals can be breathed into the lungs, or spread on the skin where they are then absorbed into the body. Although the levels entering via the skin and lungs tend to be lower than those consumed with food, chemicals ingested in this way can be more toxic. This is because they have effectively bypassed the digestive system, which is normally responsible for breaking down certain chemicals, and have gone straight into the bloodstream.

Since most people spend so much of their lives at work, we need to keep our exposure to chemicals at work as low as possible. As with your home, you need to have good ventilation, particularly if you work with chemicals. If you work in a traditional office, it is a good idea to keep inks, carbon paper and correction fluid in sealed containers.

Bringing a plant or an air filter into your office will help reduce the level of air pollution. And if the chemicals used to clean the office are overpowering, find out whether these can be changed or used more sparingly. (A good argument you can use is that this will save your employer money.) It may also be a good idea to find out more about whether any pesticides are regularly sprayed in the building.

Most people in offices tend to spend a great deal of time working in front of a computer screen. Unfortunately, all electrical goods emit extremely low-frequency electromagnetic fields. To avoid getting exposed to these potentially cancer-causing emissions, put a screening shield over your computer screen.

I do accept that in certain professions (such as hairdressing, and painting and decorating) it may be particularly difficult to reduce the level of chemicals you are exposed to. However, if there were no difference in cost, what would stop your company using products that contain fewer chemicals? It could even be a positive selling point.

How green is your garden?

Once you have chucked out all your herbicides, weed-killers, insect sprays and other noxious substances (responsibly, of course), you will have significantly lowered your potential future exposure to chemicals. The next process will take a little longer, as you need to discover new techniques to discourage weeds and pests naturally.

Since agriculture was around long before chemicals were invented, there is already a mountain of information on traditional practices. Much of it has been ignored for years, but a growing number of farmers are reviving older methods to farm their land and raise their animals organically.

If you take your gardening seriously, there are lots of books available on organic horticultural techniques. More good information can be found at the website www.organicgardening.com

Shed/garage – a chemical hot spot

The garden shed, garage or anywhere that you store building and gardening materials can be a huge source of chemicals. Old cans of paint and varnish are highly volatile and can contain a large number of synthetic chemicals such as plastics, surfactants, lead, styrenes and solvents. These storage areas can also contain toxic adhesives for use all over the house as well as wood preservatives for garden fences and furniture. On a warm day these toxic substances evaporate into the air more quickly and give off powerful fumes. If your garage is linked to your house you must ensure that it is well ventilated, otherwise these chemicals will waft straight into your living area.

It is possible to find environmentally friendly alternatives to many of these chemicals, but owing to the vast range of potential items found in these places, this will require a bit of research on your part. Unfortunately, there is just not the space to go through all the relevant options here.

Chemicals at the dentist's – clearing the mercury from your mouth

Thanks to advances in dentistry and dental awareness, we tend to keep our teeth for much longer than our ancestors did. To achieve this, dentists now use a whole range of substances to patch up or replace broken teeth. The problem is that any substance applied to our teeth is likely to be ground up and swallowed with the rest of our food.

More quicksilver than silver

The major substance in 'silver' amalgam fillings is mercury, not silver. Mercury makes up about 50 per cent of the compound (approximately one half gram per filling and as much as is found in a mercury thermometer). The other materials found in amalgam are silver, tin, copper and zinc. In the words of Professor Boyd Haley of the University of Kentucky, that is a 'colossal' amount of mercury in scientific terms. When mercury enters the blood after leaking out of an amalgam filling, it only remains there for a few minutes. Henceforth it is locked into the cells of the body as we excrete far less than we absorb. This is called 'Retention Toxicity'. Once in our organs it can stay there for decades. Whilst mercury tends to settle in the brain, no body tissues are safe as mercury is known to invade every known organ in the human body.

European countries ban amalgam dental fillings over safety fears

Amalgam fillings – which contain mercury – are thought so toxic that they have been banned in several European countries. Sweden banned mercury amalgam dental fillings in January 1997, after determining that at least 250,000 Swedes have immune and other health disorders directly related to the mercury in their teeth. Denmark banned mercury amalgams in January 1999. Austria is also phasing out mercury fillings, and in Switzerland and Japan the dental schools no longer teach amalgam use as the primary form of dental care.

In 1991, Germany's Health Ministry recommended to the German Dental Association that no further amalgam fillings be used for children, pregnant women, or those with kidney disease. In 1993 this was extended to include all women of child-bearing age, pregnant or not. The Health Ministry is now considering whether to ban its use entirely.

Furthermore, any rise in temperature from, say, drinking a hot drink, or any form of physical provocation, such as chewing, brushing with a toothbrush, and of course any dental work simply speeds up the mercury leakage even further.

Most of the materials used by dentists as temporary fillings or sealants contain a mixture of heavy metals, chemicals and plastics. The materials used to make dental impressions are also plastic, white fillings contain plastic, and amalgam fillings contain heavy metals such as mercury. Even if you choose the safer option of having your teeth repaired with porcelain, the repair is usually attached with plastics, unless you request otherwise. Even false teeth are made with plastics! And children are given 'treatment' with the known brain toxin fluoride.

Mercury's chequered past

In order to understand the current situation, we need to look back 150 years. Mercury amalgam was first introduced from China at a time when the only serious options open to people with tooth disease were tooth extraction without anaesthetic (since at that time modern anaesthetics had not been invented) or by the pouring of extremely hot gold into teeth. Since mercury amalgam fillings were not only cheap and extremely durable, but could be made up and put into the tooth at room temperature, it was hardly surprising that use of this material quickly took hold. For the first time dental treatment was affordable for the masses.

However, even back then, physicians' concerns were raised about the increasing usage of mercury due to its well-known links with dementia and loss of motor co-ordination. The familiar phrase 'mad as a hatter' originated from hat makers who were rendered 'mad' as a direct consequence of being exposed to high levels of mercury in treated cloth. This resulted in a ruling from the existing main dental body in the US – The American Society of Dental Surgeons – to adopt a resolution in 1845 that its members sign a pledge never to use mercury amalgam. Despite the ensuing suspensions and cases of malpractice in many of its members, the economic advantages won out.

Declining membership of the American Society of Dental Surgeons soon after caused it to disband, and in its place arose the American Dental Association (ADA) who, not surprisingly, promoted amalgam as a safe and desirable tooth filling material.

Mercury – The Facts

- Well over 4,000 academic research papers indicate mercury to be a highly toxic, health-damaging substance.
- Mercury has been described as being possibly the second most deadly toxin on the earth.
- According to the US Agency for Toxic Substances and Disease Registry guidelines, the average amount of mercury leaking out of just one filling is higher than the 'safe' minimal level at which long term exposure is known to result in brain damage.
- The World Health Organization (WHO) has concluded that there can be no safe level of mercury in the body and has not approved mercury amalgam as a safe tooth filling material.
- Dental amalgam has never been approved as a restorative material by the American Environmental Protection Agencies (EPA).
- The US Food and Drug Administration (FDA) do not and never have certified mixed dental amalgam as an implant material.

This stance has also been taken by the British Dental Association – a factor no doubt instrumental in the average UK citizen now having several amalgam fillings in their mouth.

While I definitely don't want to stop you going to the dentist, it is worthwhile asking your dentist about the options open to you and choosing the safest treatment.

Just one more thing before you rush off and make your appointment. It is vitally important to have existing fillings removed by a professional who specialises in this field, one of the many dentists nationwide who specialise in mercury-free dentistry. A list can be found at www.amalgam.ukgo.com/ukdent. This is because if the right procedures are not followed, then removal of the amalgam could be highly risky due to the increased degree of mercury released during the procedure. Not only will a 'mercury-free' dentist have the equipment and the know-how to remove unwanted amalgam fillings safely, they will also only use the safest dental materials to replace them.

I have had all my mercury fillings replaced and have benefited in many ways from it, particularly from a greatly increased level of energy. Indeed, after all my years of research in the field of toxicology, I would go as far as to say that if you have mercury fillings and want to do a one-off thing to improve your wellbeing, the greatest health benefits would most probably be achieved by getting your mercury amalgam fillings removed by a dentist specialising in mercury-free dentistry.

Scrap dental amalgam is classified as hazardous waste by the American Environmental Protection Agency, and by law must be stored in unbreakable, sealed containers, and handled without touching.

Finally, for anyone with a strong nerve who wants more information on the subject, go to the website www.iaomt.org where you can watch a highly disturbing, but extremely informative, brief 'smoking teeth' video made by Dr David Kennedy of the International Academy of Oral Medicine and Toxicology. In it you can see how even at body temperature mercury vapour is constantly evaporating from amalgam fillings, contaminating surrounding air at levels more than 1,000 times higher than current safety standards set by the Environmental Protection Agency (EPA) allow for the air that we breathe.

Your surrounding environment

You can do quite a lot to lower the level of chemicals in your home, but there is relatively little you can do about pollution outside. If you are planning to move, the best areas to live are those well away from large factories, big cities, major roadways and areas of intensive horticulture.

However, there are some things you can do to reduce your existing exposure. If your house is surrounded by fields that are regularly dosed in chemicals, make sure that the farmer tells you when he intends to spray so that you can stay in and keep your windows closed. Never walk through a field during or just after spraying. If you have children, going to parks may be a regular event for you. Try to find out if your local park uses lots of pesticides to control weeds. If they do, steer clear of the areas where they spray, and stay away altogether while the spraying is going on.

When driving in your car you can be exposed to a large volume of chemicals from the other traffic. The best answer may be to get an air filter for the car. Also try to stay more than four car lengths behind the car in front of you, as this allows time for the exhaust fumes to disperse.

Detox Yourself

'In the USA some genetically modified crops are regulated under pesticide regulations.'

SUE MAYER, GENEWATCH

New problems require new solutions

Our health-care system has not kept up with the dramatic changes taking place in our environment, and neither have our methods of treating illnesses. As a result, modern treatments have been designed to deal with the symptoms of disease and not the factors underlying it. So while modern medicines can forcibly change the way the body works once a disease has been established, they completely fail to prevent these diseases from occurring in the first place. *This helps to explain why we are seeing ever-greater numbers of people getting twenty-first century diseases.*

Owing to the slowness of modern medicine in adapting to the rapidly changing situation, people have accepted that the responsibility for their health lies in their own hands. Many people now recognise that ignorance in this new and rapidly evolving area of medicine may not just be putting their health at risk, it could be killing them.

The recent boom in complementary medicine is evidence that people have turned in a new direction to look for new answers to their problems. But the lack of official guidance from most GPs means that people are often faced with a bewildering array of complementary and alternative treatments.

In this chapter I will be outlining the most effective and safest treatments on the market for tackling the new health problems. I will start by suggesting a basic daily detox supplement programme to counteract twenty-first century chemicals. I will explain why this programme is so necessary, and follow by outlining additional ways to treat a wide range of different twenty-first century illnesses using the following methods:

- Nutritional therapy (see also Appendix B.1 to B.4)
- Detox (see also Appendix B.5)
- Exercise
- Herbal treatments (see also Appendix B.6)
- Homeopathy
- Massage therapy
- Acupuncture
- Diet

This chapter concludes with an easy-to-follow seven-day detox plan, designed to help you kick-start your detox and start shedding your existing body burden of twenty-first century chemicals, while learning the principles to continue this throughout your life.

The basic detox supplement programme

While chemical avoidance plays a critical role, starting a long-term daily detox programme is vital if we are to deal with our existing body burden of chemicals, and be protected from future chemical exposure. Many studies show that the most effective way of detoxing is by fortifying and powering the body's natural detoxification systems. Our detox systems rely on a wide range of nutrients to be fully functional, so we need to ensure that our levels of all the most important ones are optimised at all times.

If you prefer, you can take all the supplements and essential fats in the morning. But if you can manage it, split the dose by taking some in the morning and some in the evening. A split dose is particularly important for vitamin C, which lasts for only about eight hours in the body. If you take the total daily amount in two doses you will give your body longer protection.

It is important not to take the supplements at the same time

Basic daily detox supplement programme

- One good multivitamin and mineral supplement (see box – Levels of vitamins and minerals needed for optimal health, page 47).
- Magnesium – 200–400 mg.
- Vitamin C – 500–1,000 mg.
- Omega-3 oils – 3–5 g (see also Appendix B.3.1).
- Soluble fibre supplement – 3–10 g, such as ground psyllium seeds and husks or fruit pectin (take before a meal together with a large glass of water). Psyllium can occasionally trigger allergic reactions. In that case, use soluble fibre such as pectin that is hypoallergenic. Other sources of soluble fibre are also acceptable such as certain gums.
- MSM-Sulphur 750–1,500 mg* (see also Appendix B.4.2).
- Probiotic supplement*.

Key: mg = milligrams; g = grams; * = optional

as the soluble fibre. This is because there is a chance that the fibre may 'soak up' some of these essential nutrients.

Ideally, you should take the soluble fibre with some water as soon as you wake up in the morning. Then, by the time you have dressed and had breakfast, you can take the supplements, leaving at least 30 minutes between the two, and longer if possible. If you want to split the vitamin doses throughout the day, taking the soluble fibre before a meal and the supplements afterwards will allow sufficient time between them. Alternatively, you could take the soluble fibre first thing in the morning, and take the supplements throughout the day.

While the detox supplement programme featured here has been designed to suit the needs of the majority of people, the variability in lifestyle, diet and genetic inheritance means that not everyone's needs are the same. As a result, some people may need higher levels of certain nutrients than others. Certain stages of life will increase the need for different nutrients. Teenagers' and children's needs for nutrients vary because of their different sizes and various growth spurts. Women of childbearing age tend to need higher levels of iron than post-menopausal women due to the blood loss during menstruation. Expectant mothers will have their own particular needs of nutrients due to an increased nutritional demand from their growing unborn child. The elderly also have their own particular needs because they generally have higher levels of accumulated body toxins and a reduced food intake.

Different diseases will also affect the individual's nutritional demands. The particular nutritional demands that different diseases pose are explained at the end of the appropriate disease chapters of this book. It is also possible for individuals to be tested privately, and so have a programme designed for their personal needs (for specialists in environmental medicine see Appendix D).

Nutritional therapy – the key to 21st century health

The prominence of nutritional supplements in the detox programme is due to the fact that the mere presence of artificial chemicals appears to have increased the need for nutrients, so much so that our requirements are now thought to exceed the levels that we can now realistically get from our diet. Consequently, when tested, most people are found to be deficient in at least one or more essential nutrient. Indeed, many

We now need more nutrients than ever before:

- To protect our tissues from chemically induced free radicals.
- To power the body's detoxification systems, allowing them to process, render safer and eliminate toxic chemicals.
- To repair damage to body tissues from synthetic chemicals.
- To replenish the loss of nutrients from our body stores, triggered by toxic chemicals.
- To use in normal body functions.

Our diets are getting less nutritious because:
- 'Conventional' farming methods tend to produce nutrient-deficient foods compared to produce grown using more traditional organic farming methods.
- Increased food storage and transportation times increase nutrient depletion.
- Food processing destroys many nutrients.
- There is a greater proportion of processed foods in our diet.

Levels of vitamins and minerals needed for optimal health (total daily intake)	
Nutrient	**Optimum intake (min–max)**
Vitamin A* (retinol or beta carotene)	5,000 IU–10,000 IUS
Vitamin C	500–1,000 mg
Vitamin D	400–800 IU
Vitamin E	400–800 IU
Thiamin	3–25 mg
Riboflavin	18–25 mg
Niacin	25–50 mg
Vitamin B6	5–25 mg
Folic acid	400–1,000 mcg
Vitamin B12	2–50 mcg
Biotin	50–300 mcg
Pantothenic Acid	25–50 mg
Calcium	500–1,000 mg
Phosphorus	350–1,000 mg
Iodine	150 mcg
Magnesium	200–400 mg
Zinc	15–30 mg
Selenium	100–200 mcg
Chromium	100–400 mcg
Iron**	15–18 mg
Co-enzyme Q10	30 mg

*If pregnant or trying to conceive, do not exceed 10,000 IU of vitamin A each day.
** Adult men and post-menopausal women may not need supplemental iron.
Key: IU = international units; mcg = micrograms; mg = milligrams; 1,000 mcg = 1 mg

people are taking supplements and still testing deficient. This is because they are taking supplements based on levels set some years ago, which did not take into account higher demands as a result of our increasing chemical body burden.

The levels suggested in the detox supplement programme are based on a very extensive amount of published research on the benefits of dietary supplementation accumulated over the past few decades in both the UK and USA. In particular, I used the research of Dr E. J. Cheraskin who, over a 15-year period, established the Optimal Nutrient Allowances for vitamins in over 10,000 Americans.[3] It is also based on Dr W. Rea's work in treating over 20,000 chemically sensitive patients at the Environmental Health Center, in Dallas, USA.[4] And finally it takes into account some of the values recommended by the UK Department of Health.

The levels needed can vary dramatically between individuals, according to need, whether they are taking medicines, their exposure to chemicals and the presence of disease. In addition, many people use nutrients over a short term for 'therapeutic' purposes and take higher levels than they might take over the long term. (See Appendix B for more information about individual nutrients and the best food sources in which they can be found.) As nutrient levels can only ever be approximate, a range of intakes is often given.

Many scientists now believe that, for health, everyone needs to increase their intake of nutritional supplements to optimise functioning and to deal with the chemical load. As well as preventing illnesses, nutrients are being used by more and more specialisms in the battle against illnesses such as cancer (see page 216). In the next section I will take a more detailed look at all the different types of supplements used to detox and to ensure the body's higher nutritional needs are met.

Micronutrients – vitamins and minerals: Our exposure to toxins has dramatically increased our demand for the nutrients commonly referred to as 'antioxidants' (see Appendix B.1 to B.2). Antioxidants are needed in ever-increasing levels because they help soak up the health-damaging free radicals released when chemicals come into contact with body tissues. The more chemicals we are exposed to, the greater our need for tissue-protecting antioxidants. This explains why people who are deficient in antioxidants are at a higher risk of developing virtually all the twenty-first century chemically linked diseases discussed in this book. Consequently, supplementation of these health protectors is highly advised. The most important antioxidants are the vitamins A, C, E, co-enzyme Q10 and the minerals selenium and zinc. Other antioxidants include the omega-3 oils and the 'detoxing' amino acid glutathione (see Appendix B.4).

The B group of vitamins, in particular vitamin B6 and B12, also play a vital part in detoxification – as our bodies need large amounts of these nutrients in order to process toxic chemicals. As a result, most people who are particularly exposed to chemicals tend to be grossly deficient in these nutrients. B vitamins also play an important role in powering our metabolism, and preventing a wide range of diseases from developing, such as high cholesterol (see page 193), so any supplement programme needs to include a good level of these vital energising nutrients.

The levels of certain minerals in our diet need to be regularly topped up as well. The most important ones are zinc, magnesium and selenium. The vital need for these minerals can be gauged by the fact that magnesium deficiency alone is so common and causes so many health problems that there is an entire medical journal dedicated to this mineral (see Appendix B.2).

The easiest way to get all the vitamin and mineral supplements you need is to purchase them combined into a few top quality products obtained from a reputable natural products company, such as *Biocare, Higher Nature* and *Solgar* (see Appendix D). That way you won't have to take too many pills and capsules. You can normally get sufficient levels of zinc and selenium in a good multivitamin and mineral supplement, but

Possible reaction to detoxing

If your body is particularly run down or nutrient deficient then, for a few weeks after you start taking supplements, you might feel temporarily worse before you feel better. This is because for the first time in years, your body will actually have sufficient resources to start dealing with the massive build-up of stored chemicals. The temporary ill-effects are thought to be caused by the increased mobilisation of chemicals that are in the process of breaking down.

Don't be disheartened if this affects you. On the contrary, you should realise that this shows the supplements are having the desired effect. Keep going and this phase will soon wear off. You will then be rewarded with much better health.

most people need to take an additional supplement of magnesium to ensure they get the full amount their body requires.

Essential fatty acids: Many people are used to taking vitamin and mineral supplements, but comparatively few take essential fatty acids (see Appendix B.3). Yet these essential nutrients are vital to good health. Omega-3 and omega-6 oils are found in every cell of our body. People deficient in these health-giving oils are not only less able to detoxify chemicals, but also much more prone to developing a wide number of different diseases. Many people have a low intake of foods such as raw nuts and fish that contain higher levels of these nutrients, particular omega-3, and so tend to be deficient in them.

Before you rush out and buy your essential oil supplements, it is important to understand that we need to hit the right balance between the amounts of omega-3 and 6 we consume in order to obtain the greater benefits.

Many years ago when our diets were much less processed, nature provided us with roughly balanced amounts of omega-3 and 6 oils. But, due to dramatic changes in our diets, accompanied by the fact that food processors dislike using omega-3 oils as they go rancid more quickly, we are now getting far more omega-6 than omega-3 oils. We now get up to 20 times more omega-6 oils in our diet than omega-3 oils.

Omega-3s and 6s are the body's yin and yang. The two vie for space in our cells, brain and nerve endings, and they produce different hormone messengers. They also compete for the same enzymes so a flood of omega-6s can keep the 3s from doing their job.

Omega-6s stimulate inflammation, omega-3s suppress inflammation; omega-6s raise blood pressure, omega-3s lower it. Omega-6s make your blood clot, omega-3s keep it from clotting; omega-6s oxidise the cholesterol in your arteries and clog them, omega-3s are antioxidant.

The more omega-6s we eat, the more they dominate our cells. Consuming more omega-3s has been associated with preventing heart disease and fatal heart attacks, improving brain and vision development (so much so that infant formulas have been changed to add omega-3s), lowering blood pressure and fighting inflammation, arthritis, asthma and, in some cases, cancer, helping the body to use insulin and fend off obesity, relieving depression and also reducing violent behaviour. That is why even the most conservative medical authorities recommend that people should eat foods high in omega-3s and take regular supplements of omega-3.

It also seems only sensible to suggest that people who take omega-6 oils – such as evening primrose – should balance this by taking an oil that contains relatively high levels of omega-3. Due to the average dietary imbalances between omega-6 and 3, it seems sensible to consume fatty acid supplements that have a higher proportion of omega-3 oils than omega-6s. (At present there is no established maximum safe level for omega-6 oils.)

Since most people tend to be deficient in omega-3 oils, and most fish or vegetable oil supplements also contain a certain amount of omega-6 oils, I have only included sources high in omega-3 oils in the detox supplement programme. However, for those few conditions that require higher levels of omega-6 oils, then a separate source of omega-6, such as evening primrose oil, could also be taken.

Vegetable oils, such as flax and hemp, tend to be relatively free from chemicals, and so make a better choice for supplementation than the more heavily polluted fish oils. Flax is one of the oldest cultivated plants; its Latin name means 'most useful plant'. However, a small group of people are unable to convert vegetable oils into oils that their body can use, so fish oils would be the best choice for them. Fish oils also contain a more concentrated form of omega-3 oils so you need comparatively less of them to meet your daily requirement. My advice is to stick with reputable suppliers that acknowledge the potential problem posed by chemical contamination, that test for these substances, and sell only 'pollution free' fish oil (see Appendix D, page 322).

Some companies remove the toxins from fish oil by distilling them out. These are the cleanest oils around and the safest to take. Whilst no oil (animal or vegetable) or indeed food is pollution free, these cleaned up fish oils appear to be as close as you are going to get to being free of chemicals.

Fibre: There are two types of fibre valuable in detoxing (see Appendix B.5). The first is insoluble fibre, commonly referred to as roughage. An example of this is wheat bran. It passes through the gut relatively unchanged, but is useful because it increases the rate at which waste products move through the bowels – reducing the risk of the body absorbing toxic chemicals.

The second, more important type, is soluble fibre. This forms a gel-like consistency with water and is found in higher levels in beans and other pulses, oats, apples and oranges. You can buy it in supplement form as ground psyllium seeds, fruit pectins and gums. You should drink plenty of fluid with all forms of fibre, and in particular with psyllium husks, which tend to absorb a lot of water.

Soluble fibre plays an exceptionally important part in my detox programme because it is among the few substances that can lower the level of virtually all the different types of chemical toxins found in the body (for example, organochlorines, and toxic metals such as mercury). This is due to its powerful ability to bind to toxins while travelling through the gut, which you can then excrete safely.

Binding substances can be so effective at binding chemicals that they could potentially bind with any medications you take, thereby reducing their effect. So check with your doctor before taking fibre substances if you have been prescribed medication, particularly contraceptive pills or thyroid hormone replacement treatment, which could possibly be rendered ineffective. (And don't forget to leave a gap of at least 30 minutes after taking fibre supplements before taking vitamins and minerals and any medication.)

pH balance: The pH balance of your body is the relative level of acidity/alkalinity and is vitally important in allowing the detoxi- fication enzymes to work properly. Unfortunately, most people's diet is high in acid-producing foods (such as meat and cheese) and low in alkaline-forming foods (such as fruits and particularly vegetables). This means that in most people the enzyme systems do not function properly. As a result, their ability to detoxify most chemicals is seriously reduced. Therefore an alkalinisation supplement is useful, as this will promote more effective and rapid removal and processing of chemical toxins.

If you already eat a diet high in vegetables and fruit, or indeed the diet in this programme, you may not need this supplement. If you want to check, you can test your urine to see whether it is alkaline or acidic by using a piece of litmus paper, which is provided with most alkalinisation supplements or can be found as part of a urine testing strip at your doctor's surgery. You should not take this supplement if you have high blood pressure (hypertension) or a kidney or heart impairment, but can drink vegetable juice instead. If you are at all unsure about taking an alkalinisation supplement, check with your doctor first.

Amino acids and MSM-sulphur: One of the problems with chemical pollutants is that they damage the way our bodies break down, absorb, use and manufacture amino acids. This is why people who are damaged by chemicals are frequently deficient in amino acids, despite seemingly adequate levels in their diet.

Certain amino acids are crucial to our ability to detoxify ourselves of chemical pollutants, particularly the harder to shift organochlorines. They include methionine, cysteine, taurine and glutathione. Glutathione is possibly the body's best built-in natural detoxifier. Not only is it vital in processing artificial chemicals, it also binds to or 'chelates' mercury and other toxic metals and then carries them safely out of the body (for more information on toxic metal chelators, see page 276). These amino acids can be found in many of the foods listed in the seven-day detox plan, but to ensure that you are receiving optimal levels you could always supplement some of them. Suggested daily levels are as follows:

■ Tyrosine (catecholamine and thyroid hormone precursor) 200–500 mg.

- L-5 hydroxytryptophan (5HTP, a natural precursor of serotonin) 25–50 mg.
- Methionine (great detoxing nutrient commonly deficient in people) 200–500 mg.
- Glutathione (antioxidant and great detoxifier, particularly of mercury) 200–500 mg (see Appendix B.4).

(These supplements tend to be hard to find, and if you do find them they tend to be combined with other amino acids. For suppliers see Appendix D.)

MSM-sulphur is a natural form of sulphur found in all organisms. It is a key component in many amino acids, particularly the ones that play a vital role in detoxing, such as gluathione. Sulphur is referred to as nature's 'beauty mineral' because it helps keep skin clear and nails strong. Due to its ability to remove mercury and other heavy metals from the body safely, it is a must-take supplement for anybody who has ever had mercury amalgam fillings or vaccinations, or who lives or works in a polluted city environment (see Appendix B.4.2).

Probiotics: Probiotic means 'for life'. This contrasts with antibiotic, meaning 'against life'. The term probiotics is now generally used to describe the living beneficial bacteria that promote the health of the digestive, vaginal and urinary tracts. Probiotic bacteria strengthen the immune system and help keep harmful micro-organisms in check.

Our gastrointestinal tract is home to more than 400 different species of bacteria weighing 1.5 kg (3½ lb) in total. Most of these are beneficial bacteria. This large quantity of working bacteria performs very important functions in the body and keeps us healthy by:

- Enhancing the absorption of minerals and vitamins and improving digestion.
- Improving our immune system by producing antimicrobial substances that protect us against dangerous bacteria, fungi and viruses. This is important because many debilitating

and degenerative diseases begin in the intestinal tract. In particular, probiotics help prevent intestinal tract infections such as *Candida albicans* and *Helicobacter pylori* (causes of candidiasis and stomach ulcers respectively).

- Increasing absorption of calcium, which is important in the prevention of osteoporosis.
- Producing B vitamins.
- Supporting healthy liver function.
- Normalising bowel elimination problems and promoting regularity.
- Alleviating bowel wind, bloating and belching.
- Assisting in cholesterol management.

When there are not enough beneficial bacteria in the body, harmful bacteria are more likely to invade, taking up residence on the lining of our intestinal tract, multiplying and spreading over more and more intestinal area. This causes symptoms such as bloating, bowel wind, indigestion, constipation and diarrhoea. Many factors lower levels of good bacteria, particularly poor diet, chemical toxins, and certain pharmaceutical drugs, especially antibiotics. Taking probiotic supplements such as *Lactobacillus acidophilus* (which helps guard your small intestines), and *bifidobacterium* (which protects your large intestines) can help sustain good health.

Food and water

The process of cooking lowers the levels of essential micronutrients in many foods. By eating nuts, fruit and vegetables raw, where possible, you benefit from a good micronutrient content, as well as a whole range of other nutrients, known as phytonutrients, which play a role in enhancing our body systems. Raw nuts, fruit and vegetables also have higher levels of enzymes thought to improve digestion of foods.

Intolerance diets: Food intolerances and food allergies are becoming increasingly common (see page 149). Foods commonly known to cause problems include milk and dairy products, gluten in cereal products, nuts, seafoods, and food additives that trigger pseudo-allergic reactions. If you react only after eating certain foods, such as nuts or dairy produce, then it can be relatively easy to cut these foods from the diet. However, in many cases it might not be so clear cut.

I would recommend specialist professional advice in determining what the particular trigger is, and to help you manage the condition. Expert help is important because people with food intolerances are generally more prone to nutritional deficiencies. This is because their gut is less able to absorb nutrients, owing to an increased level of inflammation, and because cutting major food groups out of the diet can further increase these risks.

Genetically modified foods: For the past few years I have tried without success to find at least one study that has looked at the long-term effects on humans of eating genetically modified foods. I have found none. What is worse, out of the few studies I have found on animals, all of them appeared to show that GM foods shortened life expectancy. Some crops, such as 'Bt corn', have been genetically engineered to create their own pesticides (see www.wordiq.com/definition/pesticide). If you consider that some genetically modified foods such as the 'Bt potato' were originally treated by the Environmental Protection Agency (EPA) as if they were pesticides and not food and as such required no labelling, this could help to explain why (see www.wordiq.com/definition/Genetically_modified_food). The very fact that many

Biopesticides – when plants are classified as pesticides

The EPA classifies pesticides produced by genetically engineered plants as 'biopesticides'. To date two classes of genetically modified (GM) plants fall under the EPA purview: plants containing Bt toxins and those expressing resistance to viruses. The EPA regulates the pesticide contained within a GM plant in the same way it regulates a pesticide applied to a plant, but not actually the plant itself.

Evidence of health damage from the pollen of a GM crop

Researchers say that villagers living near a GM maize field in the Philippines have suffered a range of illnesses. The director of the Norwegian Institute of Gene Ecology, Professor Terje Traavik, said that there is hard evidence of a threat. He revealed details of a study apparently showing that villagers from a Filipino farming community close to GM maize fields suffered fevers, breathing problems and intestinal and skin ailments. He said blood tests indicated that the symptoms resulted from inhaling mutated maize pollen that had been carried in the wind. The GM maize involved had been modified to include a pesticide called Bt within the plant.[5]

are treated under pesticides rules and guidelines means that the people registering them must have believed from the start that they would be potentially dangerous to our health.

Due to the increasing reports of toxicities from GM foods, and the absence of published peer-reviewed safety studies on the effects these foods have on humans, together with the fact that some of these foods have been treated as pesticides and not foods, I continue to take the precautionary principle and avoid all GM foods.

Water: It is vitally important to drink water in sufficient quantities to help wash out toxins from the system. I would suggest an intake of at least 2–3 litres (3½–5 pints) per day. Don't forget, if your body becomes mildly dehydrated by just a few per cent, your energy levels can drop by 20 per cent.

Exercise

I think that deep down most of us already know that exercise brings a whole host of health benefits. Exercise plays a major role in my programme because it speeds up detoxification by mobilising toxins from your fat, increases the metabolic rate, and helps replace hormones damaged by chemical toxins. Thus it improves general mood, aids weight loss, enhances the figure and boosts fitness levels.

But before embarking on an exercise routine you should agree your proposed activity level with your doctor if you have been physically inactive for six months or longer, are diabetic, or if you have a history of any of the following: heart disease, high blood pressure, asthma, emphysema or other lung disease, or joint disease such as arthritis that might worsen with exercise.

A regular exercise regime: Exercise can be broadly divided into two main categories: aerobic exercises such as walking, jogging or dancing, which improve your stamina and fitness, and resistance exercise, which builds muscle strength and tone.

Aerobic exercise: Aim to exercise 'aerobically' for sustained periods of 15 to 30 minutes at a time at least three times a week. This means exercising at a level that raises your pulse and breathing rate and leaves you slightly sweaty. But avoid getting breathless – that indicates you are exercising too hard. The ideal level of intensity allows you to hold a 'breathy' conversation with a friend, or to sing or recite poetry out loud. If you can't talk as you exercise you are not exercising aerobically and should slow down. As your stamina improves you can steadily increase the exercise period and/or intensity. Simple forms of aerobic exercise include brisk walking (wear suitable shoes and aim to plan a route that includes a slight gradient at some point), jogging (wear trainers and jog on grass rather than tarmac, if possible, to avoid damaged joints), swimming and cycling (always wear a helmet).

Out and about
- Walk or cycle rather than use the car.
- Leave the bus or tube train one or two stops before a destination and walk the rest of the way.
- Walk up and down escalators.

At work
- Use the stairs, rather than the lift (at least part of the way).
- Go for a brisk walk during lunch breaks.

Calories Burned per 15 Minutes of Activity

Activity	Calories burned per 15-minute activity
Running (6-minute mile)	280
Jogging (9-minute mile)	193
Rowing	123
Rambling	105
Swimming	105
Dancing	80
Cycling (5.5 mph)	70
Golf	70
Walking briskly (4 mph)	70
Frisbee throwing	53

■ Cut down on emails and phone calls and deliver messages personally.

In your leisure time
■ Join a gym and encourage friends to do the same so that you motivate each other.
■ Set up your own health group with friends and exercise together (following the instructions in a book or video on exercise).
■ Go for long walks at the weekend and on holidays.
■ Choose a sport or other active pastime that you enjoy – ideally one with a club in your area that you can join.

Other therapies
There are a number of other therapies that can be of value in helping people to recover from their twenty-first century illnesses. They include herbal remedies, homeopathy, massage therapy and acupuncture.

Herbal remedies: The herbal industry is growing. More herbs are available than ever before, and more and more people are embracing their use. They differ from nutritional supplements as they are not 'essential' and so our bodies don't have to have them. Despite that, a growing number of studies reveal that they offer many benefits in preventing disease and treating existing ones (see Appendix B.6). They can, in some cases, act more like drugs. So here are some tips to help enhance proper use of herbals.

- Be an informed consumer. Research the product to determine: safety, validity of claims, dosage, most effective form, part of plant used, species, how long to use it, side-effects, any adverse effect when combined with other supplements or medications, and reasonable price.
- Inform your doctor, pharmacist and other healthcare professionals of any herbs you are considering or that you routinely use. Consult them with any questions. However, few doctors are trained in herbal lore, so you must take ultimate responsibility if you use them.
- Pick good brands that have been tested for consistency in dosage.
- Read the product label and follow the instructions.
- Use herbal products only for minor conditions and only for limited periods of time, usually ranging from weeks to months depending on the individual product. If a condition is serious or chronic, consult your doctor.
- Discontinue herbs immediately if you experience any adverse side-effects.
- Chinese herbs and medicines can be contaminated with toxic chemicals and pesticides so ensure you obtain them from a reputable source.

Homeopathy: Homeopathy is a system of medicine based on the Law of Similars or 'Let like cure like'. It is a principle that has been known for centuries. A German physician called Samuel Hahnemann developed the principle into a system of medicine called homeopathy, and it has been used successfully for the last 200 years. The concept of homeopathy differs from that of conventional medicine in that it attempts to stimulate the body to cure itself.

Homeopaths work on the principle that all symptoms, no

matter how uncomfortable they are, represent the body's attempt to restore itself to health. Instead of looking upon symptoms as something wrong that must be set right, they see them as signs of the way the body is attempting to help itself. For example, rather than simply trying to stop a cough with suppressants, as conventional medicine does, a homeopath will give a remedy that would *cause* a cough in a healthy person. This stimulates the body to restore itself. A person who takes a suppressant for a cough is not undergoing a cure but is only controlling the symptoms. Homeopathy's aim is the cure. (To find a registered homeopath, see Appendix D.)

Massage therapy: The massage therapist works by providing hands-on treatment that consists of mechanical manipulation of the soft tissues in the body such as muscles, tendons, ligaments and connective tissue, and mobilisation of the joints. Properly administered, this is thought to help healing and increase activity of the circulatory and lymphatic systems. It can also serve to relax and refresh muscles, relieve pain and help maintain healthy skin. Massage therapy also helps calm the nervous system, promoting a sense of relaxation and renewed energy, and assists in reducing tension and relieving fatigue (see International Federation of Aromatherapists, page 332).

Acupuncture: Acupuncture is the gentle insertion of extremely thin needles into specific points on the body to stimulate the flow of one's 'Qi' or natural healing energy. Acupuncture has been used in China for over 5,000 years. Acupuncturists have successfully treated chronic pain, disorders of the immune, endocrine and neurological systems, and many other conditions. (To find a registered acupuncturist, see Appendix D.)

The seven-day detox

This seven-day detox plan has been specifically designed for those who want a swift and effective way of kick-starting the body's detox and health systems into shape. I have included some great detoxifiers packed with loads of soluble fibre, and super foods bursting with essential detoxing and health-enhancing nutrients. This plan will give your body the best start possible. If you adopt some of these habits into your usual routine (after having completed the initial seven-day detox) you will be starting the rest of your life fully prepared to defend yourself from anything and everything that the twenty-first century can throw at you.

It is best to eat organic foods, of course, but for many this is not possible owing to restricted availability or expense. So the best advice is to avoid the most polluted foods (see page 25) and reduce the chemical loading of conventionally grown foods by washing and peeling fruit and vegetables and cutting excess fat off meat (fat tends to contain far more chemicals than the meat itself).

To make things as easy as possible, in addition to the diet guidelines, I have also drawn up a seven-day menu plan, which includes suggested times at which to take the supplements. This is a practical guide designed to make the whole detox programme as easy as possible.

Seven-day detox plan

Proteins: choose at least 300 g (12 oz) each day of the following meats or high protein foods (preferably organic): lean beef/venison/chicken/turkey/vegetable-based proteins such as soya and Quorn/white fish (maximum of one fish meal every week)/eggs. (Remove all visible skin and fat from meat and fish when preparing for cooking and don't eat the skin or fat on cooked meats.)

Oils: one tablespoon of flax seed oil a day (taken as a supplement), *and*

one tablespoon of any of the following unprocessed vegetable oils: walnut oil, pumpkin seed oil (all used cold in salads as heating destroys the nutritional content of these oils), olive oil (which can be used for cooking)

or

25 g raw nuts or seeds, or 25 g of a combination of raw nuts and seeds (particularly pumpkin seeds and walnuts)

or

one small avocado.

Optional: up to 100 ml (4 fl oz) each day of semi-skimmed milk or unsweetened soya milk.

Vegetables: unlimited amounts of the following vegetables, eaten raw, steamed or as fat-free vegetable soup (organic for preference): asparagus, aubergines, baby corn, bamboo shoots, beansprouts, green beans, beetroot, broccoli, Brussels sprouts, cabbage, carrots, cauliflower, celery, Swiss chard, Chinese cabbage, courgettes, cucumbers, endive, green leafy vegetables, leeks, lettuce, mangetout peas, mushrooms, okra, onions, green, red and yellow peppers, radishes, sugar snap peas, tomatoes, watercress, yellow squash, water chestnuts.

Detoxing, soluble fibre-rich foods: each day take 160 g (approx 6 oz) of cooked pulses such as lentils or split peas, kidney beans, peas (could be eaten raw), chickpeas, haricot beans
  or
  50 g (2 oz) dried weight oats
  or
  4 small oat cakes.

Fruit: four portions of fresh fruit a day. A typical portion is: an apple, an orange, half a grapefruit, 2 medium plums, a nectarine, a peach, a small banana or 100 g of any other fruit.

Fluids: at least eight large (225 ml) glasses of freshly filtered or bottled water a day. As well as keeping you well hydrated, drinking plenty of water will help to flush away unwanted chemicals released by your weight loss. To enhance detoxification, drink mineral water flavoured with lemon or lime juice. Coffee substitutes, herbal teas and filtered water can be drunk freely. Drinks (or other products) using artificial sweeteners should be avoided.

Flavourings: the following flavourings can be used at any time –

Foods and drinks to avoid

There are some foods that you should definitely avoid on the seven-day detox because they slow down or impair your ability to detoxify. They include:

■ Caffeinated drinks, because they disturb the production of energy-forming and detoxing hormones and create carbohydrate cravings.

■ Alcohol, as it slows down detoxification.

■ Foods high in trans-fats. Trans-fats are created when polyunsaturated oils and fats are heated in cooking. Food fried in sunflower oil, for example, is high in trans-fats; so is most deep-fried food. Limit yourself to cooking with olive oil from your allowance, as this is a mostly monounsaturated oil.

■ Foods very high in chemicals (see Chapter 3).

indeed, use of fresh herbs with garlic and yeast extracts is positively beneficial! Herbs, spices, mustard, chillies, garlic, pepper, salt, soy sauce, lemon juice, vinegar, Worcestershire sauce, yeast extracts, stock cubes, fat-free vegetable soup.

Supplements: take the levels as recommended earlier in this chapter. Leave at least half an hour between taking fibre supplements and other vitamins.

Putting it all together

So, now you know what you can eat every day. Next is a seven-day plan that will hopefully inspire you by suggesting many ways in which you can create tasty and interesting daily menus from the food allowances provided. So *bon appétit* and happy detoxing to you all!

Menu One

First thing	Fibre supplements
	Large glass of water
Breakfast	Tofu scramble (tofu, onions and herbs fried in 1 teaspoon of olive oil)
	Multivitamins and mineral supplement, magnesium, vitamin C, and 1 tablespoon of flax oil (taken at least half an hour after fibre supplements)

Mid-morning	1 portion of fruit
Pre-lunch	Fibre supplements
	Large glass of water
Lunch	Chicken, apple and beetroot salad with red leaves topped with a teaspoon of sliced almonds
Afternoon	2 plums
Pre-dinner	Fibre supplements
	Large glass of water
Dinner	Roast lamb
	Curried chickpeas: slice onion, garlic, a chilli pepper and a courgette, and fry (pan covered) in 1 teaspoon of olive oil. When soft, add a small tin of chopped tomatoes, 150 g of cooked chickpeas and cook for 5–10 minutes. Flavour with a pinch of salt and pepper, garam masala, cumin seeds (ground or whole). Add chopped fresh coriander to garnish, and serve.
	A slice of melon
	Any additional supplements

Menu Two

First thing	Fibre supplements
	Large glass of water
Breakfast	Porridge (made with water and with milk from allowance)
	Multivitamins, etc., as for Menu One
Mid-morning	1 portion of fruit
Pre-lunch	Fibre supplements
	Large glass of water
Lunch	Roast chicken cold cuts
	Mixed salad with red and green peppers and unlimited vegetables, dressed with lemon juice and herbs
	1 orange
Afternoon	1 portion of fruit
Pre-dinner	Fibre supplements
	Large glass of water

Dinner	Grilled steak
	Green beans
	Apple, walnuts (25 g/1 oz) and green salad, dressed with lemon juice
	Any additional supplements

Menu Three

First thing	Fibre supplements
	Large glass of water
Breakfast	Banana and mango 'smoothie'
	Two oat cakes
	Multivitamins, etc., as for Menu One
Mid-morning	Cucumber and other raw vegetable sticks
Pre-lunch	Fibre supplements
	Large glass of water
Lunch	Grilled or steamed white fish
	Steamed broccoli and carrots
	2 oat cakes
Afternoon	1 portion of fruit
Pre-dinner	Fibre supplements
	Large glass of water
Dinner	Lamb, green pepper and onion kebabs
	Mediterranean salad of sliced tomato, cucumber, avocado with a sprinkling of coriander and olives
	1 portion of fruit
	Any additional supplements

Menu Four

First thing	Fibre supplements
	Large glass of water
Breakfast	2 eggs scrambled with herbs and tomatoes (cooked with 1 teaspoon of olive oil)
	1 small glass of freshly squeezed orange juice
	Multivitamins, etc., as for Menu One
Mid-morning	1 portion of fruit
Pre-lunch	Fibre supplements
	Large glass of water

Lunch	Slices of lean meat
	White bean, tomato, rocket and onion salad dressed with lemon juice and seasoned with salt and pepper
Afternoon	1 portion of fruit
Pre-dinner	Fibre supplements
	Large glass of water
Dinner	A slice of melon
	Spicy tofu stir-fry (using seasoned tofu, garlic, onions, mushrooms, chillis, red peppers, courgettes, tomatoes stir-fried in 2 teaspoons of olive oil)
	Any additional supplements

Menu Five

First thing	Fibre supplements
	Large glass of water
Breakfast	Sugar-free muesli with milk from allowance, topped with a sliced banana
	Multivitamins, etc., as for Menu One
Mid-morning	1 apple
Pre-lunch	Fibre supplements
	Large glass of water
Lunch	Beef or venison burgers
	Orange, raw grated carrot, pumpkin seed (25 g/1 oz) and green leaf salad, dressed with lemon juice
Afternoon	1 portion of fruit
Pre-dinner	Fibre supplements
	Large glass of water
Dinner	Consommé or clear soup
	Grilled chicken breast
	Tomato sauce with steamed leeks and mushrooms
	Fresh fruit salad
	Any additional supplements

Menu Six

First thing	Fibre supplements
	Large glass of water
Breakfast	Porridge (made with water and with milk from allowance)
	Multivitamins, etc., as for Menu One
Mid-morning	Small bunch of grapes
Pre-lunch	Fibre supplements
	Large glass of water
Lunch	Warm turkey, roast garlic, spinach and pinenut salad (roast 4 cloves of garlic for about 15 minutes in 1 teaspoon of olive oil until slightly brown. Immediately mix with warmed pieces of turkey and pour over baby spinach leaves, then sprinkle with 1 teaspoon of pine nuts and flavour with lemon juice, salt and pepper)
	1 banana
Afternoon	1 portion of fruit
Pre-dinner	Fibre supplements
	Large glass of water
Dinner	Grilled beef steak
	Vegetable bake (sliced tomatoes, courgettes, yellow pepper, mushrooms and garlic; brush with olive oil and bake)
	1 pear
	Any additional supplements

Menu Seven

First thing	Fibre supplements
	Large glass of water
Breakfast	Banana and pineapple 'smoothie'
	2 oat cakes
	Multivitamins, etc., as for Menu One
Mid-morning	Raw carrot and cucumber sticks
Pre-lunch	Fibre supplements
	Large glass of water
Lunch	Grilled chicken breast

Mixed green leaf and herb salad (place in a bowl prepared green salad leaves and a mixture of chopped fresh herbs, add cherry tomatoes, dress with lemon juice and 1 tablespoon of olive oil, season with salt and pepper, and serve)

Afternoon	1 apple and 2 oat cakes
Pre-dinner	Fibre supplements
	Large glass of water
Dinner	Slice of melon
	Grilled lamb chops
	Braised/steamed mangetout (or sugar snap) peas, baby corn and carrots
	Any additional supplements

5

25 Top Tips to Enhance Your Health

'The European Union has admitted that 99 per cent of the volume of chemicals on the market are inadequately regulated; 21 per cent of Europe's highest volume chemicals have no safety data publicly available, and 86 per cent have less than the minimum amount of data publicly available to make even a basic safety assessment.'

WORLD-WIDE FUND FOR NATURE WEBSITE (WWW.WWF.ORG.UK)

To help you on your way to achieving the best of health, I have combined the advice given so far into 25 excellent tips designed to help rid your life of chemicals. Whilst you certainly don't have to do everything on this list, the more you can achieve the better. The key is to do *what* you can *when* you can, as every one will help you to detoxify over the long term.

1. Avoid contact with any sort of pesticide. This includes any substance using artificial chemicals to kill any form of animal life (such as fly sprays, flea preparations, head-lice shampoo) or plant life (such as weed-killer). Look up alternative chemical-free ways to deal with your problem. For instance use fine-tooth combs to rid hair of head lice.

2. Maximise the proportion of organically produced foods in your diet – especially fish, soft fruit and vegetables and lean

meat. Go to your local fishmonger and ask for wild, not farmed, fish.

3. Take daily supplements to ensure you are getting enough nutrients to cleanse your body of artificial chemicals (see Chapter 4).

4. Always filter or distil tap water before drinking it. If you use bottled water, buy it in a glass bottle rather than a plastic one. If you can, install a household water filter to reduce the chemicals absorbed from bath or shower water.

5. Wash and peel non-organic fresh fruit and vegetables before eating.

6. Reduce your intake of animal fats.

7. Avoid farmed salmon (more and more supermarkets now sell organic salmon) and limit your intake of tuna (due to potential contamination of mercury and organochlorine pollutants). If you do eat these foods, combine them with foods high in soluble fibre, such as beans or pulses, or take soluble fibre supplements. These measures will greatly reduce the amount of toxins absorbed from a meal.

8. If you plan to eat out, take soluble fibre supplements in advance to absorb any chemicals in the meal.

9. Use environmentally friendly household cleaning products.

10. Choose organic cosmetics, hair products and toiletries whenever possible. And if you can't find an alternative product, just try to use less of it.

11. Avoid storing fatty foods in plastic containers, or acidic foods in aluminium containers, or drinking colas in aluminium cans. These storage materials can all contaminate foods and drinks.

12. Don't microwave or heat up foods in plastic containers, particularly if they have a high fat content, as the heat will make the chemicals in the plastic rapidly migrate into the food.

13. Take regular exercise to help to strengthen your detoxification system. For example, aim to walk where you would normally ride.

14. If getting vaccinated, insist on vaccines that do not contain mercury or aluminium.

15. Try to increase the proportion of whole raw nuts, fruits and vegetables in your diet as they provide beneficial nutrients, many of which you can't get from supplements.

16. Eat foods which contain larger natural amounts of soluble fibre, such as beans, pulses like lentils, oats, apples and oranges. These will help you to detox naturally.

17. If you have highlights or other chemical treatments at the hairdresser, take some extra antioxidants, such as vitamins C and E, and soluble fibre supplements just before your visit. This will help protect your body from chemical damage.

18. Take antioxidant vitamins and soluble fibre supplements before going swimming, as this will help your body deal with the chlorine absorbed from the water.

19. Avoid mercury in dental fillings. Opt for porcelain fillings, or if this is not possible, select white fillings (although these contain plastics they are considered by most dental experts to be far less toxic than amalgam. To get the safest plastics go to a mercury-free dentist as they will be more aware of the whole issue regarding safety of dental materials and will know the best materials available).

20. Seek out fluoride-free toothpaste. Fluoride is a known and registered brain poison that lowers children's IQ. Also avoid any fluoridisation treatment offered by your dentist.

21. Avoid using deodorants that contain aluminium. Other types are available that are both natural and highly effective. Regular washing with soap and water removes the bacteria that feed on the perspiration to cause the unwanted odour. It's also a good idea to cut your intake of caffeine in drinks, as this will reduce the amount you perspire.

22. Ventilate your home by regularly keeping the windows open to clear the air of chemicals given off by household cleaners, plastics, dry-cleaned clothes, and objects treated with fire retardants.

23. Get rid of as much plastic as practical, especially the softer kinds such as clingfilm, wrapping and carrier bags. The more strongly a particular item smells of plastic, the more polluting it will be.

24. Keep house plants, such as spider plants, which can absorb a lot of airborne pollutants.

25. When renovating your house, try to source more natural, environmentally friendly products.

6

Looking Good, Feeling Great

'When I found the first paper showing that one of the most commonly detected pesticides in our food, known as an organophosphate, was actually used as a growth-promoter to fatten up animals, I knew I was on to a winner. It's one matter to find that chemicals cause a fattening effect in animals but quite another to discover that they have been deliberately used for this purpose in real life.'

THE DETOX DIET, PAULA BAILLIE-HAMILTON

The best form of defence is attack

There has to be some sort of carrot for anyone to change their lifestyle and habits in the ways I have just outlined. For most people reading this book, their incentive will be an improvement in their disease symptoms (see Part Two). However, in cutting out disease-triggering toxins and by feeding the body the increased level of nutrients modern living now demands, they could start to experience other hugely beneficial and morale-boosting health benefits they may not have initially expected, such as weight loss, improved body shape, greater energy levels and a heightened level of fitness. This is because it has become apparent that tackling toxins provides a real breakthrough in all of these problem areas. So, to find out how this book could help you achieve the body beautiful, maximise your fitness prowess, boost existing energy levels and improve your health – read on!

Achieving the body beautiful – losing fat and gaining muscle:
While it's good to be fit, what drives many to the gym is a burning desire to improve their looks. Glance at any glossy magazine and you will see images of dozens of gorgeous people with impossibly beautiful bodies plastered on each page from cover to cover. No prizes for guessing the important position good looks and a great body hold in our highly image-conscious society. Rather than helping to win athletic competitions, keeping lean and toned helps some people to win in life.

For all these reasons, it is totally understandable that many people spend much of their free time and efforts in working at shaping up. You can't stop men from wanting more muscle and women from wanting to have curves in the right places – and indeed why not? *Vive la différence* I say! However, many do not realise that exposing their bodies to toxic chemicals could be making them fatter and less shapely.

We all know that the food you eat plays a major part in determining how you look and feel. However, few realise the effects that our ever-increasing exposure to toxic chemicals are having on our looks and fitness levels. I only discovered the full extent to which we are being affected myself several years ago when researching my first book, *The Detox Diet*. I was astounded to discover the extent to which the majority of toxic chemicals make us fatter.

What controls our body weight and shape: Our weight and shape are largely determined by our natural and highly evolved weight control systems. This is a complex network of processes made up of the brain, hormones and metabolism that is designed to keep our weight stable throughout our lives. This acts as a natural slimming system.

What appears to be happening is that this natural slimming system is being poisoned by the toxic chemicals we encounter in our everyday lives, and this damage is making it increasingly difficult for us to control our weight. The result is that not only do we gain weight, but that this weight tends to be in the form of fat and not muscle.

The hormones that control our body shape are also targeted by the toxins. In men, this damage equates to smaller muscles and more fat, particularly around the stomach.[6] In women, this appears to translate to more fat accumulating around the stomach, waist and thighs.[7] In light of this, and the indefatigable rise in the production of toxic chemicals, it is no wonder that so many studies have found our body shape to have significantly changed over the past few decades.

Which chemicals are the most fattening? After stumbling across this powerful chemically-induced fattening effect, the next step for me was to find out what types of chemicals possessed it. It wasn't long before I discovered that virtually all the twenty-first century chemicals we are exposed to in our food and environment possess some sort of weight-altering effect, even at very low levels. These include a wide range of pesticides, medicines, heavy metals, plastics, solvents, environmental pollutants and fire retardants.[1]

Taking pesticides as an example, the deeper I looked into each of the dozens of different synthetic chemicals found as pesticide residues in food, the clearer it became to me that these chemicals – used to kill a huge variety of different forms of life – were the same as or very similar to ones being used to promote growth in animals. These were also associated with weight gain in humans, and were even regularly used as medicines to treat a whole range of human illnesses.[1]

How pesticides make us fatter

So how does this group of chemicals promote fattening? At low doses, organophosphates appear to fatten up animals by severely reducing their ability to use up existing fat stores. As a consequence, they gain weight more quickly, since they can't burn off body fat as well as they previously could. Their food needs fall too, as less food appears to go further. Although the use of organophosphates as growth promoters has now been banned, these former weapons of mass destruction are still one of the commonest pesticides found in many of our foods. They are also commonly used in the manufacture of rubber and plastics, and in petrol and lubricating oils as additives.

It really doesn't matter how you are exposed, whether it is from a can of fly spray or from pesticide residues in food, once they get into your body the chances are they will proceed to damage your weight-control systems, making it just that little bit harder to lose weight in the future. For more information on the chemical causes of the obesity epidemic, please see *The Detox Diet*.

How to lose weight and shape up: Fortunately, these toxin-induced body-shape-damaging effects can be reversed by following the principles described in Chapters 3 and 4 of this book. So, if your exercise efforts are having only limited success in improving your shape, you should combine this with the detox programme detailed in Chapter 4.

If you want to look at weight management in much greater depth, why not read my first book – *The Detox Diet*? This explains where the most fattening chemicals can be found in our environment, and offers a selection of specially designed diet plans.

Maximising your fitness

No serious athlete can afford to ignore the fact that chemical toxins may be damaging their overall competitiveness. Even if they are not exposed to chemicals on a daily basis as part of their job, the toxins athletes are getting in their food and from the environment could make all the difference between winning and losing.

So, how can cutting out toxins give athletes that critical edge over their competitors? To understand this, you first need to know what makes one athlete better than another. For most sports, the three key factors determining who wins or loses are:

■ Muscle size.
■ Muscle strength.
■ Muscle endurance.

The bigger the better! Bigger muscles are a great indicator of someone's overall fitness. Unfortunately, the maximum size to which our muscles can grow is largely predetermined by our genetic makeup and our hormones, so that even by exercising at maximum levels, you could not build them up beyond a certain predestined size without the benefit of illegal and highly dangerous anabolic steroids.

However, looking on the bright side, it may be possible to increase muscle size naturally. This stems from the fact that our current levels of chemical exposure could be preventing the muscles from growing to their true potential. Chemicals do this by lowering the naturally high levels of muscle-growth-promoting hormones, by damaging nerves responsible for stimulating muscle, and by damaging the muscle themselves.

So, if someone is on the brink of sporting success, detoxifying and reducing their body burden of these muscle-shrinking chemicals could give them the competitive edge that they have worked so hard to achieve – leaving their competitors with muscles struggling under their heavy toxic chemical burden.

Stronger muscles with more staying power: While muscle strength depends to some extent on the amount of muscle you have, the strength of the contraction also depends on the maximum amount of energy your muscles can muster.

Energy is produced by tiny cylindrical structures called mitochondria. They are responsible for converting the food we eat into a molecular form of energy that the whole body can easily use – known as ATP (adenosine triphosphate). Our muscles have an immense appetite for energy, so they are packed with millions of these little powerhouses. The number of mitochondria in our muscles and their efficiency ultimately determine muscle strength and endurance.

Unfortunately, the mitochondria appear to be exquisitely sensitive to a wide range of chemical toxins, which reduce their numbers and dramatically impair their effectiveness. Worse still, chemical damage can reduce the body's ability to produce the exact foods needed to fuel the mitochondria. So, not only can chemicals reduce muscle strength, but they can also lower muscle endurance by limiting production of the food supply. This translates to weaker muscles that get exhausted more readily.

Fortunately, mitochondria are very resilient structures. So, a good detoxification and nutritional programme can potentially restore your body to its full complement of mitochondria, as well as upping muscle strength for sprinters and endurance for long-distance runners alike.

The programme in Chapter 4 can provide you with a totally natural, safe and legal competitive advantage – to help you turn your dreams into reality.

Raising your energy levels

Not only athletes but everyone can join in on this free-for-all energy bonanza. And we certainly need it, with demands on our energy levels at a record high, owing to our new-found stressful 24/7 lifestyles. It's not surprising that increasing numbers of us now suffer from feeling 'tired all the time'. Consequently you would be hard pushed to find anyone who would turn down the offer of increased energy levels.

Indeed, many studies show that the number of us complaining of a lack of energy has reached epidemic proportions, with many constantly fighting against a permanent state of exhaustion. And it's not surprising when the average person's day goes something like this:

After waking up, you need at least one cup of coffee or tea to kick-start your body into action. Skipping breakfast, you leave for work, where you spend the day drinking more caffeinated drinks and eating sugary snacks that keep you going from energy boom to bust. Possibly you may find five minutes to wolf down a sandwich or burger at lunch time. By the time you have done a full day's work and got home, you are far too tired to go to the gym or take any other form of exercise, so you end up collapsing in front of the TV to eat your dinner. Then, after doing a few chores such as reading your emails, you crawl into bed. The next day this vicious circle starts all over again.

As you can see, most people use the rapid energy blast that caffeinated drinks provide us with to boost their energy levels temporarily. However, this comes at a price, because after the high comes the low – as it takes time for the body to restock its supplies of energy-boosting hormones. When energy levels collapse, most people at this point reach for the coffee pot again to get their next temporary fix. It's only when the body crashes, once people finally take time off work, that the true state of their hormonal imbalance is finally exposed.

Boost your energy levels by ridding your body of energy-draining toxins: Fortunately there are many simple ways in which you can help yourself to break out of this vicious circle. For example:

- Cut down on stimulants such as alcohol and caffeinated drinks by switching to decaf – or better still replacing them with fresh juice, herbal teas and water. It might hurt at first but it gets easier with time. Soon you will lose these highs and lows for a steady level of energy throughout the day.
- Take nutritional supplements, which allow the body to maximise energy production.
- Eat complex carbohydrates such as starches (pasta, rice, potatoes and wholegrain bread), as they release energy-giving sugars gradually throughout the day.
- Take regular exercise, as this increases levels of energy-enhancing hormones.
- Drink at least 2 litres (3½ pints) of water a day (as even mild dehydration causes fatigue).
- Lower the levels of energy-draining toxins in your body.

While the first five of the above suggestions are widely known, few realise that one of the major causes of low energy is the high level of toxins in the body. These toxins are a highly efficient drain on energy. Consequently the body is actually producing far less energy than it was originally designed to do. So, while most of us tend to get by on what we have got, we are functioning way below our real capacity.

By following the principles set out in this book – lowering levels of energy-draining chemicals from your body, cutting down on caffeine, taking a walk where you may have previously gone by car and letting your body luxuriate in all the nutrients it needs to create energy – you can boost your energy levels to heights you may never have known before and start living life the way it should be lived – looking good and feeling great.

part two

21st Century Diseases: How to Fight Back

7

Strengthen Your Immune System

'Many compounds introduced into the environment by human activity have the potential to disturb the immune system of wildlife and humans.'
WWW.OURSTOLENFUTURE.ORG/CONSENSUS/WINGSPREADIMMUNE.HTM

Immune system meltdown

The body's natural defences – the immune system – is one of the most important safeguards we have for protecting our health. Unfortunately, the exponential increase seen in immune system-related diseases suggests that this aspect of the body has become one of the major casualties of our twenty-first century world.

Owing to the sheer number of people with immune-system diseases, this problem is taken very much for granted. It is only once you step back and take a historical perspective that you can see the real impact that twenty-first century living is having. Asthma, which was relatively unheard of at the beginning of the twentieth century, now affects between 100–150 million people worldwide. This is roughly equivalent to the entire population of the Russian Federation. It is also clear that far from stabilising, the situation is in free-fall, in light of a World Health Organization (WHO) report that the number of those affected by asthma in Western Europe has doubled over the last 10 years.

Common diseases associated with a malfunctioning immune system

- Allergies
- Arthritis (eg rheumatoid arthritis)
- Asthma
- Autoimmune disorders
- Cancer
- Connective tissue disorders (eg Sjögren's syndrome)
- Diabetes
- Eczema
- Infections
- Urticaria (nettle rash)

To discover why we have become more susceptible to immune system-related diseases, we need to look briefly at what our immune system is, what strengthens it and what can damage it.

What is our immune system and why do we need it? We live in a hostile world filled with a bewildering array of infectious agents of diverse shape, size and composition. These would all quite happily use us as a rich sanctuary for propagating their selfish genes had we not also developed a series of defence mechanisms at least their equal in effectiveness and ingenuity. As well as giving us immunity against many different infections, our immune system seeks out and destroys the abnormal cells that our body regularly produces and that could turn cancerous if not kept in check.

To help achieve this we have throughout the body an entire network of fluid-filled tubes and nodes, running parallel to our blood vessels, that all connect together to form the lymphatic system, a major part of the immune system. The main immune system function of the lymphatic system is to filter out infectious organisms from the lymph fluid as it drains out of the tissues, trapping them in the lymph nodes, before returning the fluid to the bloodstream.

Other important tissues making up this immune system include the spleen and bone marrow, which produce infection-fighting white blood cells and proteins called antibodies. These travel throughout the body, into the bloodstream and in and out of the tissues, mopping up infectious organisms.

The immune system normally springs into action when the body senses that an invading micro-organism has breached its external defences. The subsequent attack normally concludes with the annihilation of the invader body as the immune cells and proteins work together to break it down.

The immune system is crippled by twenty-first century chemical toxins: By looking at the overall picture it is clear that changes in the environment and our diet must be at the heart of the new immune-system disease epidemics, because the changes are far too rapid to have arisen solely as a result of changes in our genetic makeup. We don't have to look too closely at what could have changed in our environment in order to find the prime suspect for the problem.

With every passing day, it becomes more and more apparent that the immune system is an easy target for toxic chemicals. Extensive research now shows that the majority of the commonest types of chemicals we are exposed to on a daily basis damage virtually every aspect of our immune system. Indeed there is now a separate branch of medicine, known as immunotoxicology, that specialises in this field.

All the usual chemical suspects are implicated: pesticides, heavy metals, environmental pollutants, solvents and other chemicals possessing powerful immune system-damaging properties. They appear to hinder the smooth functioning of the immune system in two main ways: either by suppressing it (immunosuppression), causing it to be underactive, or overstimulating it so that it is overactive. Most chemicals trigger a mixture of the two effects.

If suppressed, the immune system cannot work properly to tackle invading organisms, and as a result the person tends to become more vulnerable to infections and is at a greater risk of developing cancer. Immune system overdrive causes a different set of problems. People become sensitive or allergic to more and more substances, experiencing symptoms such as urticaria, runny nose, wheezing and, in extreme cases, anaphylactic shock. This also increases the long-term chances of developing an auto-immune system disorder (see page 98).

Nutrients to power your immune system: If we weren't in enough trouble from toxic chemicals, the immune system faces another challenge – a lack of nutrients. Judging by the number of nutrients vital to our immune systems, and the poor diet most people now eat, it is almost a miracle that they work at all. So what are these nutrients and what happens if we don't get enough in our diet?

The main nutrients involved are the vitamins A, B6, C, D, E, biotin and folic acid; the minerals magnesium, zinc, iron, copper and selenium; the omega-3 oils; and a sufficient and high-quality supply of proteins. Although they are all needed for the immune system to work properly, some of these nutrients are more vital than others, especially magnesium, zinc, iron and vitamin A. Unfortunately, these are among the commonest nutrients found lacking in the diet in the developed and developing world. What's more, these nutrients only have to be at slightly lower, or 'sub-optimal', levels to reduce the functioning of the immune system. This means that the vast majority of the non-supplementing population, as well as many of those taking inadequate levels of supplements, are effectively putting themselves at risk.

So what happens if the level of a vital nutrient falls? Curiously, the responses seen appear to mimic those of chemical poisoning as described above, either by suppressing the immune system or making it overactive. And if nutritional deficiency continues for any length of time, this too tends to lead to an increased risk of developing one of the many autoimmune diseases.

How to turn the situation around: The beauty of the detox approach taken in this book is that by lowering the body's exposure to chemical toxins, and by giving the immune system the nutrients it needs to work properly, you will be treating the problem by strengthening the immune system naturally and letting it work the way that nature intended. Not only should this dramatically increase one's resistance to infections, but it should also make the immune system less reactive to harmless substances, such as pollen or foods. It can also reduce many of the distressing symptoms, such as inflammation, caused by many of the autoimmune diseases.

Tackling the cause of inflammatory conditions will also help reduce dependence on powerful drugs such as corticosteroids that are commonly used to suppress an overactive immune system. Unfortunately there is no magic bullet or single nutrient that can sort everything out. For our immune system to work properly, we need to have good levels of all the above nutrients. But the good news is that not only will taking the right supplements help you to fend off these problems, it seems that higher or 'pharmacological' levels of nutrients can actually enhance the functioning of the immune system.

Now that we have covered the background of immune system disturbances, we will take a closer look, in the following pages, at the main types of diseases that they cause:

- Allergic reactions
- Vaccine-triggered immune system damage
- Autoimmune diseases
- Asthma
- Allergic rhinitis (including hay fever)
- Eczema
- Food allergies (see page 149)

Beat infections naturally – tackling a suppressed immune system

If you are fed up with catching every flu bug doing the rounds, or constantly seem to be afflicted with a cold, the probability is that your immune system is not working as nature intended. Having an underactive immune system is a very common problem faced by our modern society because many factors associated with twenty-first century living are known to weaken

AIDS

AIDS is a classic example of a disease characterised by virus-induced suppression of the immune system. Not only are people with AIDS at much higher risk of all the common infections, but they also succumb to diseases that are normally harmless to most people. AIDS victims also have a tendency to develop cancers that are linked to a weak immune system, such as the previously very rare Karposi's sarcoma.

the immune system. In addition to chemicals, many other factors can affect it such as long working hours, chronic stress, poor nutrition and infections. If our immune system is in good working order we may get the occasional cold or cough but other than that we are likely to remain disease-free and enjoy a lower risk of cancer.

When the immune system is not working properly, the body is unable to properly defend itself. At the very least, those with a mildly underactive immune system have a greater tendency to develop coughs, colds and other common infections. At the other extreme, a severely suppressed immune system carries a dramatically increased risk of succumbing to a life-threatening infection or diseases such as cancers.

The overlooked role of chemical toxins in immunosuppression:
If you go to your local doctor, he or she will probably be able to name quite a few non-chemical factors that are well known to suppress the immune system. However, the significant role chemicals play in suppressing the immune system is relatively overlooked. This is a major problem in light of a World Resources Institute (WRI) report that came to the staggering conclusion that pesticides are a likely cause of immune suppression for millions of people throughout the world.[8] (The World Resources Institute is an environmental research and policy organisation that creates solutions to protect the earth and improve people's lives. They are based in Washington, DC.)

This is of great relevance to all of us because we are exposed to these immune system-suppressing pesticides at every turn, from the food that we eat to the fly spray that we use around the house. However, it is not just pesticides in current usage that cause these problems. Some of the worst were banned decades ago – but owing to their persistence and longevity, they are still found in our food.

A classic example of this type of chemical is the organochlorines – chemicals previously designed as pesticides that are now a widespread environmental pollutant. They are found in particularly high levels in certain fish, and sea mammals such as whales. To illustrate the extent to which polluted foods can cause real damage to our immune systems, we need to turn to a study that took place in a remote part of the Canadian Arctic.

Despite being a non-industrialised area, researchers found that the resident women and their offspring had relatively very high levels of organochlorines, heavy metals and other toxic chemicals in their bodies, absorbed from the seafood that makes up a large proportion of their diet. The resistance-lowering capacity of these chemicals was illustrated by the fact that babies exposed to higher levels of pollutants in the womb had a higher incidence of ear infections as infants.[9]

There are many other drugs that suppress the immune system – indeed certain chemical compounds are so good at causing

Substances known to cause immunosuppression

- Pesticides: particularly organochlorines and organophosphates
- Environmental pollutants: PCBs and dioxins
- Toxic metals: mercury (in vaccinations and amalgam dental fillings), nickel, lead, cadmium and organotin (a highly toxic substance used in antifouling paint on boats, which ends up contaminating seafood)
- Fluoride and chlorine
- Solvents
- Medications: steroids, antimalarials, certain antibiotics, certain HIV drugs (such as AZT), immunosuppressive drugs (azathioprine and cyclosporin), non-steroidal anti-inflammatory drugs (NSAIDs)
- Recreational drugs
- Infections: malaria, HIV and salmonella
- Cancer treatments, such as chemotherapy

Do we build up resistance to toxic chemicals over time?

This is a commonly held belief that needs to be put to rest here and now. Chemicals are very different from infections, such as viruses and bacteria, which the immune system has been designed to fight. Instead of continual exposure resulting in the body building up a resistance to them, these chemicals accumulate in the body, and actually seem to target and cripple the immune system itself. Consequently, the more chemicals you are exposed to over time, the more damaged your immune system will become.

immunosuppression, they are used in medicine for this very reason. For example, corticosteroids possess such powerful immunosuppressive actions that they are used in organ transplantation to prevent tissue rejection. Problems arise when corticosteroids are used to treat other conditions, such as cancer. The accompanying suppression of the immune system is, in this instance, a very unwanted side-effect, since it increases the risk of life-threatening infections.

Indeed it has been suggested that some of the drugs used to treat HIV suppress the immune system so much that they could actually bring on symptoms of the full-blown virus-triggered syndrome in their own right! This growing controversy was highlighted on 18 March 1996 in 'A Ray of Hope' when the BBC flagship current affairs programme *Panorama* dedicated a complete programme to the controversy around the approval and use of the 'anti-HIV' drugs such as AZT (zidovudine, Retrovir).

Detox to restore and strengthen a suppressed immune system: Whether your aim is to strengthen your immune system to reduce the number of coughs and colds you are getting or to increase your ability to fight cancer, it makes sense to lower your overall exposure to known immune system-suppressing chemicals, whether they are in the form of pesticides or medication.

I am not for one moment suggesting that you stop medical treatment for potentially life-threatening problems. What I am suggesting is that you only take drugs which you have been prescribed. Then, of the non-prescription medications, you should only take those thought to be essential for your health.

As well as lowering your exposure to toxic chemicals, it is vitally important to ensure that you are getting enough nutrients. I was staggered at the profound effect that even slightly lower levels of certain nutrients can have on the overall efficiency of the immune system (see page 88).

Low levels of the mineral zinc can reduce the ability of certain parts of the immune system to work properly by up to 70 per cent.[10]

Moreover, nutrients such as some amino acids, omega-3 oils, and some vitamins such as E, C and A appear to have remarkable immune system-boosting effects when taken in amounts in excess of what are needed to prevent nutritional deficiency.

At the Department of Surgery, College of Medicine, University of Cincinnati, Ohio, several of the above vitamins and other nutrients in levels in excess of those needed to prevent deficiencies were given to patients admitted for surgical procedures. They found that not only did this reduce infectious complications in these surgical patients by approximately 75 per cent but they also reduced the hospital stay by more than 20 per cent.[11]

Dietary and other ways to strengthen your immune system:
Follow the diet suggested in this book. Eat lots of fresh and raw fruit and vegetables and vegetable proteins such as beans and other pulses, but try to limit dairy proteins. Drink plenty of water and herbal teas.

In addition, there is a whole range of natural and herbal medicines that can enhance the immune system. These include echinacea, garlic, ginger, goldenseal, aloe vera, elderberry and many others. Many appear to be very effective. However, I would suggest you make sure that you are getting all the nutrients you need first. Once any nutritional deficiencies are sorted out, you can then move on to herbal remedies.

Allergies – calming down an over-reactive immune system

If contact with certain substances makes your skin red, inflamed and lumpy, or rapidly affects your ability to breathe, you are not alone. Chances are that you are one of the huge population of people who suffer health problems from allergies caused by an overactive immune system. Allergies are potentially fatal, so having an overactive immune system can prove just as serious a problem as having an underactive one.

Allergy symptoms may follow only brief contact with a particular substance and can make the body react in a dramatic and often alarming way. These substances are known as allergens. Those who experience severe allergic reactions to foods, such as nuts, will be very careful to exclude them from their diets. Those who have previously gone into anaphylactic shock after being stung by a wasp will avoid these creatures like the plague.

While most doctors tend to concentrate on discovering what triggers these allergies and suggest ways in which to avoid them, this does not begin to address the reasons why the underlying immune system has become increasingly intolerant over the years. On the positive side, if you know what makes a situation worse then you can take steps to improve it. This section explores what is underlying this explosion in allergies, and offers new ways in which it can be tackled. When the alternative is a lifetime of powerful drugs and strictly limited diets, there is very little to lose.

Substances that commonly trigger allergic reactions (allergens)

- Foods
- Tree and grass pollen
- House dust
- Chemicals (additives, medications, environmental pollutants, latex (rubber), pesticides)
- Fur and feathers
- Insect stings
- Physical factors (cold, heat, ultraviolet light)

How allergic reactions are usually tackled: When an allergic reaction is triggered, contact with the allergen prompts the release of histamine into the tissues. This causes immediate swelling, inflammation and itching.

In most instances, this reaction is limited to the surface of the skin. This is known as urticaria (nettle rash). The symptom is a red, blotchy, swollen and itchy skin that can last for a few hours. In some cases the reaction is more extensive, resulting in lumps and swellings appearing under the skin. The name for this more serious reaction is angioedema. In extreme cases, the allergic reaction is not confined to the skin as the entire immune system goes into overdrive, sending the body into the very serious and potentially fatal medical emergency known as anaphylactic shock. When this happens, the air passages go into spasm and blood vessels dilate excessively, causing the person affected to collapse.

Up to 24 per cent of the US population may experience at least one episode of urticaria and/or angioedema in their lifetime.[12]

Once you work out what triggers the problem you may be able to avoid it. But if the allergy is triggered by something you cannot avoid, what can you do? The usual answer is to take medications that tackle the symptoms. Antihistamines provide a fast-acting and effective remedy. Corticosteroids are also very effective but take hours rather than minutes to work. In the case of anaphylactic shock, adrenaline is the treatment of choice and is a highly effective lifesaver. (Many allergy sufferers who are at risk of this severe reaction carry adrenaline with them at all times.)

Chemicals and poor nutrition make the immune system over-excitable: Avoidance of allergens that trigger these often-dramatic responses and the use of all the above treatments are justified, but they fail to tackle the problem of what makes the immune system over-react in the first place.

Symptoms of immune system damage are minimal compared to the high drama of an allergic reaction, so the health of the immune system itself has to be taken into account. As a malfunctioning immune system can increase both the risk of getting

Chemicals and the immune system

Chemicals that can directly trigger allergic reactions, from urticaria and angioedema to anaphylactic shock, include:

■ Pesticides (particularly synthetic pyrethroids, organophosphates, carbamates and organochlorines)
■ Rubber (latex)
■ Food preservatives, colourings and other additives
■ Sun screen, perfumes and other toiletry components
■ Medications (such as aspirin, antibiotics, painkillers and insect repellents)
■ Toxic metals (such as mercury and nickel)
■ Cigarette smoke
■ Wood preservatives
■ Plastics (including bisphenol A)
■ Surgical prosthetic implants
■ Solvents (such as formaldehyde and xylene
■ Chlorine in drinking water and swimming pools
■ Fluoride in water and dental treatments

Chemicals known to cause long-term underlying damage to the immune system, making it increasingly sensitive to allergens, include:

■ Environmental pollutants (such as dioxins and PCBs)
■ Pesticides (organochlorines such as DDT)
■ Toxic metals (such as mercury and aluminium)
■ Fluoride and chlorine

allergies and the severity of symptoms experienced during an attack, we ignore this issue at our peril.

The number of people developing allergies has increased dramatically over recent years, so it is safe to assume that the cause can be found in today's environment or our diet, rather than in our genes. Research suggests that the responsibility lies with our increased exposure to toxic artificial chemicals, in combination with an increasingly nutrient-deficient diet.

Vaccines – using toxic metals to stimulate the immune system: Daily exposure to chemicals can cause marked long-term immune-system damage that increases the risk of allergies developing in the first place. Indeed, some chemicals are so good at causing the immune system to go into overdrive that they are actually used for this same purpose. One example is their use in vaccines (see Appendix C).

For over 60 years, chemicals have been added to vaccines to boost the immune response to the 'headline' germ or pathogen (such as tetanus or flu) that is used in the vaccine. These chemicals are known as adjuvants. One of the commonest ones in use is the toxic metal aluminium. Unfortunately, not only does the addition of the toxic metal boost the response to the desired pathogen, it also has the side-effect of stimulating many other mechanisms of the immune system. One academic study which examined the uses of adjuvants mentioned that they were used to help the antigen to produce an early, high and long-lasting immune response. Because of this, less antigen would be needed and, as this component was the most expensive, the use of adjuvants would make vaccines cheaper to produce.

This heightened stimulation of the immune system induced by non-specific toxic metals could explain why mercury and aluminium have been so widely used as vaccine additives, despite the number of safer alternatives available. The worry is that, owing to the ever-increasing numbers of vaccines children are subjected to, the greater the build-up of toxic metals in the body. Over the long term, this results in an over-stimulated immune system, which is more prone to developing the entire range of allergic disorders. So, is it any surprise that more children than ever before are allergy sufferers?

As listed on page 96, toxic metals are by no means the only chemicals known to overstimulate the immune system. Cutting down on all chemicals will help to reduce the number of chemically triggered allergic reactions you might get, and will help to stabilise the entire immune system. In this way the immune system will become less likely to react to the entire range of allergens. This means fewer allergic episodes and less-severe symptoms.

Poor nutrition can exacerbate the problem: As even slightly sub-optimal levels of a whole range of nutrients can overstimulate and destabilise the immune system, nutrient supplementation helps to rebalance the immune system. Taking nutrients can also

Case history

A good friend of mine complained of having a red blotchy face for a month and a half, owing to a longer-lasting form of urticaria. Despite taking powerful antihistamines, it was proving impossible to shift and was causing her increasing embarrassment, particularly as her job involved lecturing and public relations work.

When I saw her the next day, I gave her some magnesium, vitamin C, a multivitamin and mineral supplement and omega-3 oils. A few hours later she called me and was absolutely delighted to tell me that her rash had totally disappeared for the first time since Christmas! Then two weeks later she was even more delighted to tell me that since taking the supplements, she had not needed to take the usual antihistamine medications at all. In addition her wheeziness had dramatically reduced, and her sinusitis had also greatly improved. Now, one year later, the previously severe eczema she has had since childhood is a thing of the past.

help suppress allergy symptoms in the shorter term, since many (such as vitamin C) act as natural antihistamines. I would like to illustrate these beneficial actions with the case history above.

What to do? Although my friend ate a 'good' diet, it was still apparently not giving her the higher levels of nutrients in the range she obviously needed. To be sure you are getting enough of these immune system strengtheners, see Chapter 4 for supplement suggestions.

Owing to the severity, speed and life-threatening nature of allergic reactions, it would be very unwise to stop taking any current medications or to avoid seeking medical advice for allergy-related problems. It is also necessary to steer clear of known allergy triggers, such as certain foods. However, if while under the supervision of a medical expert you combine all this with a good nutritional programme and reduce your exposure to chemical toxins, you will have the best of both worlds.

Autoimmune diseases – the chemical connection

Our immune system is highly effective at killing foreign bodies, such as harmful bacteria. While the effectiveness of this killing mechanism has ensured the survival of the human race until now, it is becoming increasingly apparent that instead of working to protect our bodies, the immune system is starting to turn on itself. There seems to be something about twenty-first century living that is making the immune system believe that its own tissues are foreign invaders. This is potentially devastating, as once a particular type of tissue is labelled as an enemy, the immune system will target the tissue for destruction and unleash its full might against the perceived 'threat'.

The name for this type of illness is autoimmune disease. With the number of autoimmune diseases rocketing year by year, we desperately need to discover what it is that is making our bodies

Types of autoimmune diseases

The type of autoimmune disease that develops depends on whether the tissue your immune system attacks is found only in one organ, or is more widespread. Starting with the organ-specific and progressing on to the more non-specific, here is a rundown of the major types of autoimmune disease:

- Hashimoto's thyroiditis
- Primary myxoedema
- Thyrotoxicosis (Graves' disease)
- Pernicious anaemia
- Addison's disease
- Myasthenia gravis
- Insulin-dependent (Type II or juvenile) diabetes
- Goodpasture's syndrome
- Pemphigus vulgaris
- Pemphigoid
- Autoimmune haemolytic anaemia
- Idiopathic thrombocytopenic purpura
- Primary biliary cirrhosis
- Ulcerative colitis
- Sjögren's syndrome
- Rheumatoid arthritis
- Scleroderma
- Wegener's granulomatosis
- Poly/dermatomyositis
- Discoid lupus erythematosus (DLE)
- Systemic lupus erythematosus (SLE)

increasingly self-destruct, if we are to have any chance of turning the situation around before it gets too late. By learning more about the causes, we can not only help those with autoimmune diseases to suppress their often distressing symptoms, but also find out the best ways to actively reduce the risk of developing these debilitating illnesses in the future.

Increase in autoimmune diseases: These once-rare diseases are now among some of the commonest health problems afflicting modern society. To discover what is making our immune systems go so desperately wrong, we need to examine what makes some people more vulnerable to developing autoimmune diseases than others.

Heredity plays an important role. Not only do autoimmune diseases tend to run in families, but people affected by one are more likely to go on to develop another. However, since more and more people getting these diseases do not have strong family links with these conditions, other factors have to be at work. Like the other previously mentioned immune system disorders, exposure to toxic chemicals appears to be playing a major part in this autoimmune system disease epidemic.

The connection between chemicals and autoimmune diseases was first noticed when people whose jobs, habits or medical treatments exposed them to larger amounts of certain chemicals were found to be at greater risk of developing autoimmune diseases. When this was examined more closely

Chemicals linked to autoimmune diseases

- Oestrogen replacement therapy in post-menopausal women has been linked to SLE, scleroderma and Raynaud's disease.
- Oral contraceptives may play a role in promoting lupus.
- Industrial exposure to silica dust increases the risk of scleroderma in men.
- Solvent exposure has been investigated as a risk factor for scleroderma.
- Mercury has been strongly linked to kidney disease.
- More than 80 drugs have been associated with triggering lupus.
- Gold, a common treatment of rheumatoid arthritis itself, appears to promote autoimmune disorders.

it was discovered that these chemicals not only trigger a wide range of autoimmune diseases, but also exacerbate existing ones. So how is this thought to have come about?

How chemicals are thought to trigger autoimmune diseases: We have seen how chemical exposure can upset the natural balance of the immune system by increasing its level of activity. As the increasing chemical contamination of our world has resulted in our overall body burden of toxins increasing, the natural balance of our immune system is becoming increasingly disturbed.

One of the consequences of long-term chemically-induced over-stimulation is that the body starts producing greater numbers of auto-antibodies. These are antibodies that mistakenly treat our own body tissues as foreign. If they attack a particular organ, such as your thyroid gland as in the case of Hashimoto's thyroiditis, the amount of thyroid hormone your body produces will be severely reduced. Although this causes many difficulties, thyroid hormone replacement therapy makes it relatively easy to deal with this situation. However, things get much more difficult if the tissues that the auto-antibodies target are more widespread, such as in systemic lupus erythematosus (SLE). This is a disease where auto-antibodies to connective tissue are created. Since connective tissue is present throughout the body, the disease symptoms will be much more widespread and difficult to deal with.

Tackling the problem: While you cannot rid yourself of an autoimmune system disease, it is possible to calm down an over-revved immune system by reducing your levels of toxic chemicals. This can be an effective way of putting the brakes on disease progression and keeping symptoms to a minimum. It will also help lower your chances of developing another auto-immune disease.

To achieve the best effects you also need to ensure you are getting all the nutrients you now need (see Chapter 4). This is because nutrient deficiencies, or even slightly low levels of nutrients, are known to increase disease symptoms as well as the

Factors thought to trigger autoimmune diseases

- Toxic metals: mercury (in vaccines, dental fillings and skin whiteners), aluminium (in vaccines and water), palladium (in rat poison, dental alloys and jewellery), gold, thallium (in rat poison).
- Drugs (for instance bleomycin chemotherapy can trigger the autoimmune disease scleroderma).
- Pesticides and pesticide synergists: organochlorines, organophosphates, carbamates, synthetic pyrethroids, piperonyl butoxide.
- Environmental pollutants: PCBs, chlorinated dibenzo-p-dioxins.
- Organic solvents.
- Silica, silicone.
- Hair dyes.
- Plastics: vinyl chloride.
- Iodine, chlorine, fluoride.
- Particulates.
- Ultraviolet radiation and ozone.
- Micro-organisms.

overall risk of getting an autoimmune disease by overactivating the immune system.

By taking nutritional supplements you can further fortify your immune system whilst simultaneously protecting your body from the harmful effects of toxic chemicals. Although it is best to take a mixture of everything, the nutrients particularly important in calming down the immune system are zinc, selenium, magnesium, and vitamins A, B, C, D and E.

Some people with health problems such as thyroid diseases may have difficulty taking supplements, particularly if they are being prescribed thyroid hormone replacements. So I would strongly advise anyone receiving medical treatment to seek their doctor's advice before embarking on a course of supplements. They could also consult a doctor who specialises in environmental medicine, as he or she will be more used to administering nutritional supplements to people with health problems and who might already be on powerful immune system-suppressing drugs (see Appendix D).

Asthma – reclaiming the breath of life

Although I have seen and treated many asthma sufferers, the all-encompassing way in which this illness intrudes on everyday life was only brought home to me after my mother developed the condition. Although she now has her asthma under control, she knows that at any moment her symptoms could suddenly erupt when she least expects.

Unfortunately, she is not alone, as asthma is becoming one of the most prevalent illnesses affecting twenty-first century society. The sheer scale of the problem, not only in the UK but worldwide, is simply staggering. The World Health Organization (WHO) recently estimated that between 100 and 150 million people around the globe suffer from asthma.

Even more worryingly, this number is rising fast. In Western Europe as a whole, asthma has doubled in 10 years. The situation is just as grim in the United States where the overall prevalence of asthma increased from 3.1 per cent in 1980 to 5.4 per cent in 1994, with the numbers among impoverished inner city children being much higher.

The combined prevalence of diagnosed and undiagnosed asthma among inner city children at nine to 12 years of age has been estimated at 26 per cent and 27 per cent in Detroit and San Diego respectively.[13]

So what is asthma? Asthma is a lung disease that attacks all age groups but often starts in childhood. It is characterised by recurrent attacks of breathlessness and wheezing, which vary in severity and frequency from person to person. These attacks are triggered by factors ranging from emotional stress, foods and pollutants, to exercise and exposure to the cold.

This condition causes inflammation of the air passages in the lungs and affects the sensitivity of the nerve endings in the airways, so that they are easily irritated. In an attack, the lining of the passages swells causing the airways to narrow, thereby reducing the flow of air into and out of the lungs.

What is behind this asthma pandemic? While scientists are struggling to find an answer, the sales of asthma suppressant drugs have never been higher. But despite being good at suppressing attacks, they can't stop someone developing asthma in the first place.

So what is the story so far? Most experts agree that asthma is a multi-factorial problem comprised of a mixture of components: hereditary, allergic, environmental, infectious, emotional and nutritional – and also including pharmaceutical drugs, cigarette smoke and exercise. While it is vital to minimise exposure to the factors that trigger these symptoms, these are only part of the problem.

Many of the artificial chemicals now present in our bodies are already known to predispose people to or trigger asthma. The existence of a more susceptible population appears to be borne out by the fact that our diets are becoming ever more highly processed and nutrient deficient. Our bodies are therefore failing to get even the basic levels of nutrients they need to work properly. The consequence of this is that people are becoming less and less able to neutralise and rid themselves of the increased load of asthma-inducing toxins that they are now being exposed to. The end result can be found in the figures revealing that more and more people are now becoming asthmatic.

Chemicals which trigger asthma: So what chemicals are best avoided if you are an asthma sufferer? Although all the usual

Toxic environment + more-susceptible population = asthma?

Professor Anthony Seaton from the University of Aberdeen medical school believes that the dramatic recent rise in asthma incidence could be due to a more 'toxic' environment and a more-susceptible population, such as those lacking sufficient levels of vitamins in their diet. (Professor Seaton holds a chair of environmental and occupational medicine at the University of Aberdeen. His research concerns the interactions of the environment and human health and he was chair of the government's expert panel on air quality standards from 1991 to 2001.)[14]

Chemicals linked to asthma

- Toxic metals (mercury, lead, platinum salts, nickel, chromium and cobalt).
- Pesticides (organophosphates and carbamates).
- Drugs (non-steroidal anti-inflammatory drugs such as aspirin).
- Air pollutants (nitrogen dioxide, ozone and sulphur dioxide).
- Solvents (diesel fumes).
- Plastics.
- Food additives (tartrazine, a yellow dye).
- Chlorine and fluoride.

suspects are implicated, toxic metals are some of the most powerful asthma-inducing agents. They do this by damaging the underlying immune system, making it over-react and hypersensitive to asthma-provoking allergens.

Mercury tends to be found in much higher levels in those who have asthma. As levels of mercury tend to increase in direct proportion to the number of fillings in the mouth, it may not be surprising to hear that people participating in a study in which mercury amalgam fillings were removed experienced a great improvement in their asthma symptoms.[15]

Pesticides increase the long-term risk of getting asthma and also trigger acute asthma attacks in their own right. Studies examining their effects on farmers have revealed that the pesticides found to have the most powerful asthma-inducing effects include organophosphates and carbamates.[16] As these are some of the most commonly used pesticides in food production, by eating certain foods you could be unknowingly exposing yourself to a small but potent shot of asthma-triggering chemicals.

Air pollution is a well-known factor linked to higher rates of asthma attacks, owing to the higher levels of solvents present from diesel and its exhaust products. The greater the air pollution, the higher the level of hospital admissions for severe asthma symptoms.[17]

Chlorine is another chemical commonly linked to asthma. To get an indication of how toxic it is to our lungs, you only need go back to the reason why it was used as a gas in the First World War. It is a powerful lung irritant that affects breathing. This is why people who regularly work around, and swim in, pools in which chlorine is used as a water disinfectant are thought to be more prone to developing asthma.[18]

As chemicals play such a powerful role in triggering asthma, it is a good idea to reduce your overall exposure to these toxins. Eating cleaner, less-processed and less-polluted foods, filtering your water, and consuming foods high in soluble fibre will help to lower the existing body burden of many asthma-inducing toxins (see Chapters 3 and 4).

Nutrients to prevent and reduce asthma symptoms: We already know that low levels of nutrients can weaken the immune system, making it hyper-react to irritants. So it is not surprising that supplementing the diet with vitamins, particularly A, B6, B12, C and E, and nutrients such as magnesium, zinc and omega-3 oils, often results in a dramatic decrease in the frequency and severity of wheezing or asthmatic attacks.

In particular, asthma tends to occur more commonly in those who have a low intake (and therefore low blood levels) of certain antioxidant nutrients, such as vitamins A, C and E and co-enzyme Q10. For instance, the risk of bronchial hyper-reactivity is increased sevenfold among those with the lowest intake of vitamin C.[19] This beneficial effect also appears to protect unborn children from developing asthma in later life as the children of pregnant mothers who had higher levels of antioxidants in their diets during pregnancy had a lower incidence of asthma.[19]

Other nutrients found to be critical in the development of asthma are vitamin B6, and the mineral magnesium, the levels of both tending to be low in asthmatics. Magnesium is seen to play an obvious role as it allows muscles to relax and stretch and helps the airways to dilate naturally, thus preventing spasm of the bronchial passages.[20] So, by taking the supplements as recommended in Chapter 4 it is possible to restore and strengthen your immune system. This is particularly important if you are on a nutritionally restricted diet as a result of having to cut out certain foods known to trigger asthma.

Conquering allergic rhinitis

On a beautiful fresh day at the beginning of summer, when the flowers are looking fabulous and there is a gentle breeze in the air, the last thing you want is to be driven mad by a streaming nose and eyes. However, for an ever-growing population, this is a regular occurrence.

Hay fever, otherwise known as seasonal allergic rhinitis, is an example of one of the commonest non-life-threatening health problems. It affects more than 20 per cent of individuals (all age groups) worldwide, 25 per cent of the US population and over 23 per cent of the UK population. Not only does allergic rhinitis drive you mad, but it has serious financial drawbacks arising from higher healthcare expenditure and decreased productivity through lost days at school or work. Some people suffer not only in spring and summer, but all year round.

As with asthma, the situation shows little sign of easing up as the incidence of allergic rhinitis has been steadily rising over the last few decades. While sales of medications are booming and look set to increase to ever-greater heights, they totally fail to tackle the real cause of the problem. Their benefits are also won at a cost because antihistamines, decongestants, anticholinergic agents and corticosteroid drug therapy typically used in the treatment of allergic rhinitis often have problematic side-effects that include sedation, impaired learning/memory and cardiac arrhythmias (abnormal heart rate). For many children, the health price paid for a dry nose could potentially be unacceptably high.

So if you don't want to spend your life sneezing, using up tissues at a rate of knots and spending a small fortune on drugs that can make you feel lethargic and not on top form, read on. Once you understand your condition a bit more, you will realise that there is actually a great deal that can be done to greatly reduce symptoms without having to resort to powerful drugs.

What is allergic rhinitis? This is an allergic condition triggered by various substances leading to inflammation of the eyes, nasal passages and sinuses, sneezing, nasal congestion and constantly dripping nose. People tend to suffer from one of two main forms: the seasonal type (hay fever) where symptoms occur mainly throughout the height of the tree and grass pollen season, and the perennial type, which can be experienced at any time all year round.

Allergic rhinitis tends to be a long-term problem, which conventional medicine has no apparent means of preventing. Few of the children who develop it will grow out of it. In fact, all modern medicine can do is suppress the symptoms by means of powerful and often toxic prescription drugs, and by advising people to avoid the triggers that make the condition worse. These triggers can range from pollen to synthetic drugs, air pollution and food sensitivities.

Addressing the cause, not just the symptoms: There is increasing evidence that our more polluted environment, in combination with a nutrient-deficient diet, is damaging our immune systems. The end result seems to be that we are becoming more prone to developing forms of allergic rhinitis such as hay fever. The upshot of this is that our immune system is more susceptible and hyper-reactive to allergens such as pollen. Therefore, reducing the overall chemical exposure can bring about short-term relief, and longer-term resolution too.

One of my friends suffered from severe pollen-induced hay fever for much of his childhood and adult life, driving him mad, along with most of his family. But once his wife started introducing more organic foods into his diet, and used fewer chemicals around the home, his symptoms started to improve. By the following pollen season he was better still and required virtually no medications at all for his hay fever. This shows that you don't have to be stuck with this problem all your life, since by changing shopping habits and lifestyle it is possible to turn things around.

Chemical triggers: The nose and sinuses are particularly vulnerable to chemical damage because these areas are often the first to be exposed to pollutants and the first to show evidence of chemical damage. Consequently, allergic rhinitis symptoms are a common initial problem for many who are sensitive to chemicals. In fact, many people with a history of hay fever or rhinitis go on to develop a more serious chemical-related disease. So if you get a runny nose after breathing in polluted air, it is important to tackle your chemical exposure before your symptoms progress to something more serious.

The types of chemicals linked to allergic rhinitis are similar to those linked to asthma. You don't have to be exposed to these chemicals in air to be affected as they can be found in foods, drinks and skincare products, as well as dental amalgam and glues.

It therefore makes sense to lower your intake of rhinitis-triggering chemicals in all aspects of your life. So, in addition to eating more organically, and washing, peeling and skinning non-organic foods to remove chemicals present on the surface, you should avoid strongly smelling chemical substances (because if you can smell them, they are already in your nose and body). Combine this with a detox programme (see Chapter 4), drink

Known triggers of hay fever

Here is a quick rundown of factors acting as short- and longer-term triggers of hay fever/rhinitis:

Biological-based allergens:
- Pollen
- Moulds
- House dust
- Foods (such as wheat, eggs and dairy products)

Chemicals:
- Solvents
- Diesel fuel
- Pesticides
- Plastics
- Toxic metals (such as mercury, lead, nickel, cadmium and chromium)
- Perfumes
- Newspaper print
- Chlorine
- Synthetic drugs

plenty of water and take soluble fibre supplements to rid your body of its existing stores of chemical toxins, and hopefully your days of suffering will be numbered.

Nutrients to tackle allergic rhinitis: Again, owing to the similarities between the two diseases of allergic rhinitis and asthma, many of the nutrients found to be effective in treating and preventing one are also valuable in treating and preventing the other.

Clear favourites are vitamin C and the mineral magnesium, as they act like natural antihistamines and are highly effective in both preventing and actively reducing symptoms.[21] They are not only cheaper, but also lack the annoying sedative side-effects that accompany regular antihistamine medications.

For best results, you need to have a balance of nutrient supplements, as suggested in Chapter 4. There are many reasons why these nutrients are so effective. For example, vitamin B6 and zinc help to balance histamine levels as well as strengthening the immune system. A good all-round antioxidant mixture that contains vitamins A, E, beta carotene, selenium and the flavonoid quercetin is also effective as these nutrients can soak up much of the damage caused by higher levels of airborne pollutant-induced free radicals. Vitamin B5 also helps to reduce symptoms. Certain amino acids, such as glutathione, can also protect the body against allergic rhinitis. Methionine, in combination with calcium, also works as an effective antihistamine. It is also vitally important to ensure you have omega-3 oil supplements as they are essential in rebalancing the immune system.

It is a good idea to limit your intake of salt, saturated fats, trans fats (as in margarine) and supplements which contain only omega-6 oils. (Although all omega-3 supplements contain some omega-6 oils, as long as sufficient levels of omega-3 are taken the presence of omega-6 oils is not usually problematic as it is the overall balance that is important.)

Eczema – more than skin deep

All my first three children developed eczema at one stage or another. So you can imagine that ever since the first one was diagnosed, I have been at great pains to discover what causes this painful and disfiguring problem, as well as seeking out all possible ways of treating it. The more I learnt about it, the easier it was to prevent. The result of my quest to date is that all my children are now eczema free, and that is without so much as a whiff of corticosteroid cream.

Eczema is now thought to affect a massive 13 per cent of people in the West at some stage during their lives, causing distress and irritation to all those whom it afflicts. If you want to discover what has turned eczema into one of the most frequent dermatological diseases of modern day life, read on. You will find that there are positive and effective ways to tackle eczema, using safe and natural methods.

Scratching the surface: Eczema, also commonly referred to as dermatitis, is a skin condition characterised by an itchy, red rash. In many cases the skin can become scaly, and can crack and weep. The itchiness is annoying, and the scratching that frequently accompanies it increases the risk of a skin infection.

In infancy, eczema is commonly found on the face, behind the ears and on the trunk. Then, in childhood, it tends to settle on the backs of the knees and the front of the elbows, wrists and ankles. In adults, the face and the trunk are once more involved. Although many children grow out of it, for others it can remain a long-term problem.

There are two main types of eczema: allergic eczema and irritant contact eczema.

- Allergic eczema: This is when the body develops eczema as an allergic reaction to certain allergens, such as a type of food in the diet.
- Irritant contact eczema: Here eczema is triggered by direct skin contact with certain irritants such as metals and chemicals.

While conventional medicine has many powerful drugs in its armoury to suppress eczema, it has few means of preventing it from occurring in the first place. As a result, ever-greater numbers of people are being subjected to powerful cortico-steroid creams, which, in addition to having the unwanted side-effect of making the skin thinner, can further increase the risk of infection owing to their immune-suppressant actions. These toxic drugs can be very effective at suppressing the symptoms in the short term, but if we are to have any chance of finding a long-term cure to this problem, we need to examine why we are becoming more and more vulnerable to this disease in the first place.

Chemicals and eczema: At the heart of these abnormal responses appears to lie a damaged immune system. Like all the previously discussed immune disorders, this problem appears to have arisen from the increased levels of chemicals in the body in combination with an increasingly nutrient-deficient diet. This combination appears to unbalance the immune system, making it oversensitive to a wide range of eczema-triggering factors, both biological and chemical.

Much of the evidence for this comes from extensive research into the large number of people who develop eczema as a consequence of handling chemicals as part of their work. Eczema from direct skin contact with chemicals is a huge problem because the skin can absorb up to 60 per cent of substances in contact with

Chemicals that trigger eczema

- Toxic metals (such as mercury, nickel, gold, cobalt and chromate)
- Pesticides
- Solvents (such as turpentine)
- Fragrances
- Plastics (resins)
- Mineral oils
- Chlorine
- Pharmaceutical drugs

it. With such a potentially large amount of chemicals entering the body through the skin, the total body load can increase, making the body more vulnerable to developing immune-system diseases such as eczema, and these chemicals can easily trigger a local response on the skin. The types of chemicals that are known to trigger eczema in this way are listed on page 112.

Out of all these chemicals, the ones that touch a raw nerve with me are the eczema-inducing mercury-based preservatives used in vaccines. They were banned from childhood vaccinations in the US following many health problems (and a multi-billion dollar law suit), yet mercury-based vaccines are still widely used in the UK, despite the many safer alternatives available on the market. Although mercury has recently been taken out of the childhood triple DTP vaccination, it remains in other vaccines that children can still be given. To give an idea of how some of these vaccines containing mercury can trigger eczema, I would like to describe a personal family incident.

After receiving her first vaccine as a baby, my niece developed a small patch of eczema that took many months to disappear. Although this made her mother more wary about subjecting her daughter to any further vaccines, an outbreak of meningitis in her neighbourhood impelled her to get her daughter vaccinated against this disease. Unfortunately, her fears were realised as, immediately following vaccination, her child's body developed a bright red, weeping, eczematous rash that affected over half her skin. If my sister had been warned about this well-documented side-effect of mercury-based vaccines, bearing in mind her child's previous history, she would certainly have insisted on a mercury-free version (see pages 10, 259 and Appendix C).

So, to minimise your risk of getting eczema, or to tackle it if you already have it, it makes sense to lower your overall exposure to the above chemicals, and also to lower their levels in your body by following the detox programme as described in Chapter 4.

Nutrients to treat eczema: Nutrients make up an essential part of any programme to rid the body of eczema. This is largely due to their ability to restore balance in a damaged immune system. For

Are our children being 'programmed' to develop eczema in the womb?

It seems likely that early damage to our immune system could be at the very heart of the recent rise in eczema rates. Evidence suggests that exposure to higher levels of chemicals while in the womb damages the immune system, making it more reactive to eczema-inducing triggers for life.[22, 23] Subsequent increased exposure to toxins can increase the risk even further. So it seems that our children can be, in effect, 'programmed' to develop eczema even before they are born. With the level of pollution on the up, it seems that the number of people getting eczema is likely to rise even higher.

best results, a good coverage of essential nutrients is important (see Chapter 4). Vitamins A and D are particularly useful as these nutrients can not only help balance the immune system, but they also are able to slow down the rapid turnover of skin cells seen in eczema. Vitamin C helps strengthen the skin while vitamin E and zinc improve skin healing.

As eczema sufferers tend to have lower levels of the antioxidants selenium and glutathione in their blood, these immune-strengthening nutrients can prove highly useful too. Magnesium is also beneficial as it reduces eczema and helpfully protects the skin from known eczema-inducing chemical triggers. Magnesium is found in higher levels in the Dead Sea, which may be why so many people with skin disorders find the water therapeutic. And iron is thought to be of benefit owing to the rapid turnover of skin cells, which results in an increased demand for iron. As B vitamins strengthen the immune system they too play a beneficial role.

Omega-3 and omega-6 oils play a valuable role as people with eczema are known to have a particular problem in processing these essential fatty acids. Many studies have confirmed the benefits of supplementing the diet with these oils.

Supplements can benefit children, too. My daughter developed eczema on her cheeks when she was an infant. This cleared up within days of her being started on a vitamin and mineral supplement designed for children, in combination with a small amount of omega oils (a teaspoon of flax seed oil). My niece's eczema also showed a dramatic improvement within days of taking a suitable supplement. As long as the nutrient levels are appropriate for the age of person taking them, supplements are beneficial. The company called Biocare (see Appendix) produce a capsule supplement which contains vitamins and minerals in powdered form. I added these to her milk alongside 50 mg of powdered magnesium (half a 100 mg capsule).

The ideal diet for eczema would include a larger proportion of foods of non-animal origin. It also helps if the diet is low in saturated fats. If you suspect an allergy to eggs, dairy or wheat, you can confirm it by avoiding these potentially eczema-triggering food groups one at a time, and seeing if there is any improvement.

8

Boost Your Brain Power

'Twenty-five per cent of the thousands of chemicals released in our environment are known neurotoxins, that is nerve poisoning chemicals.'

ANGER, 1984

Poisoned minds

The brain is the most important part of the body; it makes us who and what we are. It controls everything we do and say and its health is fundamental to our survival. Unfortunately, the massive recent escalation of health problems involving the brain suggests that there is something about twenty-first century living that has quite literally poisoned our minds.

In the past, scientists have blamed this massive increase in disease on an ageing population. However, people are getting these illnesses at an ever-younger age, and this fact, coupled with a dramatic rise in childhood brain disorders such as autism, suggests that other influences are causing our brains to malfunction.

Clues can be found by looking to our new environment. A sizeable number of the chemicals that we and our children are increasingly being bombarded with are known brain and nerve toxins. If you put this together with the fact that the brain is increasingly being starved of the nutrients it needs, it should come as no surprise that all sorts of brain diseases are on the increase.

The good news is that we can do a lot to improve the current situation and to prevent these diseases from happening in the first place. To find out why our central nervous system (CNS) is so sensitive to toxins and nutrient deficiencies, we need to understand more about what it is and how it works.

Common 21st century brain problems

- Alzheimer's
- Autism
- Behavioural problems, in children and adults
- Brain cancer
- Dementia
- Depression
- Dyslexia and other learning disorders
- Epilepsy
- Memory loss
- Multiple sclerosis
- Parkinson's disease
- Schizophrenia

What is our central nervous system? The brain and nervous system together form the central nervous system (CNS). They are our mental 'hardware'. They consist of an incredibly complex network of neurons (nerve cells) connected by axons (nerve fibres) covered by fatty myelin sheaths. These nerve fibres, which can often be several feet long, connect the brain with different parts of the body. They transmit messages from one part of the body to another by sending tiny electric currents along the fibres and via neurotransmitters, which are chemical messengers released by one nerve cell and received by the nerve cell they are effectively 'talking' to.

As each individual brain cell can form tens of thousands of connections with other brain cells, this allows the possibility of very complex co-ordinated actions. This is vital to the way we work, as we multi-task on a regular basis.

Owing to all these many responsibilities, the brain is one of the most active parts of our body. It works 24/7. To keep it working properly it needs a continual supply of nutrients, with its preferred food being the simple sugar glucose. The excellent blood supply to the brain ensures a continual source of this vital brain food. For protection, it has a highly developed blood–brain barrier, formed by the modification of brain capillaries (small blood vessels) which are packed so tightly together that they effectively block unwanted natural hazards, such as infections, from entering the brain from the bloodstream.

What makes our central nervous system so vulnerable to chemical toxins? The brain is able to control the body remarkably well, but it is a sitting duck when it comes to defending itself from the raft of toxic chemicals it is now exposed to on a daily basis.

The excellent blood supply the brain receives means that it is exposed to a higher level of blood-borne toxins, while its high fatty content acts as a sponge – soaking them up. Once these chemicals arrive at the brain they quickly take up residence and are then very hard to shift. Not only is the blood–brain barrier unable to prevent these modern artificial chemicals from entering, they can actually make the barrier much less effective, so allowing more chemicals, plus other unwanted substances, to enter.

Once there, they are comparatively harder to neutralise or remove. One reason for this is the relatively low level of anti-oxidant nutrients present in the brain. This means that there are fewer antioxidants to neutralise the higher levels of tissue-damaging free radicals triggered by the presence of these chemicals. This, in combination with the limited defence mechanisms present in brain tissue and our less nutritious modern diets, magnifies the amount of brain damage chemicals can cause.

How do I know if I am being affected by these toxins?

The range of symptoms and signs people experience from brain-damaging toxins is very wide and can include the following:

- Headache
- Migraines
- Depression
- Impaired concentration
- Memory defects
- Suicidal tendencies
- Collapse
- Behavioural problems
- Pins and needles
- Skin numbness
- General weakness and fatigue
- Anxiety
- Panic attacks
- Learning difficulties
- Speech difficulties
- Reduced dexterity
- Reduced intelligence
- Seizures
- Movement difficulties
- Paralysis
- Dizziness
- Balance problems
- Deafness and visual problems

Added to this is the fact that nerve cells appear to be very delicate structures. Unlike other parts of our bodies, once damaged, most are not able to regenerate. Many toxic chemicals are highly effective nerve poisons, which in addition to killing nerve cells outright, can also prevent growing brains from developing properly and can reduce levels of neurotransmitters and hormones.

As a result this continuous poisoning by twenty-first century toxins, in conjunction with increasingly nutrient-deficient diet, appears to be a major factor behind the growing number of people affected by brain diseases.

What chemicals are known to trigger nerve damage? There are many different types of chemicals that can damage the nervous system. Some are more harmful than others. The following include some of the more powerful nerve-damaging chemicals:

- Pesticides – particularly organophosphates, organochlorines, carbamates and synthetic pyrethroids
- Environmental pollutants – organochlorines, dioxins
- Heavy metals – particularly mercury
- Solvents – these highly fat-soluble chemicals rapidly penetrate the brain
- Chlorine and fluoride

Early recognition of this damage is vital. The earlier the appropriate treatment is started, the less risk there is that problems such as memory loss will progress to a permanent disease such as dementia. Even if diseases have already developed, it is sometimes possible to slow down disease progression and even alleviate certain devastating symptoms by taking the right combination of supplements.

Nutrients vital in powering your brain and nerves: Numerous studies show that mental wellbeing is affected by substandard levels of nutrition. This all stems from the fact that we are not getting enough of the right nutrients to feed the brain in the way it requires.

Essential fatty acids are a prime example. Approximately half the fats in our brains are made up of polyunsaturated fats. However, these fats, commonly found in nuts, seeds and fish, are becoming more and more of a rarity in our diets. Consequently, this lack of essential fats can damage the fundamental way the brain is designed to work, making it much more prone to chemical damage and to virtually all forms of brain and nerve diseases.

Owing to the constant level of activity going on in processing information and controlling body functions, the brain has a high need for nutrients such as vitamins and minerals. Inadequate intake of these nutrients not only makes the brain more vulnerable to damage from toxic chemicals, but also reduces the levels of neurotransmitters vital to the healthy functioning of the brain. This is why low levels of nutrients can affect intelligence and behaviour.

For instance, the low level of nutrients in the average child's diet is known to lower IQ. Fortunately, this effect can be readily improved by adding vitamins, minerals and essential oils in the form of supplements to children's diets.[24] Other studies show that young people in prison commit 35 per cent fewer violent offences after just two weeks of getting supplements of vitamins, minerals and essential fats.[25] So just think what would happen to the crime rates if supplements were given to all those in prison. The bottom line is that you have to give the brain what it needs if you want it to work properly, and if you don't, you can't be too surprised if things go wrong.

Although there are a great number of twenty-first century brain problems linked to chemical toxins and poor nutrition, I have chosen to focus on the following:

- Memory loss
- Depression
- Multiple sclerosis
- Parkinson's disease
- Behavioural disorders (ADHD), (see page 263)
- Autism (see page 269)
- Dyslexia and other learning difficulties (see page 277)

Memory loss – clearing the brain fog

If you ever have trouble remembering a name, or lose your train of thought in the middle of a sentence, you may be experiencing brain fog. Brain fog sufferers usually have one or more of the following symptoms: forgetfulness, spaciness, feelings of confusion and inability to focus. This is a major problem in today's world, where being alert and having a good memory are vital. Consequently, any lapse in memory can cause major ripples throughout your life.

Unfortunately, poor memory and concentration are becoming more and more commonplace. But unlike diseases such as full-blown dementia, a poor memory is not treated as a separate condition for which there are well-known treatments. Therefore it tends not to be taken seriously as a 'real' problem – most doctors are simply not able to deal with it.

Although reports in the medical press suggest that the incidence of this condition is dramatically increasing, the fact that brain fog is not recognised as a problem in its own right means that it is very difficult to judge exactly how many people are suffering with this condition. In my personal experience, I have found a poor memory to be an increasing problem in many young professionals. So what causes brain fog, and why is it on the increase?

What is behind the rise in memory problems? The number of people suffering from officially recognised memory-loss diseases such as Alzheimer's or other forms of dementia is very much on the up. The number of people expected to develop full-blown dementia is expected to more than double by the midpoint of the twenty-first century.[26] However, while many experts have tried to explain this rise away by suggesting it is merely due to our ageing population, it is becoming increasingly clear that many other 'environmental' factors are involved.[27]

In fact, there are a whole range of factors that can result in poorer concentration and memory, such as infection, trauma, and hormonal upsets such as diabetes and low thyroid hormones. However, I will concentrate here on dealing with the ones caused by toxins, because many of the factors listed are well

Factors known to impair brain functioning

- Nutrient deficiencies
- Anaemia
- Post-operative complications (particularly following major surgery)
- Blood-sugar regulation problems
- Toxins (such as pesticides, pollutants, toxic metals and solvents)
- Food sensitivities
- High homocysteine levels
- A diet high in saturated fats and meats, but low in vegetables and fruit

known to cause memory problems. For instance, it is pretty obvious if memory loss developed immediately after a head injury from a car accident but perhaps much less so if it was caused by the presence of mercury fillings in your mouth.

A patient of mine had been plagued for years with a poor memory and brain fog. But she just put this down to diabetes, even when her sugar control was relatively good. However, after half of her copious fillings were removed she called to thank me as her brain fog was on the wane. And by the time they had all been taken out she was extremely relieved to discover that she was shot of this problem for the first time in almost a decade. Not only that, but her previously failing kidneys, which she had been told were only working at 60 per cent of their normal capacity, started to recover. One year on they appear to be normal. This is probably because, in addition to being a known powerful brian poison, mercury is a well-known kidney toxin, and removing the source allowed her kidneys to recover.

Thinking requires complex activity between many different parts of the brain, so damage to one part can have an effect on overall brain functioning. The fact that a massive 25 per cent of industrial chemicals are known to possess widespread brain-damaging actions suggests that our ever-increasing exposure to chemicals could be a major factor underlying brain fog. In fact, brain fog is often one of the first signs of a recognisable sensitivity to toxic chemicals. Considering the presence of these chemicals in our everyday lives, it is no surprise that our minds are becoming more and more confused!

Which toxins are known to target our memory? The most common toxins associated with brain fog and memory loss are:

- Pesticides
- Solvents
- Toxic metals

From Auschwitz to Alzheimer's: Organophosphates (ops), one of the most commonly used groups of pesticides, were originally created as nerve agents. Their lethality to humans was first proven by testing the op known as tabun on prisoners at Auschwitz. Following the Second World War, they started to be used as pesticides as they made highly effective bug killers. They are now commonly found on our food and in many other non-food products such as household fly sprays.

However, their ability to poison human beings has not been forgotten as they are still being used as highly effective chemicals of mass destruction by terrorists or other organisations, usually in the form of the ops known as sarin, tabun, VX or soman. For instance, tabun and sarin were among the agents used by the previous Iraqi government on the Kurds, and sarin was the agent

Ban on dichlorvos in insect killers after cancer alert

'Almost 50 makes of insect killer were ordered to be removed from shop shelves yesterday amid fears that they could cause cancer. The Government, acting on scientific advice, decided to suspend from sale a list of products, including some from household names such as Boots, Superdrug and Vapona.

'The decision makes it illegal to sell, advertise or supply the products concerned. Health chiefs stressed that it was a precautionary move until further chemical tests had been conducted.

'The 47 products on the suspended list include fly, moth, wasp and cockroach killers. The decision was taken after advice from the independent Advisory Committee on Pesticides (ACP) which said it could not rule out a cancer risk from a chemical called dichlorvos, which all the products contain.

'There are fears that long term exposure to the chemical could be linked to skin, liver and breast cancer. Critics say dichlorvos is one of the organophosphates linked to nervous disorders.' (http://news.bbc.co.uk/1/low/uk/1939569.stm)

used in the Tokyo subway terrorist attack in 1995. Even in the people who were not killed in Tokyo (and the people sent to help them), exposure to these chemicals resulted in long-term memory loss, with the greater the exposure the more severe the memory loss.[28, 29]

In the light of this, I was staggered to discover that organophosphates had actually been given FDA approval to be used to 'treat' patients with Alzheimer's disease in the USA. Yes I did say treat.[30] Not surprisingly, in this role they are referred to, not as organophosphates, but as acetylcholinesterase-inhibiting drugs. The organophosphate, sorry, anti-acetylcholinesterase chemical used for this purpose, metrifonate, is converted into a chemical called dichlorvos once in the body. Dichlorvos is the active metabolite (breakdown product) and is thought to be largely responsible for the drug's 'therapeutic effect' (see box opposite, Ban on dichlorvos in insect killers after cancer alert).

Fortunately, the pharmaceutical company which had applied for FDA approval of the drug metrifonate has recently suspended its application to use it, seemingly following serious side effects. However, some of the drugs currently used to treat Alzheimer's possess similar anti-cholinesterase actions as organophosphates, such as the drugs known as donepezil and tacrine.

Secondly, let us consider solvents. These highly fat-soluble liquids, some of which are commonly used as anaesthetics, with powerful mind-altering actions, are strongly linked with Alzheimer's itself. A study carried out by Dr Walter Kukull in Seattle, Washington, USA found that people who had worked with organic solvents, such as benzene, toluene, phenols, alcohols and ketones, in the past were more at risk of developing Alzheimer's disease.[31] (Dr Kukull is professor of epidemiology and director of the National Alzheimer's Coordinating Center at the University of Washington.)

Finally, the toxic metals. People who have Alzheimer's disease are found to have higher levels of certain metals in their brains, and in their bloodstream. These include metals such as aluminium, mercury, iron and copper. This is thought to be due to an underlying problem in the way the brain stores metals.

Consequently, higher levels end up being stored in brain tissue than should be there. Other people at risk of memory problems include workers exposed to higher levels of lead, as the greater the lead exposure, the greater the memory loss.[32]

By generally lowering your exposure to chemical toxins and by starting a suitable detox programme (see Chapters 3 and 4), you can do your bit to 'de-fog' your brain and lower the odds of developing a more severe memory loss problem in the future.

Brain food for thought: As the brain is highly dependent on a minimum level of nutrition to function properly, it will stop working as nature intended if it doesn't get what it needs when it needs it. This is why when many people with brain fog are given nutritional supplements, they find that the fog evaporates. Not only that, but they regain most of their previous mental sharpness. If nutrient deficiency is the problem, a significant improvement can be made in weeks.

Kicking off with antioxidants, memory problems can arise because of a higher level of oxidative stress, that is too many free radicals from toxins and diseases. Not only can antioxidants prevent toxin-induced brain damage, but they can also reduce the risk of getting Alzheimer's disease and other forms of dementia.[33] Beneficial antioxidants include vitamins C and E, selenium, the herb ginkgo biloba, alpha-lipoic acid (Solgar) glutathione and N-acetylcysteine (to source these supplements see Appendix D for companies such as mynutrition.co.uk).

The lack of other nutrients such as vitamins B6, B12 and folic acid is known to cause blood atherosclerosis. As a good blood flow is important in ensuring that the brain is well supplied with these nutrients, people with a deficiency in their diet tend to have a greater degree of blood vessel disease and a higher incidence of mild memory loss, age-related memory loss, vascular dementia and Alzheimer's disease.[34] So by ensuring the body gets enough of these, and other nutrients such as omega-3 oils, the risk of developing these conditions can be reduced.

Other ways known to be of benefit in maximising memory include the following:

- Reduce your intake of processed foods (particularly those high in refined carbohydrates and sugars).
- Reduce your intake of saturated fat (animal fat).
- Eat more vegetables, whole cereals and legumes, including soya products containing beneficial phyto-oestrogens (soya-based products are good in moderation for men although too much could affect normal sex hormone balance).
- Cut down on stimulants such as coffee, tea, fizzy drinks and alcohol.
- Stop taking drugs (including unnecessary prescription drugs), but only in consultation with your GP.
- Discover whether you have any food sensitivities and, if so, eliminate those foods from your diet.

Natural highs – beating the 21st century blues!

Despite the obvious benefits to our everyday lives that modern-day living brings, in the form of electric lighting and a highly sophisticated communications network, the stress accompanying today's round-the-clock lifestyle appears to be decreasing our ability to enjoy life to the full.

This, combined with our ever-increasing use of mood-altering substances such as stimulants, prescription medications and drugs, our increased exposure to toxic chemicals and our highly processed and less nutritious diet, is linked to an increase in depression and other mood disorders.

Moderate to severe depression is now one of the most common diseases of our time with nearly 3 per cent seeking treatment. And that figure is thought to greatly underestimate the real numbers since only a third of sufferers ever go to a doctor. The good news is that there is a great deal you can do to enhance your mood, and make yourself far more resilient to the stresses and strains that life will inevitably throw at you.

What makes us depressed: All of us at some stage experience periods of intense sadness, but true depression can be completely

Common symptoms of depression:

■ Overpowering feelings of hopelessness and suicidal thoughts
■ Disturbed eating and bowel habits
■ Excessive weight loss or weight gain
■ Inability to concentrate
■ Increased anxiety
■ Inability to enjoy anything in life
■ A tendency to burst into tears
■ Sleep disturbance, such as waking up too early in the morning
■ Low self-esteem

overwhelming and totally disabling, causing the affected person to withdraw from participating in everyday life. True depression affects people in different ways with symptoms ranging from increased anxiety, to overpowering feelings of hopelessness and suicidal thoughts. Some people with manic depression (otherwise known as bipolar disease) have periods of low mood interspersed with periods of tremendous elation, known as mania, in which their thinking processes are clearly disturbed.

These powerful feelings are thought to be caused by imbalances in the level of mood-enhancing neurotransmitters, such as catecholamines and serotonin. These are our 'happy hormones'. In fact, the main conventional drugs targeted at alleviating depression are thought to work by artificially boosting or interfering with levels of these neurotransmitters.

Tackling the cause of these imbalances would seem to hold the key to treating this debilitating disease, or alternatively preventing it from occurring in the first place. If you look at the following factors known to underlie depression, you will see that you actually have control over some of them. They include:

■ Genetic predisposition (family history of depression)
■ Outside stresses and events beyond your control such as bereavement, illness and job loss
■ Drugs (recreational drugs and prescription medications)
■ Chemical toxins
■ Poor nutrition

How prescription medications could get you down

Dozens of prescription drugs are known to cause depression. They do so by lowering levels of the brain's 'happy hormones', catecholamines and serotonin.[35] Because many illnesses are caused by imbalances in these hormones, many medical drugs have actually been designed to target their production. They include drugs used to control blood pressure and treat heart rate problems and infections. However, they can also trigger depression. Consequently, in lowering the levels of catecholamines and serotonin to treat one health problem, they have, in effect, created a new one. These drugs are becoming so widespread that some scientists think that the general increases in depression rates could be partly due to their increased use.[36] These drugs include some long-term antipsychotics, certain oral contraceptives, some antihypertensives (reserpine, alpha-methyldopa betablockers) and some antibiotics (metromidayole sulphonamides).

As many pesticides found in our foods are made of similar chemicals to those used as catecholamine-altering prescription medicines, you could be unknowingly exposed to these same mood-depressing chemicals just by eating conventionally grown foods.

The first three are commonly recognised and widely acknowledged in the medical community, but the real breakthrough comes from the discovery of the vital role that chemical toxins and poor nutrition play in the development of depression. So despite being much researched in the academic world, these last two factors have been relatively ignored by the medical profession, who tend to base their treatments on easy-to-prescribe but potentially harmful medications. A far safer method of alleviating depressive symptoms and reducing the risk of future depressive episodes is to let your body boost production of these essential 'happy hormones' naturally.

Which chemicals cause depression?: Up to 90 per cent of the commonest types of toxic chemicals in our food and environment are known to alter levels of catecholamines and/or serotonin. Indeed the link between toxic chemicals and depression appears to be so strong that it seems incredible that it has been virtually ignored by conventional medicine and, to some extent, by complementary medicine as well.

Chemicals known to be linked to depression

- Pesticides (especially organophosphates)
- Toxic metals (such as mercury, lead, antimony)
- Solvents
- Medications (such as barbiturates, tranquillisers, sleeping pills, heart drugs that contain reserpine, beta blockers, high blood pressure-lowering drugs, ulcer drugs, systemic corticosteroids, anticonvulsants, antiparkinsonism drugs, antibiotics, and certain painkillers and arthritis drugs
- Environmental pollutants

One way of illustrating this link is to look at people who use chemicals on a regular basis, for example farmers and others who work with pesticides. People in this group not only have higher rates of depression, they are also more likely to commit suicide.[37, 38] But it's not just pesticide workers who are at risk. Over a two-year period ending in 1996, the organophosphate pesticide methyl parathion was sprayed by unlicensed pest control operators in more than 1,500 homes and offices, despite the fact that this chemical was only licensed for use on food crops and indoor use was prohibited. This led to the deaths of many household pets, and many associated health problems in the residents, who had to be temporarily relocated. In addition, over half the victims interviewed reported depressive symptoms at levels suggesting probable clinical levels of depression.[39]

Heavy metals, such as mercury, lead and vanadium, appear to be another major source of depression. One study showed that people with mercury poisoning symptoms caused by their amalgam fillings also had above normal rates of mental strain and depression.[40] Another study showed that the removal of mercury fillings resulted in health improvements in 70 per cent of those who suffered from mercury-linked problems, which included depression.[41] The link between lead and depression can be clearly seen in metal foundry workers who are exposed to lead as part of their jobs. When their blood levels of lead were measured, it became clear that the higher the lead levels, the greater the chance of developing depression. Those with higher levels of lead in their body also had a greater degree of other mood-related problems.[42]

Vanadium is a naturally occurring trace mineral, but is also released into the air by burning petroleum or petroleum products. Whilst at low levels it appears to be essential to the diet, at high levels it appears to be toxic. Vanadium levels may be elevated during manic-depressive episodes, leading some experts to suggest that following a low-vanadium diet may be helpful for people with bipolar disease. Foods with the highest levels of vanadium are mushrooms, shellfish, black pepper, parsley, dill weed, sweeteners, grain and grain products.

Solvents are a very common mood-altering substance, and we are all in contact with them in our everyday lives. Of these, alcohol is perhaps the best known depressant. In a study of people who were exposed to solvents as part of their work, 50 per cent had evidence of mood disorders including depression.[43] But again it's not just people affected by chemicals at work who are in the firing line. Use of the insect repellent solvent DEET (N,N-diethyl-m-toluamide) has been known to trigger manic depression.[44]

By lowering your body's chemical burden by following my detox programme (see Chapter 4), and by limiting your future contact with toxins (see Chapter 3), you can do a great deal to increase your own natural ability to banish the blues. But to get the best results, you also need to know about mood-enhancing nutrients as they also play a critical role.

Nutrients can give you natural highs: Unfortunately for the millions of people with depression, the medical profession is so wrapped up in conventional antidepressants that it seems as though their knowledge of the mood-enhancing actions of various nutrients has actually fallen behind that of the ordinary man or woman in the street. This has been confirmed by a report that shows that the public tend to give much more favourable ratings to vitamin and mineral supplements, special diets and self-help books for dealing with depression, than do doctors, who tend to favour potentially harmful pharmaceutical medications to treat depressive conditions.[45]

The ability of nutrients to reduce the symptoms of depression is confirmed in a growing number of academic studies. They are thought to do this by boosting production of the body's natural 'happy hormones'. Indeed, the link between nutrition and depression gets stronger if you consider that a low level of body nutrients such as vitamins, minerals and essential fatty acids can predispose people to:

■ Major depressive illnesses, including manic depression.
■ Increased depression after bereavement.
■ Increased depression and mood changes associated with premenstrual syndrome.
■ Increased depressive symptoms in alcoholism.
■ Increased depressive symptoms in multiple sclerosis patients.
■ Increased post-natal depression.

Many prescription medications can also induce certain nutrient deficiencies that increase the risk of depression still further. For instance, the contraceptive pill is known to deplete the body of many essential nutrients such as vitamin B6, and a low level of this vitamin is strongly linked to depression.[46] All in all, this shows that the general public's preference for natural antidepressive nutrients is correct.

Higher levels of supplements in treating depression

Supplements appear to offer dramatic benefits in treating different forms of depression. A study was carried out at the University of Calgary, Canada, in which people who suffered from manic depression were given higher levels of vitamins and minerals. The findings were astonishing. For those who completed the minimum six-month open trial, symptoms reduced by 55–66 per cent, and their need for prescription antidepressant medications decreased by more than 50 per cent. In some cases, the supplements replaced antidepressant medications completely and the patients remained well.[47]

Which nutrients help the most? Many nutrients appear to have a positive mood-boosting action. Antioxidants appear to be particularly effective. For example, people with higher levels of antioxidants, such as vitamins A, C and E, in their diets tend to have lower levels of depression.[48] Other vitamins and minerals known to be mood-enhancing, or helpful in preventing depression, are the B vitamins B1, B2, B3, B6, B12 and folic acid, vitamin D, inositol, zinc, iron, calcium, magnesium, copper, manganese and chromium. The B vitamins and zinc in particular play a crucial role in preventing depression.

The essential fatty acids, in particular omega-3 oils, also play a vital part in the prevention and treatment of depression. This could be related to their ability to transport some of the 'happy hormones' into the brain.

Certain amino acids, such as tryptophan and l-phenylalanine, are important as they are the precursors of one of the 'happy hormones', serotonin. Another amino acid, tyrosine (sometimes called L-tyrosine), a precursor of catecholamines such as noradrenaline (another 'happy hormone'), can be of value as a dietary supplement. (To source this nutrient see Appendix D, page 321 for www.mynutrition.co.uk. The company Solgar produce tyrosine in supplement form, L-tyrosine – 500 mg.)

Other beneficial substances include phosphatidylserine, a natural substance derived from an amino acid, which also affects mood-enhancing neurotransmitter levels in the brain. The powerful natural antioxidant alpha-lipoic acid can be of benefit to some. There are several herbal therapies, such as St John's Wort, Siberian ginseng and ginkgo biloba. Some supplements, such as St John's Wort, have side-effects and can't be taken at the same time as some prescription medications. So, before embarking on a course of herbal supplements, it would be advisable to consult a herbal specialist. (Contact the National Institute of Medical Herbalists, see Appendix D, page 332.)

The following factors can also cause depressive symptoms, so it is wise to reduce them where possible:

- Disturbed blood sugar balance – and excessive intake of refined sugar.
- Overuse of stimulants (such as tea, coffee, chocolate, cola drinks, cigarettes and alcohol).
- Intolerance to wheat and dairy products.

Multiple sclerosis

When one of my colleagues recently told me that he had pins and needles down one side of his body, I have to admit that I was concerned because I was listening to someone I knew well describe a typical symptom of multiple sclerosis (MS). Although he recognised it as a problem he was not aware of the potential seriousness of the situation. Three weeks later he had a brain scan and my fears were proved groundless when no evidence for this diagnosis was found. However, this and a few other mild but as yet unexplained symptoms still remained.

Shortly afterwards he consulted Dr Jack Levenson, author of *Menace in the Mouth* and an expert on mercury-free dentistry. The doctor was shocked by the number of mercury fillings in my colleague's mouth. Indeed his first comment on seeing all those fillings was that if that environment was a workplace it would be closed down for being too toxic. Further tests prompted him to say that there was a high probability that my colleague's symptoms were a direct result of mercury poisoning from his amalgam fillings. After going through the major procedure of having his fillings removed – by no means pain-free and certainly not cheap – to his great relief my colleague's symptoms improved.

Two inches – the short road from mouth to brain: Mercury levels in the brain have been shown to be present in direct proportion to the number of tooth surfaces covered by amalgam fillings. The brain and nerves are highly vulnerable targets for mercury and are significantly damaged by chronic, long-term exposure to mercury vapour from amalgam fillings. Mercury vapour passes through the lining of the mouth and nose and is transported directly to the brain. From here, mercury is transported to all parts of the brain and spinal cord. Symptoms depend on which part of the brain is most affected.

One year on, my colleague has accepted the fact that he will be left with some residual symptoms, but as he is otherwise very fit and they have not limited his abilities in any way, it is something that he can easily live with. This might not have been the case if the mercury had been left in his mouth to poison his body for much longer, as he might have ended up developing multiple sclerosis or indeed another of the many diseases triggered by mercury.

What is multiple sclerosis? MS affects over 1 in 2,000 of the population in many developed countries, and is one of the commonest neurological causes of long-term disability. And there are no signs of the problem abating as, like many other twenty-first century diseases, the number of people being diagnosed with this disease has, in some countries, more than doubled in a 20-year time frame.

MS can affect any part of the body, but the most commonly reported symptoms are double or blurred vision, pins and needles in the extremities, slurred speech, difficulty in walking, dragging of either foot, loss of coordination and balance, and loss of sensation anywhere in the body.

The clinical progression characteristically involves episodes of relapse and recovery when the symptoms get worse and then improve. The symptoms and signs of the first attack usually improve within one to three months, but after a variable interval they may recur. Some people never see any improvement and continue to deteriorate. Although the main problem originates from damage to the myelin sheath around the nerves, symptoms vary widely, exposing the fact that the term 'multiple sclerosis' is now thought to cover a collection of quite disparate problems.

How nerves get damaged: MS occurs because of damage to the myelin sheath – the thin protective layer of fatty membrane that surrounds the nerve fibres in the brain and spinal cord.

The myelin sheath acts like insulation and also speeds the transmission of nerve signals. Any damage to this protective layer can cause deterioration in nerve function.

In MS this damage is caused by inflammation of the nerve fibres and loss of myelin covering (a process known as demyelination). Hard scar tissue then forms over these damaged patches, or lesions, and multiple sclerosis (which literally means 'many scars') is the result. These patches of demyelination (known as plaques) can occur on any nerves, which explains the wide-ranging symptoms experienced by people with MS.

Twenty-first century poisoning causes nerve damage: The entire gamut of twenty-first century toxic chemicals and other factors in our environment appear to conspire to slowly poison our nervous systems.[49] Although MS has a very strong genetic component, as evident in many families affected by MS, there is growing evidence that our environment is

Factors linked to multiple sclerosis

MS appears to be a multi-factorial disease linked to the following:
- Food additives.
- Artificial sweeteners – such as aspartame in 'diet'/'low-sugar'/'sugar-free' foods and drinks – and flavour enhancers e.g. monosodium glutamate.
- B12 deficiency.
- Climate and geography.
- Environmental toxins (such as organochlorines).
- Previous history of allergies.
- Genetic predisposition.
- Toxic metal poisoning.
- High-fat diets.
- Infections.
- Radiation.
- Low levels of essential fatty acids.
- Low levels of vitamins and minerals.
- Medications including overuse of antibiotics.
- Pesticides.
- Solvents.
- Vaccinations.

Aspartame lawsuits accuse many companies of poisoning the public

6 April 2004: lawsuits were filed in three separate California courts against 12 companies who either produce or use the artificial sweetener aspartame as a sugar substitute in their products. The suits alleged that the food companies committed fraud and breach of warranty by marketing products to the public such as Diet Coke, Diet Pepsi, sugar-free gum, Flintstone's vitamins, yoghurt and children's aspirin with the full knowledge that aspartame, the sweetener in them, is neurotoxic.

playing a major role in the triggering and development of MS disease.

Of the twenty-first century factors listed opposite, chemical toxins appear to be particularly strongly linked to MS. Many chemicals seem to trigger the onset of this disease or exacerbate the symptoms. Some, such as the artificial sweetener aspartame, commonly found in diet drinks, even mimic the symptoms.

Indeed, Dr Russel Blaylock, a retired neurosurgeon, has even authored a book – *Excitotoxins: the taste that kills* – in which he claims that aspartame and multiple sclerosis are closely related as aspartame not only mimics symptoms of MS but can also trigger it and worsen the symptoms in those with existing MS.

We already know that 25 per cent of industrial chemicals are nerve poisons. However, to find which chemicals are most likely to trigger or exacerbate MS, we need to review the existing evidence. Concern that MS may be caused by some sort of toxic overload from man-made poisons first arose when 'outbreaks' of MS occurred following local cases of environmental pollution with heavy metals.[50] One of these episodes occurred in Key West, Florida, USA between 1983 and 1985. During that time up to 40 people developed MS. This was eventually linked to the dumping of toxic debris containing high levels of mercury and lead.[51]

What makes this link with mercury more compelling is that the mass population vaccination in France with the Hepatitis B vaccine (in which mercury was used as a preservative) triggered an outbreak of hundreds of cases of MS.[52] Another common source of mercury is dental amalgam, so it may not be too surprising to hear that the health of MS patients can significantly improve after mercury fillings have been replaced with a non-metallic, less toxic substitute.[53] Whilst some countries like Sweden have banned the use of amalgam fillings – since 1991 the Swedish Government even pays 70 per cent of the costs towards their removal – they continue to be widely used in the UK.

Solvents, such as organic solvents and VOCs (see Glossary), also appear to be strongly linked to MS, as those working with these substances are at greater risk of developing this disease. Those particularly at risk are painters, construction workers and food processing workers.[49] There is also evidence that people with MS have higher levels of solvents in their bodies. This may be the result of higher levels of exposure or a relative inability to process and expel these chemicals – which are highly fat soluble and so can enter and damage the myelin sheath.

Like most of the other twenty-first century diseases, pesticides – in particular the highly fat-soluble organochlorine types – are also linked to MS. One academic paper described how a man with no previous medical complaints developed neurological symptoms characteristic of MS after being exposed to organochlorine pesticides on just two occasions. These symptoms progressed until his death. At autopsy, his brain showed the classical signs of multiple sclerosis.[54] People with MS tend to have more than double the levels of organochlorine pesticides in their bodies than those without MS.

MS patients have up to five times the overall number of artificial chemicals in their bodies than normal. This suggests that as well as being exposed to more toxic chemicals, people who develop chemically linked MS are less able to process and expel these chemicals, which then accumulate in the body. This relative inability to process toxins may be due to many things, including a genetic inability to detoxify, as well as increased exposure to chemicals and poor nutrition.

So by reducing your future exposure to chemicals and by embarking on a good detox programme, as in Chapters 3 and 4, you could not only help reduce existing symptoms and the number of relapses, you could also decrease the risk of developing this debilitating disease in the future.

Nutrition and MS: Most patients with MS tend to be deficient in a great number of different vitamins, minerals and other nutrients such as omega-3 and omega-6 oils.[55, 56] Furthermore, the more nutrient-deficient the person is, the faster the disease progresses.[57] These nutrient deficiencies also appear to get worse during MS attacks, possibly because higher levels of nutrients are used up in trying to suppress inflammation.

So with this many problems associated with a lack of nutrients, you can see why a good nutritional supplementation programme can help to clear up acute attacks[58] and help prevent relapses from occurring.[59] Many of these nutrients are vital in the detoxification processes and for preserving the health of the nervous system and the fatty nerve sheath. So it is not surprising that people who have poorer nutrition, or who need more nutrients owing to a higher level of chemicals or an inability to process them, end up developing MS.

Some of the more important nutrients include vitamin B12 (very important indeed), magnesium, vitamin D, folic acid, selenium, and vitamins C and E and other antioxidants. Other useful nutrients are MSM-sulphur (MSM stands for Methyl-sulphonylmethane – a natural form of organic sulphur found in all living organisms, see Appendix B.4.2), and the amino acids glutathiamine and L-phenylalanine. Other steps you can take include the following:

- Have yourself checked for mercury poisoning from your fillings.
- Cut down on diet drinks or other 'sugar-free' products that use artificial sweeteners.
- Check for nutritional deficiencies and take the appropriate supplements.
- Cut down on saturated fats, as a diet low in saturated fat greatly slows down the rate of deterioration of MS.

- Root out any food allergies, which are thought to be relatively common among MS suffers. These include milk and gluten (cereal) products, tannin (in tea), caffeine and citrus fruits, as well as food from the nightshade group – potatoes, tomatoes, aubergines and peppers. Cocoa products are also suspect.
- Seek out alternative therapies – such as the herb ginkgo biloba, and the homeopathic remedies *Buthus australis*, *Thallium metallicum* and *Argentum metallicum*.
- Consider self-help groups for emotional support and to help you keep up to date with the latest 'breakthroughs'.
- Relaxation exercise can also be beneficial.

Parkinson's disease

When the ever-youthful Michael J. Fox, well known for his role in *Back to the Future*, developed Parkinson's disease (PD), public perception of this disease changed overnight. Far from being confined to older people, it was now realised that this illness could affect people supposedly in the prime of life. The revival in interest about this disease led to the uncomfortable discovery that the age at which people were developing Parkinson's disease had dramatically fallen.

In fact, in the space of a couple of decades, a totally new group of people getting PD had emerged – those who developed this condition under the age of 40. Further investigation revealed that people in this younger group tended to have a higher exposure to environmental chemicals, such as insecticides, from living in a fumigated house or in an agricultural area. Their disease also tended to be more aggressive than that found in older people. This is particularly distressing in view of the fact that there is currently no known cure.

This revival of interest in PD caught the public's attention to such an extent that the popular US soap *ER* even incorporated a young medical student with PD into a story line. To fully understand why this problem is increasing, we need to know more about PD and how it develops. Only once this is understood can we move forward and find ways to prevent this disease from occurring in the first place, or minimise symptoms and help to slow down disease progression.

About Parkinson's disease: Parkinson's disease is a neuro-degenerative disorder, or brain-wasting disease. Two hundred years ago it was very rare, but now it is the second most common neuro-degenerative disorder, affecting 1 per cent of people over 60 years old. For some reason, nerve cells that produce the neuro-transmitter dopamine, located in the part of the brain that controls movement (the substantia niagra), start to die. As the number of nerve cells falls, so does the level of dopamine produced.

Dopamine production in this part of the brain plays a major role in initiating and controlling our body movements. The subsequent low levels of dopamine cause the muscular symptoms characteristic of PD, such as tremor, muscle rigidity and a generally reduced level of movement. Unfortunately, once this process starts, it appears to be progressive.

Current methods of treatment are based on prescription medications. However, while they can help initially, they tend to

Parkinson's disease and parkinsonism

People with symptoms of parkinsonism do not necessarily have full-blown Parkinson's disease. Those with parkinsonism have many of the features of PD, but their symptoms are known to be caused by other factors such as drugs, viral diseases, Wilson's disease, brain tumours, heavy metal exposure, environmental toxins and head injury. Consequently, more people suffer with parkinsonism than with Parkinson's disease itself. Parkinson's disease is known to be progressive (symptoms increase in severity over time), whereas this is not necessarily the case with parkinsonism. As some 20–25 per cent of people diagnosed with Parkinson's disease will eventually be discovered to have some other form of parkinsonism, it is important for all those diagnosed with Parkinson's disease to see a neurologist who has experience diagnosing and treating this disorder. Since there are many causes of parkinsonism, some of which can be treated, this disorder can often be treated more easily. Depending on the cause, such as drug-induced parkinsonism, the symptoms can even be stopped. (Drugs that can cause parkinsonism include some used to treat blood pressure, vomiting and seizures.)

become less and less effective with time. In addition, they have their fair share of side-effects, some of which can be debilitating in their own right. Although there are surgical methods being developed to treat Parkinson's disease, at present they are very much in their infancy.

Chemicals and Parkinson's disease: To date, there are many things known to trigger PD. But out of all the known or suspected factors, exposure to toxic chemicals ranks as one of the highest. Not only has a previous exposure to toxic chemicals been found in those developing Parkinson's disease at an earlier age, this factor also increases the risk of developing the condition in later life. Chemical poisoning can produce many of the symptoms experienced by PD sufferers and can also trigger the disease itself. In fact some chemicals are so effective in triggering parkinsonism that they are used to create 'animal models' of this disease for research purposes.

In the light of the extensive body of research that shows many toxic chemicals target and reduce dopamine production, this is perhaps not so surprising. Approximately 25 per cent of the industrial chemicals we are exposed to on a daily basis are known to poison nerve cells, so it is perhaps surprising that more people are

Causes of Parkinson's disease and parkinsonism

- Ageing
- Drinking well water (probably related to water contaminants)
- Medications (such as reserpine, phenothiazine and butyrophenones)
- Genetic factors
- Head injury
- Toxic metals (such as aluminium, copper, iron, cobalt, manganese, lead and mercury)
- Immunological abnormalities
- Infections
- Rural living
- Pesticides (such as organophosphates, organochlorines and synthetic pyrethroids)

MPTP, pesticides, PD and parkinsonism

In the 1980s, a synthetic chemical known as MPTP (1-methyl-4-phenyl-1,2,3,6-tetrahydropyridine) was found to be a potential neurotoxin affecting dopamine-producing cells. This was discovered following the observation that humans accidentally exposed to this chemical developed irreversible clinical, chemical, and pathological alterations that mimic those found in Parkinson's disease and parkinsonism. Since then this chemical has been used to reproduce an almost perfect model of PD and parkinsonism in animals.

The problem we now face is that substances containing MPTP-like fragments are used as herbicides and intermediates in the synthesis of many artificial compounds, including some drugs. Our increased exposure to MPTP-like pesticides and contaminants is thought to be one of the factors behind the recent increase in Parkinson's disease.

NOT developing Parkinson's disease. The chemicals implicated can be found by looking at the people who are most likely to get Parkinson's disease. Farmers and agricultural workers working with pesticides are at higher risk, as are toxic metal workers.

Exposure to toxins at an ever-earlier age tends to weaken the body's systems, and the number and levels of chemicals in our environment is rising. These factors work in combination to increase the adult susceptibility to these pesticides, and the damage they do. Those less able to deal with chemical toxins and who have less well-developed detoxification systems appear to be most at risk.

This increasing sensitivity to chemicals could be why far greater numbers of younger people are developing Parkinson's disease. Not only are people who work with chemicals vulnerable, but anyone who is exposed to larger amounts of these chemicals in their everyday life seems more and more at risk. This higher exposure to ever greater amounts of chemicals known to target dopamine-producing cells could ultimately result in the destruction of the substantia nigra.[60]

While PD tends to be progressive once it has developed, it makes sense to avoid and rid the body of chemicals that speed up the destruction of the remaining dopamine-producing nerve cells. In addition to reducing the risk of developing PD and parkinsonism, this should have the effect of slowing down disease progression and maximising the body's natural production of dopamine.

Nutrition and Parkinson's disease: A wide range of nutrients is known to play an important role in protecting the body against PD. Antioxidants are particularly useful as they soak up the free radicals triggered by toxic chemicals that attack the body's dopamine-producing nerve cells. Research shows that a high intake of antioxidants can actually protect the body from the toxic nerve-damaging effects of chemicals. Indeed, nutritional supplements have been successfully used to reduce toxic side-effects from certain PD drugs.[61]

However, recent research shows that the source of the antioxidants is just as important as the nutrients themselves. At the annual meeting of the American Academy of Neurology held in Honolulu in 2003, a strong correlation was revealed between high fruit and fruit drink consumption and risk of Parkinson's disease. This increased risk was not thought to be due to a higher intake of vitamin C, as this is known to protect against PD, but was believed to result from the higher levels of pesticides and herbicides that accumulate on these foods. So, in this instance, the unfortunate conclusion is that the benefit of eating more nutrient-rich foods appears to have been outweighed by the increased presence of food-borne brain-damaging pesticides that now accompany conventionally grown foods.

Because of this, it seems prudent to ensure that as well as avoiding chemicals you should also take nutritional supplements, as shown in Chapter 4. In addition to the supplements recommended, the antioxidant amino acid glutathione can prove particularly beneficial in protecting dopamine-producing nerve cells. (To source glutathione, see Solgar on page 322.)

9

Digestive Health

'Let food be your medicine.' HIPPOCRATES

Your gut in the firing line

We all know that you are what you eat. So if your diet is full of nutritionally deficient foods, you will eventually end up paying the price in terms of faulty digestion, poor absorption, gut infections, bloating and inflammation. However, few realise that many so-called 'healthy' foods, such as salmon, apples and strawberries, could also be damaging your gut. The main problem lies not with the food itself, but rather in the levels of chemicals that they contain.

Agriculture has changed so dramatically over the past 100 years that some of the foods previously considered the healthiest are now often the most contaminated with artificial chemicals.

The Trojan Horse effect

For most people, the majority of chemicals they are exposed to tend to enter their bodies concealed in the food that they eat, rather like the ancient Greek army that invaded the city of Troy by means of a large wooden horse. A Greek soldier told the Trojans that the horse was a sacred offering to the goddess Athena. The Trojans believed that story and innocently towed the horse into the city. Once that Trojan Horse was safely within the city walls, the Greeks hidden inside crept out at night and opened the gates, allowing their army to enter and destroy that beautiful and proud city. You too are innocently consuming the foods that you are told are good for you. Why should you suspect that these foods harbour poisonous chemicals?

Gut problems linked to chemical exposure

- Bad breath
- Coeliac disease
- Colitis
- Dry mouth
- Food absorption disorders
- Gastric and duodenal ulcers
- Gastritis
- Cancer
- Haemorrhoids
- Heartburn
- Irritable bowel syndrome
- Leukoplakia
- Mouth ulcers
- Pruritus ani
- Regional enteritis

Unfortunately, when we eat these contaminated foods, the chemicals that enter our gut poison any part of the digestive system that they subsequently come into contact with. This is because the toxic effects of such chemicals don't conveniently turn off once eaten (see Chapter 3). Therefore the gut is directly in the firing line of food-borne twenty-first century toxins.

Some people say that not much has changed as the gut has been vulnerable to attack by natural toxins in foods for millions of years. But over the millennia, our bodies have gradually developed finely tuned detoxification systems to cope with many of these natural toxins. One hundred years is not nearly long enough for the body to adapt to the onslaught of huge quantities and thousands of different types of artificial chemicals. The failure of the body's detoxification system to deal with the majority of these new chemicals is at the heart of the ever-increasing problems of chemically-linked gut diseases. To understand more about the ways in which chemicals are increasing our risk of succumbing to bowel diseases, we need to take a closer look at the digestive system.

What is our digestive system and why is it so vulnerable to chemical damage? The digestive system starts with the mouth, continues with the oesophagus and stomach, carries on into the duodenum and small intestine (small bowel) and ends with the large intestine (large bowel or gut). The main function of our digestive system is to break down food so it can be used by the body. The breakdown of food starts the moment it enters our mouth and continues through the rest of the system. Once the food is broken down into its basic components, our bodies are then able to absorb it through the gut wall, where it can be converted into energy or stored as fat, or used to build tissues or repair damaged parts of the body.

The main part of the digestive system is made up of the large and small bowel. This is, in effect, a long muscular tube, up to 8.5 m (27½ ft) long. The small bowel is mainly responsible for churning out 10 litres (17½ pints) of digestive juices per day to break down food. The large bowel is crammed with billions of bacteria, which play an essential role in breaking down foods and in creating nutrients, such as certain vitamins. Once the food is broken down, the nutrients can then be absorbed into the body through the gut's huge surface area, which is approximately the size of a tennis court.

All these actions taking place in the gut are coordinated by extremely complex control mechanisms involving the brain, hormones, nerves and all the other major digestive organs such as the liver and the pancreas.

The problem we now face is that all of the tissues making up the digestive system are known to be extremely sensitive to damage from artificial chemicals. The gut tends to get more than its fair share of contamination because of the additional burden of chemicals in the food we eat. As these food-borne chemicals will not yet have been processed and to some extent neutralised by the liver, they are likely to be even more dangerous. However, most synthetic chemicals are never completely broken down, so may be stored in some poisonous form in the body.

Consequences of chemical damage to our gut: To understand the role these chemicals could be playing in bowel disease, it helps to know more about the many different ways in which chemicals can damage the digestive system. Once these are known it becomes easier to understand the potentially major role chemicals are having in triggering twenty-first century gut diseases.

Chemicals are known to:

- Damage the inner wall of the gut, reducing the overall ability to absorb essential nutrients from the food.
- Trigger inflammation in the bowel wall.
- Destroy nutrients such as vitamins present in the gut.
- Increase or reduce production of digestive juices and hormones produced throughout the gut (reduction can result in undigested foods and overproduction can result in ulceration).
- Reduce the thickness of the protective mucous layer that protects the bowel wall from powerful digestive juices, thereby increasing the risk of ulceration.
- Kill many of the good bacteria in the gut, upsetting the microfloral balance and making it easier for harmful bacteria, viruses and fungi to multiply. This could result in ulceration and infections such as candidiasis. Bacterial imbalance can also affect food breakdown and the ability of bacteria to produce essential vitamins.
- Damage the parts of the brain and the hormones that control digestion.
- Poison the underlying immune system, which increases the chances of developing a food allergy or intolerance.
- Make the muscles in the bowel wall go into spasm (causing cramp and diarrhoea) or to relax (leading to excessive dilation and constipation).
- Increase the risk of cancer.

The good news is that if the general principles described in this book are used to lower the level of toxins in food and the overall body burden of chemicals, this could help prevent or ease the symptoms of many chemically linked digestive system diseases.

Detoxification and good nutrition are the cornerstones of good digestive health: Owing to the fact that exposure to chemicals can seriously reduce the level of nutrients we are now able to get from our food, it is becoming clearer that if we want long-term good health we need to avoid toxins (see Chapter 3) and detoxify on a regular basis. We must also make doubly sure that our bodies are getting enough nutrients (see Chapter 4) as one of the consequences of poor nutrient absorption is a subsequent reduction in our ability to digest food. This acts like a vicious circle.

In addition to eating a good diet made up of a large proportion of whole, raw and less polluted foods, which tend to be more nutritious, the effects of chemicals can also be reversed to some extent by taking probiotics. These boost numbers of beneficial bacteria in the gut, which are regularly depleted by synthetic chemicals, and in so doing provide a natural living barrier to infections and toxins in the gut. They help nutrient absorption, too, a vital process which is also damaged by artificial chemicals.

The overall level of dietary fibre is particularly important for gut health. Soluble fibre helps to lower the body burden of chemicals. Some forms also feed the good microflora. These forms of fibre are called probiotics. Insoluble fibre (roughage) helps reduce the time that waste products spend in the gut, thereby lowering the chances of chemicals being reabsorbed.

By paying attention to our digestive system, we find that energy levels improve, the skin becomes clearer, the problem of body odours is reduced and the immune system is strengthened. This will also help us to tackle the following twenty-first century digestive system diseases that are affecting an ever-increasing number of people. These include:

- Food intolerances (such as food allergies, lactase intolerance and coeliac disease).
- Inflammatory bowel disease (such as Crohn's disease and ulcerative colitis).
- Irritable bowel syndrome.

Tackling food intolerances

There can be few things more terrifying for a mother than to see her young child experience a potentially life-threatening reaction to a food. I witnessed this first-hand when a friend's young son

---

Types of food intolerances

■ Food allergies
■ 'Pseudoallergic' reactions (adverse reactions to chemicals in the food, such as food additives)
■ General food intolerances (non-allergic and lactose intolerance)
■ Coeliac disease

---

developed a dramatic reaction after eating a mouthful of food that contained uncooked egg – a food he was allergic to. His skin started to swell up, then his tongue, and if we hadn't had certain medications immediately to hand that saved his life, the outcome could have been very different. This dramatic, life-threatening reaction is known as a severe food allergy. It is at one extreme of a wider spectrum of digestive system disorders, which occur when people react to certain foods in their diet. These reactions are known collectively as 'food intolerances'.

The statistics covering those affected by these different forms of food intolerance make uncomfortable reading. The number of people with food allergies has more than doubled in the last 10 years, and is currently thought to comprise a massive 7–10 per cent of many populations. Up to 20 per cent of children are thought to have pseudoallergic reactions to food, with reactions to additives thought to be responsible for up to 2 per cent of these.[62] Coeliac disease is now one of the most common chronic diseases children can get. The number of children developing coeliac disease in Sweden alone increased by a factor of nine between the years 1970 and 1988. This trend of ever-increasing numbers of people getting food intolerances shows absolutely no signs of slowing down.[63]

About the different types of food intolerances: Food intolerances are frequently quite difficult to diagnose. This is not only because many of the symptoms are general ones and not specific to the gut, but also due to the common lack of medical understanding about these similar, yet different, conditions. The relative lack of specific tests makes it that much harder to clinch a diagnosis, even when one of these problems is suspected. Owing to the lack of readily available information on the subject, I will start by describing the main types of food intolerances that affect us.

True food allergies: 'True' food allergies are triggered by consuming tiny amounts of certain foods, most commonly cow's milk, eggs, peanuts, wheat, fish and shellfish. Eating a food one has an allergy to can provoke any or all of the following symptoms: an itchy red lumpy skin (urticaria, angioedema, see page 95), eczema (see page 111), wheezing from constriction of the airways (see page 103), (allergic rhinitis (see page 107), gastrointestinal symptoms such as cramp and diarrhoea, and cardiovascular symptoms, which at their worst can develop into anaphylactic shock (see page 95). Food elimination diets are the best way of managing true food allergies.[64] This means identifying and removing the problem food from the diet. The good news is that most children tend to grow out of their childhood food allergies (with the possible exception of nut allergy).

Pseudoallergic reactions to food additives and other chemicals: Pseudoallergic reactions to food can be triggered by chemicals in and around food products, such as colourings, preservatives and flavourings. Although the symptoms can overlap with those of true food allergies, the mechanisms that bring them about are thought to differ.[64] Again, avoidance of these additives is the best management tool.

General food intolerances (non-allergic and lactase intolerance): A larger group of children, who have reactions to many of the above foods, are found to be 'intolerant' to those foods, rather than being truly allergic.[65] The most common symptom of general food intolerance is a skin rash. But gut symptoms, such as diarrhoea, constipation and tummy cramp, and in some cases breathing difficulties, can also occur. These varied reactions arise from a variety of different problems involving food digestion, absorption or metabolism. As with food allergies, symptoms of food intolerances can be lessened by identifying the food the body is reacting to, then removing it from the diet.[66]

A particularly common form is lactose intolerance, an adverse reaction to cow's milk due to a deficiency of lactase, an enzyme needed to break down the main sugar found in milk. Although a deficiency of this enzyme is often inherited, more and more people are developing this problem during late childhood or adulthood.

Coeliac disease: Coeliac disease is yet another example of a food intolerance. It arises when the body reacts to a food component known as gluten, a protein commonly found in wheat, barley, rye and oats. This disease tends to reveal itself in early childhood when affected infants fail to thrive, develop anaemia, have pale bowel movements and develop a swollen abdomen. Management involves eliminating gluten from the diet for life – which, as you can imagine, proves a great hardship for all those affected.

Something in our current environment is making us react to foods we could previously tolerate. Only this could explain why the number of people with, say, peanut allergies has doubled in some populations over six years, despite a steady level of peanut consumption.

What is causing more and more people to become intolerant to food? The reason as to why we are increasingly starting to react to our food is challenging many scientists. However, Claudia Miller from the University of Texas Health Science Center, at San Antonio, USA has published a very interesting academic paper that provides a credible explanation.

She has suggested that the rise in food intolerances could be due to an early exposure to chemical toxins such as pesticides, solvents and indoor air contaminants.[2] This is because people who are more exposed to these substances are much more likely to react to foods that they could previously tolerate. So how are chemicals thought to bring about this effect?

Synthetic chemicals are thought to be involved in food intolerance reactions in two main ways:

- They damage the immune system, making it over-react to substances it could previously tolerate.
- They trigger a food intolerance reaction in their own right.

If we start by tackling the first issue of chemical damage to the immune system, this is a well-known consequence of chemical overexposure. The ability of chemicals to excessively stimulate the immune system, making it over-react to substances such as foods that it could previously tolerate, appears to be common. The number of chemicals causing these immune system-damaging effects is very extensive and includes all the major types of toxic chemicals, such as pesticides, heavy metals and solvents.[2] Although damage to the immune system appears to be linked to all forms of food intolerances, the exact form that develops will depend on many different factors, such as the type of chemical involved, genetic makeup, and a person's general nutritional state.

The second main way chemicals are linked to food intolerance reactions is to trigger these reactions in their own right. In this way, additives such as food colourings, additives, flavourings, fragrances and preservatives are thought to bring about pseudoallergic food intolerance reactions.[64]

This suggests that a reduction in the overall body burden of chemicals from food and other sources would reduce all types of food intolerance reactions. Not only would this mean fewer people developing these reactions, it would also help ease the symptoms of those already affected. In addition to cutting down on one's general exposure to chemicals, it would also make sense to embark on a long-term detox programme designed to effectively tackle the existing chemical body burden (see Chapter 4).

Nutrients for healing an irritable gut and a damaged immune system: People with food intolerances have been found to benefit greatly from taking regular nutritional supplements. One of the most important appears to be zinc. Low levels of zinc are

Case study

The value of a detox programme in combination with nutritional supplementation is highlighted in a book called *Chemical Sensitivities* by Professor William Rea. He gives an example of a child treated in his hospital whose mother was exposed to fumes from an oil refinery throughout her pregnancy. The infant suffered from chronic diarrhoea and vomiting. Months later he developed sinusitis, recurrent ear infections and anaemia, as well as allergies to 24 different foods and various moulds, dusts and chemicals. However, the whole situation was turned round in a programme that included a reduction in his exposure to chemicals, a course of nutritional supplements, and avoidance of problematic foods. After several months, there was a marked improvement in the child's general health and allergic symptoms as well as in his ability to tolerate different foods.

regularly found in many people with food intolerances.[67] Zinc supplementation reduces gut inflammation and, if given in the first few months of life, it can strengthen the immune system and lower the lifetime risk of allergic disorders.[68, 69]

Other nutrients of value are the antioxidants vitamins C and E, and selenium[70, 71, 68] as they appear to reduce the chemically induced immune-system damage that is so commonly found in people with food intolerances. Magnesium is also vital owing to its ability to suppress immune system overactivity. Vitamin B6 is good for strengthening the immune system while omega-3 oils suppress bowel inflammation.[71, 72]

If food intolerances continue for long periods of time, or if milk products are cut from the diet, the levels of vitamins B2, B3, D, iron and calcium can decline, leading to a deficiency in these nutrients. Consequently, any multivitamin and mineral supplement taken needs to contain adequate levels of these nutrients.[73, 74, 75] Lastly, probiotics can also improve the bacterial balance of the gut, helping to reduce inflammation.

Food avoidance: It is especially important to discover and avoid the foods that the body has difficulty in tolerating. If the problem is thought to arise from contact with cow's milk then this should be eliminated from the diet. If it is gluten, then gluten-free foods should be selected. However, there can be real diffi-culty in determining which food is causing the problem, so I would strongly recommend seeking specialist professional help in discovering the particular trigger and in managing the food allergy or intolerance.

Individual management is particularly important in the light of the fact that people with food intolerances are generally more prone to nutritional deficiencies. There are two main reasons for this. First, their gut is less able to absorb nutrients due to an increased level of inflammation, and second, cutting major food groups out of the diet can further increase the risk of nutrient deficiencies.

Controlling inflammatory bowel disease

My first inkling of a chemical link to inflammatory bowel disease was a little too close to home. Several years ago, immediately following one of my son's routine vaccinations (MMR), he went from being a happy, vocal child who was progressing very well to a more withdrawn child who developed copious green, offensive, mucous diarrhoea. As the weeks turned into months, I was so concerned that I had a stool sample sent off to check for bowel parasites and even seriously considered requesting a bowel biopsy to see whether he had an inflammatory bowel disorder. All drew a blank until, out of desperation, I went to an alterna-tive therapist, something I had never previously done, who told me that the vaccine was the most likely cause. The therapist gave me a range of supplements to give him, which, to my great surprise and relief, cured him.

In the light of my current knowledge on toxins, I am greatly relieved, not only that the problem was so effectively resolved, but also that he did not go on to develop autism, something I know now to have been a real possibility. From that moment, my family has been vaccine free and I am delighted to report that there have been no similar episodes.

Unfortunately, many hundreds of thousands of people around the world every year are now touched by inflammatory bowel disease. With one Scottish study showing a threefold rise in child-hood Crohn's disease between 1968 and 1983, and a recent follow-up revealing further rises[76] it appears to be one of those twenty-first century illnesses that is very much on the increase.

What is inflammatory bowel disease? For diagnostic purposes, doctors tend to divide inflammatory bowel disease (IBD) into two categories: Crohn's disease and ulcerative colitis (UC). Crohn's involves all the layers of tissue in the bowel and can affect any part of the gastrointestinal tract from the mouth to the anus, while ulcerative colitis affects only the lower part of the gut – the colon or rectum.

Despite this superficial division, there is a compelling argument that they represent two different poles of the same disease. This is because of the marked similarity between these two conditions, reflected in the fact that no single test is sufficient to diagnose either disease. Indeed in 10–20 per cent of cases it is almost impossible to differentiate between the two. As such, both diseases will be considered together.

Generally speaking, the symptoms, which can be life threatening, depend on the region of gut affected and the severity of disease. They include abdominal pains, diarrhoea, mucus and/or blood in the stool, and weight loss.

In Crohn's, the entire wall of the bowel can be involved, and becomes thickened and swollen. Deep ulcers can form, and penetrate through the bowel wall to become abscesses. Fistulas (an abnormal connection between two surfaces) can develop between adjacent loops of bowel, other organs and even to the skin. In ulcerative colitis, the inner layer of the bowel tends to bleed more readily, to form ulcers. If the condition becomes really severe the entire wall of the gut can become very thin and may even rupture.

The hidden triggers: According to conventional medicine, inflammatory bowel disease is an incurable condition, the cause of which is as yet unknown. However, evidence is building that IBD is brought about by a combination of genetic and environmental factors.[77] The growing importance of the environmental aspect is particularly apparent if you consider that certain populations, such as the Japanese, previously free from this disease, have been more prone to develop it as they increasingly adopt Western habits.

While genetic inheritance is a strong factor in the development of this condition, the number of additional triggers has grown to include the following:

- Infections (for example *Mycobacterium paratuberculosis*, found in milk)
- Poor nutrition
- Food allergies
- Stress
- Synthetic chemicals
- Toxic metals
- Urban living
- Smoking
- Preservatives and food additives
- Solvents
- Vaccinations (such as measles)
- Conventional medicines (antibiotics, nonsteroidal antiinflammatories, and the contraceptive pill, gold and sulphasalazine.[77, 78, 79, 80, 81, 82]

Whatever the trigger, the overriding opinion is that IBD is autoimmune in nature. At the heart of the problem is a malfunctioning immune system, which for some reason is sent into overdrive, and as a result attacks and inflames the body's own tissues (see page 99). This is reflected in the fact that the majority of treatments used by conventional medicine are targeted at suppressing the immune system. However, while these drugs can often suppress the disease, they do not alter the long-term prognosis, very probably because they fail to tackle whatever it is that causes the immune system to malfunction in the first place. This is what interests me, as I believe that determining the factors that cause this immune system chaos holds the key to solving the mystery of IBD.

IBD – the chemical connection: The first clue as to what could be underlying this hyperactive immune system syndrome came about with the discovery that this illness was first described in 1913 – a decade or two after synthetic chemicals were first developed. This is highly relevant, as in retrospect we now know that many toxic chemicals have the ability to unbalance the immune system, increasing our propensity to develop autoimmune diseases.[83] Indeed, some synthetic chemicals are so good at this that they are actually used to induce an animal model of inflammatory bowel disease.[78]

Many chemicals are known to trigger IBD. This may happen when an already chemically damaged system is exposed to high levels of one toxin, which tips the balance, resulting in the development of disease. The ultimate responsibility probably lies with a combination of chemicals and other factors, rather than just one.

To help show the link between toxins and IBD, I will now highlight two areas in which we are commonly exposed to toxins: vaccination and smoking. Starting with the controversial link between IBD and vaccines, few people realise that when they are getting a vaccine, not only are they getting a dose of the 'named' antigen or disease they are being vaccinated against, such as diphtheria, but also a mixture of highly toxic and cancer-promoting chemicals thrown in as preservatives and 'adjuvants'. The aim of an adjuvant is to increase the body's immune response, thereby increasing the number of antibodies produced to protect against the disease (see page 10 for chemicals used in vaccines and page 97 for adjuvants).

Aluminium is an adjuvant component that appears to be common to most vaccines. One of the main reasons for using this adjuvant seems to be cost cutting. The use of adjuvants in boosting the immune response is thought to reduce the amount of antigen required to get an immune response, thus saving on vaccine production costs.[84] However, the general 'revving up' effects on the immune system appear to damage the gut. This could help to explain the many studies showing that vaccination can trigger inflammatory bowel disease.[81, 85]

This link between aluminium and IBD is strengthened by the fact that increased intake of aluminium in the form of food additives can also increase the risk of developing Crohn's disease. Furthermore, when these additives are cut out of the diet, symptoms of Crohn's are significantly improved.[86] As urban living exposes us to increased amounts of aluminium, this could partly explain the observed link between the urban diet and Crohn's disease.[87]

Other chemicals known to be associated with Crohn's include some of those found in cigarette smoke, such as benzene, cadmium, arsenic, nickel, chromium, 2-naphthyl-amine, vinyl chloride, 4-aminobiphenyl and beryllium.[88] The increase of free radicals induced by exposure of the gut to cigarette smoke has been shown to heighten the allergic and inflammatory response of the bowel.[78] Lastly, since pesticides, other toxic metals (especially mercury and lead), plastics and solvents can also fundamentally damage the immune system, they too could be contributing to the underlying problem.

So in summary, owing to the role that chemicals are playing in triggering IBD, it would be a sensible move to reduce your daily exposure to these autoimmune-triggering chemicals, as well as to improve the body's ability to shift its existing chemical load.

Nutritional support: Nutrient deficiencies are one of the main problems experienced by those suffering from IBD. These are due to:

- A tendency to eat less nutrient-rich food.
- An inflamed gut, which is less able to absorb nutrients.
- A smaller surface area through which to absorb nutrients, as a consequence of previous abdominal surgery.

These deficiencies commonly include the vitamins A, B6, B12, C, D, E, K and folic acid, the minerals iron, selenium, zinc and magnesium, the omega-3 oils and the amino acid glutathione. Consequently, these and other nutritional deficiencies need to be tested individually and treated by healthcare professionals.

The good news is that in treating the nutrient deficiencies, you will also help suppress the symptoms of inflammatory bowel disease. This is because supplementation is known to strengthen the bowel wall and make it less leaky.

Other supplements of benefit include the amino acid methionine, owing to its ability to help restore a damaged detoxification system. Omega-3 oil supplementation reduces low-grade inflammation while helping the body to overcome an often impaired fatty acid metabolism. Prebiotics and probiotics can be helpful in restoring the natural microflora of the gut, helping to protect against harmful bacteria and toxic substances.

Studies have shown that psyllium seed husks benefit many with IBD, as they appear to protect the bowel wall and lower the levels of substances that exacerbate inflammation. However, care needs to be taken here, as those with active inflammation may need a low-fibre residue-free diet – particularly if they develop sub-acute or acute bowel obstruction. Before taking any form of fibre or vitamin and mineral supplement, you should discuss your individual needs with your healthcare professional, as what works fine for one person may not be suitable for another. In addition, some people are allergic to psyllium, so other sources (such as fruit pectin) may be a better choice.

Other measures which can prove beneficial include the following:

- Reducing your intake of refined sugars.
- Reducing your intake of saturated fats.
- Reducing your intake of animal-derived proteins.
- Reducing your intake of omega-6 oils.
- Testing for food sensitivities (cereal, dairy and yeast products being among the most common allergens).
- Eating more fruit and vegetables.
- Eating more organic produce.
- Stopping smoking.
- Avoiding unnecessary medications (but consult your doctor first).
- Cutting down on processed foods.

- Drinking more water.
- Cutting down on coffee and fizzy drinks (some of the additives and substances in these can also trigger gut inflammation).

Eliminating irritable bowel syndrome

One day when I was working out at my local gym, a health worker came up to me and thanked me for curing her irritable bowel syndrome (IBS). As I had never seen her professionally, let alone treated her for this complaint, this came as a bit of a surprise. However, I soon discovered that this improvement occurred after she had followed the programme in my first book, *The Detox Diet*, which involved reducing chemical exposure and taking nutritional supplements. Before she started the programme, she had just been put on the waiting list for a full set of investigations for her irritable bowel syndrome which was greatly troubling her. By the time she was due to have the investigations several months later, all her previously distressing sysmtoms had gone.

She was by no means alone in having irritable bowel syndrome, as it appears to be one of the commonest health problems in the world. In the USA up to one in five people have this condition. If you suffer from a general range of bowel problems that don't fall under any neat category, chances are that you too may have irritable bowel syndrome.[89]

Confirming your diagnosis: IBS is currently defined by the Rome II criteria. However, this condition is also known by several other names, such as spastic colon, mucous colitis and non-inflammatory bowel disease.

Those affected by IBS usually have variable periods of relapse and remission. Common symptoms experienced are bloating, abdominal pain, gas, alternating diarrhoea and constipation, excess mucus in the faeces and urgency to defecate.

But before a diagnosis of IBS can be made, other testable causes of bowel disease which possess similar symptoms may need to be ruled out as IBS is a so-called 'disease of exclusion'. These include coeliac disease, diverticulitis, lactose intolerance, laxative abuse, intestinal parasites, Crohn's disease, ulcerative colitis, hormonal imbalance, antacid use and sometimes even metabolic disorders such as diabetes mellitus.

Conventional tests usually fail to reveal any obvious physical abnormalities. Internal examination of the gut using colonoscopy can often reveal a 'normal looking' gut but with an abnormally high level of muscular contraction (along with increased gut spasms). So, if there are no obvious physical abnormalities, what could be causing this extremely common problem? Could this heightened activity of the gut shed any further light on the situation?

Is IBS all in the mind? Owing to the lack of provable pathology using conventional tests, and because of its known link to stress, IBS has been viewed by many in conventional medicine as a 'psychosomatic disorder'. There has also been an association with hypochondriasis or depression. However, while a link with depression may be true for some, it is not true for the vast majority of suffers.

Despite this lack of understanding of the causes of IBS in conventional medicine, most naturopaths have been treating it for years. They have found that true IBS can be triggered by many different factors, such as food intolerances, followed by neurological problems (as opposed to neurotic problems!), with poor diet and nutritional deficiencies also being common.

Although IBS triggers appear to vary greatly, the fascinating thing is that most of them can be linked to an underlying reaction to chemical toxins. This is the conclusion reached by Professor William Rea. He has treated over 20,000 patients in his Dallas Hospital which specialises in the diagnosis and treatment of environmental diseases. He found that IBS appears to be strongly linked to environmental triggers, such as chemicals. The good news is that symptoms can often be eliminated by removing these triggers, together with lowering the body's total pollutant load.

Factors associated with irritable bowel syndrome

■ A raised blood level of organochlorine pesticides
■ Certain inhaled allergens (such as mould, animal fur, and pollen from weeds, trees and grasses)
■ Foods (the worst offenders being wheat, sugar, milk, yeast, beef, pork, coffee and orange juice)
■ Chemical exposure (to such as formaldehyde, phenol, ethanol, chlorine, pesticides and car fumes)
■ Prescription drugs (such as antibiotics and corticosteroids)
■ Gut infections and infestation with intestinal parasites
■ Stress
■ Low level of digestive juices

How chemicals trigger IBS symptoms: The gastrointestinal system is extremely vulnerable to the harmful effects of chemicals. It seems that chemicals can totally disrupt the smooth functioning of virtually every aspect of bowel functioning. The gut is exposed to chemicals in the diet, together with the background exposure that all the organs get from the existing body burden of chemicals. This means that our intestines tend to be exposed to higher levels of chemicals than other parts of the body.

But rather than listing all the chemicals involved, it is more helpful to understand how the gut works and the ways in which chemicals can interfere with this system. This information makes it easier to understand how chemicals can produce the wide range of symptoms so commonly experienced by IBS sufferers.

The layer of muscle in the bowel wall controls the diameter of the bowel. When the muscle in the gut wall contracts, the diameter of the gut decreases. When the muscle relaxes, the bowel becomes dilated. The degree of contraction and dilation is regulated by a number of different hormones, nerves, mineral levels and overall body pH. Toxic chemicals can damage all these controlling factors.

Chemicals can also alter the rate and extent of gut muscle contraction, prompting the gut to go into either spasm or prolonged relaxation – a possible cause of the change in gut activity commonly seen in IBS sufferers. This muscle spasm or dilation could also lead to symptoms of bloating, diarrhoea and constipation. Another way in which chemicals may produce symptoms of IBS is by altering the levels of mucus secretion, increasing it or decreasing it. Chemical damage caused to the balance of gut microflora results in excess wind. The range of symptoms experienced largely depends upon which part of the gut is affected, as well as the particular damage done.

So you can see that toxic chemicals can induce the range of symptoms experienced by IBS sufferers. But this form of damage does not usually show up in conventional tests because doctors don't actively look for it, which could explain why these tests tend not to be able to find a physical cause.

Treating IBS: As chemicals are known to induce symptoms of IBS, then any programme designed to ease these symptoms should include an element of both chemical avoidance and detox. This is why the detox diet in my first book was so effective in the case of the health worker with IBS. And if this chemical reduction takes place in combination with an avoidance of the known trigger factors, such as allergens, and certain foods, this will prove to be even more effective.

Nutritional therapy can speed up this process as it actively lowers the existing body chemical load. All of the nutrients suggested in the detox programme in Chapter 4 should be beneficial. Out of all of these nutrients, magnesium is particularly useful as it can help relax the muscle in the gut and help avoid spasms caused by chemically induced mineral imbalances.

Probiotics can also help restore the gut bacterial balance, and digestive enzyme supplements may be of benefit if indigestion is a problem.[90]

Soluble fibre such as psyllium seed husks may be beneficial too. Soluble fibre also helps in rebalancing the microflora of the gut, since it acts as a food source for them. Care should be taken with insoluble fibre such as wheat bran, as some IBS sufferers find it can irritate the gut, particularly in those who are sensitive to wheat.

Other steps that can help include lowering stress levels by learning a relaxation technique, taking up yoga or going for long walks. Avoiding coffee, alcohol and spices may also ease symptoms.

10

Hormonal Health

'Endocrine disrupting chemicals (EDCs) are substances which can mimic, block or interfere with hormones such as oestrogen, androgen and thyroid, affecting wildlife and humans alike. As a result, they can hijack normal biological processes and may cause neurological, behavioural, developmental or sexual defects.'

WORLD-WIDE FUND FOR NATURE WEBSITE (WWW.WWF.ORG.UK)

Hormonal havoc

The spiralling number of people developing hormone-related health problems, such as diabetes, thyroid disease and infertility, indicates that there is something about modern-day life that appears to be playing havoc with our hormones. Hormones play an important role in every aspect of our lives, so this increasing disruption in hormonal health presents us all with a very serious problem.

Coincidentally, it was the discovery of hormone-altering chemicals in the environment that originally drew me to this subject some years ago. A chance reading of an article revealing how toxic chemicals appeared to be affecting the fertility and reproductive health of our wildlife rang alarm bells in my head. If these chemicals, which I had previously not even heard of, were already making animals infertile, sterile and in some cases wiping out whole species, the chances are that humans, with our greater exposure to chemicals and our similar body systems, are also being affected in some way.

Some time later, after much research and time spent fitting the jigsaw of evidence together, it became clear to me that our hormones are being affected by virtually all the chemicals that we are exposed to in our environment. Indeed, every single synthetic chemical that I have looked at to date possesses the ability to affect levels of at least one type of hormone. With a new chemical being created and introduced into the environment every 20 minutes, and with overall chemical production continuing to rise to ever greater levels, the current situation is set to get even worse.

But things are looking up. Despite the failure of many specialists in conventional medicine to acknowledge the true unfolding state of affairs, a growing number of scientists specialising in environmental medicine are putting more effort and resources into assessing the extent to which our lives are being affected, as well as trying to find out ways of improving the situation. Indeed, their work has enabled me to write this book. So, if you are one of those who are affected, be reassured as there are many things you can do to help yourself.

Our hormones control all aspects of our lives: Firstly, it helps to know what hormones are and why they are so important. Our hormones are natural chemical molecules that act as internal messengers. They are produced in glandular tissue and, when released, carry information and instructions around the body, enabling one part to communicate with another. Although only minuscule amounts of hormones are produced, they help control virtually all the body's functions, such as growth, reproduction, metabolism and weight control.

Levels of these hormones are themselves controlled by a complex regulatory system that involves a degree of feedback from the brain. The flexibility of the system has allowed humans to adapt to a wide range of situations and environments. But this same flexibility appears to have opened us up to attack, as a blockage in one part of the system can have serious repercussions on the smooth running of the rest.

Unfortunately for us, modern chemicals do not damage just one part of the hormonal system. They possess an ability to interfere with the entire system, from the brain that triggers

Why hormones are vulnerable to chemical damage

Chemicals appear to be able to bring about this damage because:

■ Hormone-producing tissues (endocrine glands) are a particular target for blood-borne chemicals, owing to their excellent blood supply.

■ Hormone-producing tissues usually contain a higher proportion of fat so they tend to accumulate the more persistent fat-soluble toxins. Therefore these highly important and sensitive tissues are among the most polluted parts of the body.

■ Chemicals can obstruct the production of hormones.

■ Chemicals can impair the release of hormones.

■ Many chemicals can mimic the action of natural hormones, but unlike natural chemicals, which can be effectively switched off, there is no such mechanism present for the artificial hormone mimics.

■ Chemicals can block natural hormones from tissues they need to stimulate.

■ Chemicals damage the normal circadian rhythm of hormone release, setting millions of subsequent reactions out of sync.

■ Toxins can dramatically change the rate at which hormones are broken down and removed from the body, resulting in lowered hormone levels.

hormone release, to the endocrine glands that create the hormones. All the major types of hormones are highly vulnerable to toxic chemical damage, including the sex hormones, thyroid hormones, insulin, growth hormone, catecholamines and corticosteroids.

Not only do all the major types of chemicals in our environment possess an ability to interfere with our hormones, but they are already present at concentrations that are thousands of times higher than the natural hormones they appear to mimic. Despite being generally many times less potent than natural hormones, they exist at damaging levels which are affecting us.[91]

How to improve hormonal health: So you can see that to obtain optimal hormonal health it is vital to start tackling the build-up of existing chemicals in the body by reducing the daily exposure to toxins, in combination with taking steps to tackle the existing body burden (see Chapters 3 and 4).

Proper nutrition also plays a vital role in optimising hormonal health. People who have nutrient deficiencies are at greater risk of developing hormonal imbalances. And people with hormonal diseases have a greater demand for nutrients. For example, those with overactive thyroid glands tend to need a higher level of antioxidants. Good nutrition also strengthens the body's ability to protect itself against the damage caused by toxins, by soaking up excess free radicals and boosting the body's ability to rid itself of chemicals. The supplement programme suggested in Chapter 4 provides a good general level of nutrients that should be of benefit to all those with existing hormonal imbalances. It will also help to strengthen the hormonal system and, in so doing, reduce the risk of future disease.

Other general ways in which to boost hormonal health include:

- Cutting down on the levels of toxins (see Chapter 3).
- Reducing your intake of stimulants, such as coffee, cigarettes and tea.
- Cutting down on refined sugar.
- Increasing the amount of regular exercise you take.

Controlling diabetes

Diabetes is one of the most important diseases in the world – not only because of the way it forces us to completely change the way we live, or the significant damage it can cause to our bodies, but because the number of sufferers has increased so dramatically. Currently some 17 million Americans and 1.2 million Britons have diabetes.

It gets worse – the World Health Organization has predicted that between 1997 and 2035, the number of diabetics worldwide will more than double from 143 million to about 300 million.[92] The importance of this disease is also reflected in the fact that the pharmaceutical company Eli Lilly & Co have now built the largest factory dedicated to the production of a single drug in industrial history – and that drug is insulin.

The reason why ever more of us seem to be getting diabetes

has baffled scientists for years. However, recent research carried out by doctors specialising in environmental medicine not only provides us with a possible answer to that question, but, more importantly, a way in which the diabetic epidemic could be turned around. Before we find out how, we need to understand more about the disease itself.

More about diabetes: Insulin is a hormone that encourages the storage of glucose, principally in the muscles and liver after eating a meal. Diabetes is a serious hormonal and metabolic disorder caused by an inability by the tissues to take up glucose, resulting in an abnormally high level of blood sugar. This is either due to a total lack of insulin, known as Type I diabetes, or a reduced ability by the tissues to respond to insulin, known as Type II diabetes.

Type I diabetes (formerly known as insulin-dependent or juvenile diabetes) is a condition in which the pancreas fails to produce any insulin. This develops most often in children and adolescents, but is being increasingly noted later in life. The classic symptoms of this are excessive urination (polyuria), excessive thirst (polydipsia), weight loss and tiredness. People with Type I diabetes are totally dependent on daily insulin injections for survival.

Type II diabetes (formerly named non-insulin-dependent or maturity onset diabetes) results from growing resistance by the tissues to the insulin produced by the pancreas. Type II diabetes is much more common and accounts for around 90 per cent of all diabetes cases worldwide. It occurs most frequently in adults, but is being noted increasingly in adolescents as well. People affected can have the same symptoms as in Type I but they are often less severe. Indeed, in many cases, no early symptoms appear and the disease is only diagnosed several years after its onset, when complications may already be present. Although 40 per cent of people with Type II diabetes need insulin injections, about 40 per cent are given oral drugs for satisfactory blood glucose control, and the rest can cope through dietary changes alone.

Complications of diabetes are often severe and include diabetic retinopathy (a leading cause of blindness and visual disability), kidney failure, heart disease (accounting for approximately 50 per cent of all deaths among people with diabetes), diabetic neuropathy (probably the most common complication of diabetes leading to sensory loss, damage to the limbs and impotence), and diabetic foot disease.

Changing pattern of diabetes: Both types of diabetes are complex diseases caused by a combination of genetic predisposition and environmental factors. Although the increase has in part been put down to population growth, an ageing population, unhealthy diets, obesity and sedentary lifestyles, many now believe that the disease process underlying diabetes has fundamentally changed and that new environmental factors are increasingly to blame for between 10 and 50 per cent of the current pandemic.[93]

One of the factors pointing towards environmental agents as one of the major causes is that people are exposed to certain chemicals in their jobs, such as nitrates and PCBs for Type I diabetes and arsenic and dioxins for Type II diabetes. Studies have suggested that the greater the exposure to these chemicals, the higher the risk of developing diabetes. Indeed it is not just those who work with chemicals who appear to be at risk as another study found a direct relationship between the level of the ubiquitous common pollutant PCB and the chance of developing diabetes.

Another factor is a change in the fundamental nature of the disease as certain groups of people have become more vulnerable to developing diabetes. For example, not only have steep rises been documented in the number of children affected by Type I diabetes but the age at which they are developing the disease has dramatically fallen. In addition, the age at which people are developing Type II diabetes is also reducing, as children are now increasingly developing this disease – previously only known to affect adults.[94]

Understanding which environmental agents could have produced the current pandemic of diabetes would be an important step to not only reversing it, but helping to minimise symptoms in those who already have diabetes.

Diabetes and chemicals

Toxic chemicals can increase the risk of developing diabetes by:
- Triggering diabetes in those with an inherited tendency to the condition.
- Altering levels of hormones that are vital to sugar control, such as insulin.
- Destroying insulin-producing cells.
- Damaging most other aspects of carbohydrate metabolism.

Triggering diabetes: It is becoming increasingly apparent that the artificial chemicals we are exposed to in our modern environment are able to trigger diabetes in their own right. And the reason that we are seeing the number of people with diabetes escalate could be a direct result of our ever-increasing exposure to these 'diabeto-genic' substances.

These chemicals appear to be so powerful at causing diabetes that they could be partly responsible for the changes that we are now seeing in disease patterns, such as a lowering in the age of those getting diabetes. This could be because chemicals tend to be far more toxic and cause greater damage to the bodies of infants than to adults. The increasing body burden of chemicals in mothers' bodies could therefore explain why diabetes is affecting people at an ever younger age. It would also explain why both children of older mothers (with their higher body burdens of chemicals), and first-born children (who tend to get the biggest load of chemicals from their mothers), possess an even higher risk of developing diabetes.

Some patients clearly have chemically induced diabetes, while others have a more hazy etiology. However, even the familiar types seem to be waiting for the right set of environmental triggers in order to activate their genetic time bomb. We have seen the onset of both Type I and Type II diabetes after exposure to a high level of pesticide or natural gas. However the 'diabeto-genic' nature of these chemicals appears to be so powerful that they can induce diabetes in those without a family history of the disease.

PROFESSOR WILLIAM REA,
EXTRACT FROM *CHEMICAL SENSITIVITIES*, VOLUME 3

Chemicals linked to diabetes

- Pesticides (such as herbicides, organophosphates and carbamates)
- Organochlorine pesticides (such as DDT)
- Environmental pollutants (such as dioxins, PCBs)
- Heavy metals (such as arsenic, mercury and lead)
- Medications (including antibiotics such as penicillin, cephalosporin and erythromycin; blood pressure medications; the heart drug nifedipine; diuretics such as frusemide and chlorthiazide; sedatives such as benzodiazepines, tranquillisers and barbiturates; and painkillers such as paracetamol)
- Cigarette smoke
- Alcohol
- Solvents (such as benzene)
- Preservatives
- Food contaminants (such as nitrate from artificial fertilisers and inorganic bromide)

Chemicals that trigger or exacerbate diabetes: Many chemicals appear to be linked to diabetes, but the most important groups of 'diabeto-genic' chemicals are the organochlorine pesticides and environmental contaminants. The higher the level of these common contaminants in the body, the greater the risk of developing diabetes.[95] Organochlorines appear to be strongly linked to this disease because of their powerful ability to interfere with normal carbohydrate metabolism.[96] The good news is that by lowering the body levels of these chemicals, much of this damage can be reversed. However, since organochlorines are stored in body fat, any form of rapid weight loss results in the mobilisation of large amounts of these stored toxins into the bloodstream, where they are transported to vital body organs and cause even greater damage. If not anticipated and properly prepared for (by taking nutritional supplements and soluble fibre), the subsequent damage could potentially double the long-term risk of developing diabetes.[97]

People working with other types of pesticides, such as herbicides and insecticides, also have a higher risk of developing diabetes.[98] As well as triggering hormonal damage, these chemicals can cause dramatic swings in blood sugar levels.[99] In fact, this 'diabeto-genic' nature of pesticides can be so powerful that one type of pesticide is actually used to induce diabetes in animals to create an 'animal model' of the disease for research purposes. Diabetic 'animal models' are also created by exposing creatures to an antibiotic known as streptozotocin. This chemical triggers the disease by poisoning insulin-producing cells.[100]

Antibiotics are not the only synthetic medicines that possess powerful diabetic-inducing actions, as a large number of pharmaceutical drugs are known to do this. This group covers a wide range of different drugs including those used to treat high blood pressure, diuretics, sedatives and painkillers.

The list of chemicals linked to diabetes extends to cover many other groups such as the toxic metals. These appear to trigger diabetes by increasing levels of tissue-damaging free radicals. The higher the level of these toxic metals in the body, the greater the apparent diabetic risk.[101] Greater exposure to chemicals from common water contaminants such as the solvent benzene, food contaminants such as inorganic bromide, and nitrates from artificial fertilisers and preservatives are also linked to an increased risk of diabetes.[102]

Nutrients that help prevent diabetes: The important part that proper nutrition plays in managing diabetes is shown by the fact that over 100 studies have now taken place into the use of nutritional supplements in treating and preventing diabetes. They appear to be highly beneficial and, unlike many medications, they also seem to be safe.[103] Not only can vitamin and mineral supplements reduce insulin requirements in Type I diabetes, but

---

Diabetic alert over blood pressure pills

A report of a study carried out on behalf of the National Institute of Clinical Excellence (NICE, www.nice.org.uk) reported that patients taking a combination of two types of the most commonly used blood pressure drugs, a thiazide diuretic and a beta-blocker, could increase their risk of developing diabetes by 20 per cent compared to other treatments.

they can also reduce the degree of insulin resistance in Type II diabetes, protect the body against developing complications of diabetes and guard against further chemical damage.[104]

Antioxidants appear to be of particular value since much of the damage brought about by chemicals is thought to be caused by increased levels of free radicals. If you consider that a high sugar level increases free radical production in its own right, the need for antioxidants in diabetics is particularly important. It is therefore not surprising that diabetics tend to be deficient in antioxidants and that diabetic control and the prevention of further chemical damage can be greatly improved by taking supplements. Antioxidants are also helpful in dealing with diabetic complications. The antioxidant alpha-lipoic acid has been used for over 30 years in Germany to treat diabetic-induced neuropathy.[105] The range of beneficial antioxidants includes vitamins A, C and E, selenium, zinc, alpha-lipoic acid (particularly good at preventing nerve symptoms), co-enzyme Q10, glutathione, methionine and cysteine.

But it is not just antioxidants that enhance the body's response to insulin – many other nutrients can help. For instance, up to 70 per cent of people with Type II diabetes tend to be deficient in vitamin D, which is important in carbohydrate metabolism. Supplementation of this vitamin has been shown to greatly improve diabetic control by reducing the degree of insulin resistance.[104] Many of the B group of vitamins (B1, B3, B6, B12 and biotin) also play an important role, as diabetics tend to use these nutrients up at a faster rate.

Minerals such as zinc and magnesium help prevent people developing diabetes and greatly improve diabetic control by lowering insulin resistance.[106] Chromium is also thought to be good at lowering abnormally high glucose levels. Vanadium is a metal that has aroused recent interest owing to its ability to enhance the effects of insulin at low levels. However, the long-term safety of this substance is as yet unknown.[107] It is also known to be toxic at high levels.

Polyunsaturated fats, such as the omega-3 oils, are also vitally important in preventing the onset of diabetes and reducing the degree of insulin resistance in diabetics.[108] Soluble fibre supplements are not only great detoxifiers, binding many of the chemicals linked to worsening diabetic control, but they can also improve diabetic control by lowering high blood glucose levels.[109] This ability to lower blood glucose has been formally recognised, as the American Diabetic Association and the National Cholesterol Education Program have updated their guidelines to increase the levels of soluble fibre recommended from 10–25 g a day.[110]

In addition to avoiding toxins and starting a detox programme (see Chapters 3 and 4), other ways in which diabetic control can be improved include:

- Adopting a diet low in refined sugars
- Weight loss (gradual not rapid)
- Increasing physical activity levels (walking for only half an hour a day reduced the risk of diabetes by more than 50 per cent)
- Avoiding exposure to foods or other substances that trigger allergic symptoms

Thyroid disease – the silent epidemic

If you are feeling tired all the time, have lost your vital spark and seem to have forgotten what it is like to feel normal, it may not be due to your age – you could be one of the millions of people whose thyroid gland is not working properly. Some specialists estimate that approximately one in five people over 55 is now affected, yet only one in 100 people ends up being diagnosed with an underactive thyroid.[111] Therefore the vast majority of sufferers are potentially missing out on a wealth of restorative treatment and a far better quality of life.

So why does thyroid disease appear to be a largely silent epidemic, with sufferers simply accepting their symptoms without looking any further for answers? The most likely explanation is that the symptoms can be very generalised and difficult to spot if you are not specifically looking for them. In addition, there has been over-reliance on blood tests at the expense of clinical examination, and so most specialists only treat those who have abnormally low levels of thyroid hormone in the blood. This rules out treatment for an increasing group of people who have all the signs and symptoms of thyroid deficiency, and who are shown to respond to replacement therapy, but are not deemed suitable for treatment because their blood levels are not below a certain arbitrary level.

In fact many people with 'normal' blood levels of thyroid hormone actually need higher levels to function efficiently. Certain conditions can also throw the readings off, including pregnancy, medications and illness. Thyroid tests can also show a high degree of inaccuracy. The result is that most doctors end up treating the blood test results and not the patient.

But it is not just the cases of underactive thyroid that are on the increase, as other common forms of thyroid disease are also becoming much more widespread. These include thyroid cancer, which in Australia has increased 30-fold in the space of four decades[112] and overactive thyroid, which in some populations has increased more than three times over the last 10 years.[113]

Symptoms of thyroid disease: To get to grips with why thyroid diseases are on the increase, we need to understand a bit more about how the thyroid gland works. The thyroid is situated in the neck and produces two types of thyroid hormones: thyroxine and tri-iodothyronine. These hormones are released into the blood periodically, where most of them bind to specially created proteins and are carried round the body to wherever they are needed. Thyroid hormones are essential because they control the metabolic rate (power metabolism, burn fat and stimulate carbohydrate utilisation), stimulate growth, play a part in weight control, allow normal brain development in babies, are essential hormones in reproduction, and enable the heart and cardiovascular system to work properly.

Natural control of the thyroid gland is a complex business, relying on many factors such as nerve signals from the brain, adequate levels of nutrition, and feedback from existing levels of thyroid hormones in the body. Because of the relative complexity of this system and the number of factors that can disrupt normal thyroid functioning, there are many ways in which things can go wrong. And when they do, the result is usually one of two conditions: hypothyroidism (abnormally low levels of thyroid hormones) or hyperthyroidism (abnormally high levels of thyroid hormones).

Those with hypothyroidism (an underactive thyroid), tend to experience some or all of the following symptoms: weakness, fatigue, muscle and joint aches, cold intolerance, constipation, weight gain, depression, hoarse voice, dry, cold and puffy skin, thinning hair and eyebrows, and anaemia. The principal conventional treatment of an underactive thyroid is to give synthetic thyroid hormone.

Those with hyperthyroidism (an overactive thyroid) tend to have some or all of the following: increased nervousness, heat intolerance, increased sweating, fatigue, weakness, muscle cramps, weight loss, frequent bowel movements, tremor of the hand, prominent staring eyes, warm moist skin, fine hair and increased levels of thyroid hormones in the blood. An overactive thyroid is usually treated by antithyroid drugs, radioactive iodine and surgery. However, all of these drugs confer serious side-effects, including bone marrow suppression, hepatitis, painful joints and jaundice. In addition, approximately half of all the people treated with radioactive iodine for an overactive thyroid end up eventually needing lifelong thyroid hormone replacement.

Environmental changes and thyroid disease: There is compelling evidence linking thyroid disease with recent changes in our environment.[93] And it's not just those working with chemicals who appear to be at risk, as current levels of environmental pollution have put us all in the firing line. Those who actually go on to develop thyroid diseases probably do so through a combination of the following factors:

- An increased genetic susceptibility to thyroid disease.
- Previous exposure to thyroid-damaging toxins.
- Chemical exposure at an early age (the earlier the exposure the greater the damage).
- Previous history of poor nutrition.

When I was researching my previous book on how chemicals affect our weight, I examined the effect on the thyroid gland of each of the major types of chemicals we are now exposed to. I was shocked by what I found, as the majority of these chemicals have some sort of thyroid-damaging action. Not only do different chemicals possess the ability to increase or decrease the level of thyroid hormone in the body, but some chemicals induce both conditions under differing circumstances.

Starting with pesticides, this group of herbicides, insecticides and fungicides commonly found in our foods contains some of the most powerful thyroid hormone suppressors known. Some are actually used for this very purpose in animals, to make them put on weight faster, and in humans, to suppress an overactive thyroid.[114, 115] The extensive use of these chemicals on our fields means that in many agricultural regions, thyroid-damaging pesticides are seeping into the water supplies.[116]

Chemicals known to damage the thyroid gland

- Pesticides (such as DDT, lindane, HCB, organophosphates and carbamates)
- Environmental pollutants (such as PCBs, PBBs and dioxins)
- Toxic metals (such as mercury)
- Medications
- Meat contaminants (such as animal growth promoters and veterinary medicines)
- Halogens (such as chlorine, bromide and fluoride)
- Food additives and preservatives
- Plastics
- Synthetic rubber
- Solvents

There is also a powerful link between the levels of environmental pollutants in our bodies, such as HCB, PCBs and dioxins, and thyroid hormone levels. In many cases the more polluted the body is, the lower the level of thyroid hormones in the blood.[117]

Toxic metals such as mercury can damage thyroid functioning by increasing the risk of developing autoimmune thyroid disease, and even thyroid cancer.[118] Synthetic compounds such as plastics and synthetic rubber also appear to add to the problem. For instance, workers engaged in the production of synthetic rubber revealed a high (35 per cent) prevalence of thyroid disease. Indeed, the longer the time spent working with these chemicals, the lower the levels of thyroid hormones detected in the blood.[119] Phthalates, the chemicals that make plastics flexible and one of the commonest types of environmental pollutants, also appear to possess powerful anti-thyroid actions.[120]

Balancing thyroid hormones naturally: Good nutrition plays a crucial role in helping to prevent the development of thyroid disease, by protecting the thyroid gland from chemical damage. Antioxidants appear to be particularly important since people with thyroid diseases tend to have lower levels of these nutrients in their blood.[121] Supplementing antioxidants not only helps reduce some of the symptoms in those with overactive thyroids, but it can also prevent or reduce chemically induced thyroid damage.[122]

Other nutrients of value include vitamin D, which is found to be deficient in 40 per cent of female Japanese patients suffering from the autoimmune thyroid disease known as Graves' disease, which is associated with an overproduction of thyroid hormone.[123] Graves' disease can also be associated with low levels of vitamin B12. Folic acid and vitamin B6 supplementation are particularly beneficial to those with an underactive thyroid.

Many minerals also play an important role in thyroid metabolism, not least iodine which in combination with the amino acid tyrosine is essential for the production of thyroid hormone. This is important as approximately one billion people throughout the world are thought to be iodine deficient. In addition, low levels of iodine also tend to make the thyroid gland more susceptible to chemical damage.[120] The minerals selenium, magnesium, zinc, iron and copper are also thought to play an important role in maintaining normal thyroid functioning.

Other potentially beneficial nutrients for the thyroid are essential fatty acids, particularly since their metabolism appears to be abnormal in thyroid disease states.[124] For those with an overactive thyroid, carnitine appears to be a natural antagonist (opposes the action) of thyroid hormone and so may be potentially beneficial. The amino acid thyrosine and kelp (a type of seaweed) can be useful in those with hypothyroidism as they help boost levels of thyroid hormone – but they should be avoided in those with an overactive thyroid.

Restoring your natural fertility

Becoming pregnant and managing to carry a child to term appears to be a growing problem in our modern world. A surprising 8–12 per cent of couples worldwide are thought to be infertile, and many top scientists predict that this number is set to increase still further.[125]

The heartache that this causes is incalculable, since few problems are as distressing as an inability to conceive. Not only can the basic instinct to have a child be very powerful, in many countries there is an additional stress as parenthood is expected and so being childless can be socially unacceptable. The burning need for children can lead to vast sums of money being spent on high-tech fertility techniques, which have very significant health risks attached.

However, after many years working in the field of environmental medicine, what really surprises me is not that the infertility rate is so high, but that so many babies are still being born at all! Indeed, the discovery that current levels of pollution are causing infertility and reproductive problems in our wildlife is what brought me into this field in the first place.

On the bright side, it does seem that by addressing the potential problems, fertility can often be improved dramatically. As an older mother of four children (the last born when I was 39) I can verify that, for me, all aspects of pregnancy and childbirth became much easier as I grew older. I strongly feel that the reason for this was my continually improving diet, which from the birth of my first child to that of my last, completely changed to one that is now largely organic, supplemented with essential nutrients.

Fertility problems – the hidden causes: Even for couples who are fertile, getting pregnant is not as easy as they may have assumed, particularly since parenthood is increasingly being delayed owing to career demands. The average length of time taken to get pregnant is six months, although a year to 18 months is not uncommon. However, even if you fail to become pregnant after 18 months, it does not necessarily mean that you and/or your partner are infertile.

Fertility and the speed of conception are reliant on many factors, some of which can be sorted out fairly easily, whereas others may require more attention. Once a couple realise that they are having problems conceiving, many seek help from their own doctor who will carry out a few basic tests. If no obviously remediable cause can be found and the couple have still not conceived, they normally get referred to a specialist, who takes the couple through a second round of tests.

Those who have run the gamut of these investigations will know that the number of tests involved reflects the numerous causes of fertility problems. This can involve both the woman and the man: reduced fertility in the man is the problem in a third of cases; in one third of cases the problem involves the woman; and in the remainder there are factors involving both partners.

The list of factors known to cause sub-fertility is much wider than is usually tested for in conventional investigations and includes the following:

- Stress (a major factor in infertility)
- Chromosomal abnormalities

■ Genito-urinary infections
■ Hormonal imbalances
■ Physical defects
■ Poor nutrition
■ Illnesses, both short- and long-term
■ Drugs
■ Irradiation
■ Toxic chemicals (such as pesticides, toxic metals, solvents and environmental pollutants such as dioxins and PCBs)
■ Smoking
■ Alcohol
■ Halogens (such as chlorine and bromine)
■ Allergies
■ Immune system problems

The chemical connection: While most of these causes are well documented and have been known about for years, more attention has recently been directed to the effects that toxic chemicals are having on our fertility. It may be no coincidence that since the 1950s, synthetic chemical production has increased fivefold, while the average sperm count has dropped by over half. In light of the known damaging effects chemicals have on sperm production, this recent dramatic fall in sperm count comes as little surprise.[126]

Despite this slump in our fertility levels, the situation can potentially be reversed by making a deliberate effort to lower our exposure to chemical toxins. This was shown in a group of organic farmers who ate a higher than average proportion of organic foods and were found to have almost double the sperm count found in the average population.

In order to reverse this situation, we first need to know which chemicals do the most damage to fertility so we can devise ways of avoiding them or minimising their toxicity. By understanding this problem, we are one step away from finding significant and effective ways of dealing with it.

Chemicals that damage fertility: Chemicals are well known for causing serious damage to every aspect of our fertility. Chemically induced changes in sex hormone levels even affect sexual behaviour: they 'feminise' boys and 'masculinise' girls. Chemicals also poison sperm and eggs, making eggs less fertile and more likely to miscarry if they are fertilised.[126]

Early warning signs indicating the damage artificial chemicals can cause to human reproduction emerged a couple of decades ago when a US fertility clinic started seeing an increasing number of male workers at a factory that manufactured pesticides. Further observations revealed that the longer the duration of pesticide exposure, the lower their sperm count. Worse still, after a couple of years of working with this particular pesticide, sperm production ceased, leaving many of them irreversibly infertile.[127] Although this particular pesticide [1,2-dibromo-3-chloropropane (DBCP)] has since been banned in the USA, it is still being used in other countries, and understandably will be continuing to devastate the fertility and the lives of the people who are exposed to it.

Other studies have looked at the level of pesticides in those women undergoing *in vitro* fertilisation (IVF) and have discovered that the higher the level of toxins detected in body fluids, particularly the persistent pesticides and environmental pollutants known as organochlorines, the lower the chances of successful fertilisation.[128] IVF fertilisation rates are also significantly lower if the male partner has previous exposure to pesticides.[129] As pesticides are designed to kill or suppress reproduction in pests, these anti-fertility effects should come as little surprise.

Increased exposure to toxic metals such as mercury and lead is also linked to infertility. These toxic metals extend the time taken to become pregnant. Unfortunately, studies show that the levels that affect fertility appear to be those to which we are currently exposed. For instance, couples who eat greater amounts of seafood tend to have higher levels of mercury, and the higher the level of mercury the lower the fertility.[130] Higher body levels of mercury are also found in people with a large

Does tap water harm unborn babies?

Water companies have been warned to limit levels of chlorine used to disinfect tap water supplies amid fears of a link to birth defects and miscarriage. Government experts said research suggests chlorine by-products may harm the developing baby in the womb. Chlorine is used to kill bugs and to disinfect recycled tap water.

The research is understood to have looked at chlorine by-product levels in three water company regions and compared the results with Health Service records on miscarriage and birth defects, such as low birth weight.

Professor Ieuan Hughes, Chairman of the Committee on toxicity, said, 'The information suggests there might be a small risk of an association between birth outcome problems and chlorination by products in water.' – Article in the Scottish *Daily Mail* (21 April 2004).

number of amalgam (mercury-containing) fillings. Fortunately, it seems that if higher levels of toxic metals are detected in the body, and if their levels are lowered by using a system of specially targeted supplements called chelation (see page 276), then the chances of conception can be greatly improved.[131]

Other chemicals that can lower fertility and increase the risk of miscarriages are solvents, cigarette smoke, plastics, environmental pollutants such as PCBs and dioxins, chlorine (used to disinfect tap water) and bromine (a food contaminant).[132, 133, 134]

Nutrients for fertility: The low level of nutrients in most normal diets is itself a common cause of reduced fertility. Even slightly sub-optimal levels of certain vitamins and minerals can cause infertility or repeated miscarriage. Poor nutrition can also increase the fertility damage brought about by toxic chemicals.

Some of the most important fertility-enhancing nutrients are the antioxidants, such as vitamins A, C and E, selenium, co-enzyme Q10, glutathione, acetyl-cysteine and isoflavones. Supplementing these nutrients can help protect the reproductive organs, eggs and sperm against chemically induced free-radical damage, and can greatly boost fertility.[135]

The minerals zinc and magnesium are also strongly linked to fertility, as they appear essential in maintaining the quantity and activity of sperm – indeed zinc is found in high concentrations in the testes and in the tail and covering of the sperm itself. Unfortunately, due to the changes in agricultural practices, together with changed eating habits, few men now get adequate levels of these vital nutrients in their diets. This helps to explain how nutrient supplementation has been shown to be so effective in boosting fertility levels and restoring sperm counts to 'normal' levels.[136, 137]

Other nutrients often deficient in the diet and therefore worth supplementing are B6, B12, folic acid, and the amino acids carnitine and arginine.[138] Omega-3 fatty oils are also useful. As a high ratio of omega-6:3 oils can lower male fertility, men should avoid supplementing with just omega-6 oils, or eating foods high in omega-6, and should only take supplements high in omega-3, as a higher intake of omega-3 will lead to a more balanced ratio of omega-6:3 oils and hence improved fertility. Soluble fibre can help bind many of the harmful toxins in the diet as well as lowering the levels of those currently present in the body.

General advice for maximising fertility: It appears clear that to optimise your chances of becoming pregnant and having a healthy baby, it would be sensible to reduce the regular exposure to chemicals as well as the existing body burden in both prospective parents. While reducing exposure to chemicals is sensible at any time and particularly during pregnancy, total fasting or very severe food restriction should not be attempted at any time by either partner because the subsequent excessive mobilisation of toxins could potentially affect the health of egg, sperm and developing foetus.

Optimal nutrition for both partners is also vital for reducing the risk of miscarriage and increasing the chances of having a healthy child. If actively trying for a baby, it is wise for the woman to take supplements specifically designed for pregnancy as the levels of certain nutrients need to be carefully controlled. For example, vitamin A should be limited to a maximum of 10,000 IU a day. As it takes three months for sperm to develop and one month for the egg to mature, good nutrition during the run up to pregnancy will boost the odds of becoming pregnant. It will also lower the risk of complications associated with pregnancy, such as morning sickness and anaemia. Studies also show that if mothers take the appropriate nutritional supplements during pregnancy, such as folic acid, their babies are at much lower risk of developing diseases such as spina bifida, asthma and childhood cancer.

11

Cardiovascular Diseases

'The dawn of a new era for stroke treatment' – a title of an academic paper reporting the proven benefits antioxidant nutrients offer in preventing stroke-induced brain damage.'

KOGURE, 2002

Is there a chemical connection with cardiovascular diseases?

When people talk about the problems caused by chemicals, the diseases foremost in their minds include the most obvious and best publicised ones such as cancer, immune system disorders and hormonal imbalances. Consequently, few would consider diseases of the cardiovascular system – such as heart disease, high blood pressure, strokes and high cholesterol – to be on that list. However, it does not take much investigation to discover that not only is there a connection, but the link appears to be of great significance.

The cardiovascular system is controlled by hormones and nerves, and made up of different kinds of muscle tissue – all known to be vulnerable to chemical damage – so it stands to reason that these systems would be affected in some way. Yet despite a well-established link between chemicals and cardiovascular damage, this particular form of toxicity gets little attention from either general physician or lay person. This has great significance for the individuals who have or are developing heart problems, as they could be failing to address potentially preventable sources of their condition.

The link between certain toxic metals, such as lead, and high blood pressure has appeared to be so powerful that the title of one academic article goes as far as to question whether lead exposure could be the principal cause of high blood pressure.[139]

This comparative ignorance of the true situation is potentially disastrous, particularly since cardiovascular diseases are now so common. Any additional knowledge on a potentially reversible problem could make all the difference between life and death for millions of people worldwide.[140] But before we can find out why the cardiovascular system is so sensitive to chemical damage, we need to know more about it.

How the cardiovascular system works: In essence, the cardiovascular system consists of the heart and blood vessels. The blood vessels form a network of tubes filled with blood, which is pumped round by the heart to all the body tissues. Blood has a dual purpose – it provides nourishment, and acts as a waste disposal system. Without a regular source of blood the body tissues would soon die.

The brain is *involved* in all bodily systems but the cardiovascular system is *largely controlled* by the blood vessels responding to the needs of the tissues.

Unfortunately, since all the major tissues involved in this process are known to be exquisitely sensitive to chemical damage, the cardiovascular system itself is extremely vulnerable to such damage.

Which chemicals appear to be involved? Numerous studies show that certain groups of people who are exposed to higher levels of particular chemicals in different aspects of their work or domestic lives are at a higher risk of developing cardiovascular diseases. The type of chemical they work with tends to determine the type of disease they will get. Chemicals implicated include all the usual suspects, such as pesticides, environmental pollutants, heavy metals, solvents, plastics, chlorine and fluoride.

As previously mentioned, high blood pressure appears to be most strongly connected to an increased exposure to toxic metals, whereas higher blood fat (lipids), high cholesterol levels and diabetes all tend to have powerful associations with increased levels of organochlorine pesticides and environmental pollutants. So while it is a good idea to reduce your intake of all toxic chemicals, if you have a particular cardiovascular disease and want to target the removal of chemicals that are known to be linked to this problem, you will find the relevant information in this chapter.

Poor nutrition increases the risk of cardiovascular disease: Good nutrition itself is also essential to keep the cardiovascular system in good working order. Those deficient in certain nutrients tend to be at a much higher risk of developing cardiovascular illnesses. For instance, lower blood levels of the vitamins B6, B12 and folic acid tend to result in higher blood levels of the protein homocysteine. Excessively high levels of this protein are linked to increased rates of heart disease and high blood pressure. Fortunately, supplementation with these nutrients brings the levels of homocysteine back to normal and so substantially reduces the risk of heart disease.[141, 142]

Nutrients with antioxidant properties also appear to play an important role in preventing and treating many cardiovascular diseases, such as stroke and high blood pressure. Other nutrients, such as minerals, amino acids and essential fatty acids, are also of great value in optimising cardiovascular health.

So, while the link between cardiovascular diseases, nutrition and toxic chemicals is currently undervalued and little understood, this book offers new ways to prevent and deal with the following:

■ High cholesterol.
■ Heart disease.
■ High blood pressure.
■ Stroke.

Natural ways of lowering cholesterol

For the last few decades, many millions of people have been waging a war against higher levels of cholesterol. Because of the strong link between increased levels of cholesterol and a higher risk of heart disease, vast sums of money have been spent on testing for, and treating, the problem.

For many people, the first step in reducing high cholesterol levels is to cut down on the amount of cholesterol in their food. However, for many, reducing dietary cholesterol alone can often make very little impact on their overall levels. To explain why, I would like to take you back five years or so to the time when I was researching my first book – *The Detox Diet*.

While investigating the relationship between chemicals and excess body weight, I looked at the effect particular toxins had on cholesterol levels. The more studies I read, the more intrigued I was, because it became increasingly apparent that the major types of toxic chemicals now found in the body can significantly increase blood levels of cholesterol – at current exposure levels.

Since then I have been looking forward to an opportunity to write about this well-researched but not widely known connection, as it opens up major new ways in which millions of people can now safely tackle their cholesterol levels. But before I discuss this further, I will briefly explain what cholesterol is, why we need it and why too much is not always a good thing.

All about cholesterol: Despite modern society's demonisation of the fat, or lipid, known as cholesterol, the truth is that we all need a certain amount of it as it is vital for life. Every cell in the body contains a certain amount of cholesterol, because it is essential for creating and maintaining cell shape and structure. Cholesterol is also an essential precursor of many hormones, including steroids such as male and female sex hormones and corticosteroids, and is a precursor of vitamin D.

Cholesterol is a component of bile, which helps break down fats in the small intestine. It also plays a vital role in transporting fats around the body, to be stored or used as fuel.

There are two main types: 'good' HDL (high-density lipoproteins) cholesterol and 'bad' LDL (low-density lipoproteins) cholesterol. The higher the level of LDL cholesterol in the blood the more likely it is that cholesterol will be dumped on the

Factors that influence cholesterol levels

The level of cholesterol in the blood, the ratio of good to bad cholesterol and levels of other blood fats such as triglycerides are influenced by the following factors:

■ Genetic makeup
■ The levels of certain hormones (such as sex hormones, insulin, catecholamines and thyroid hormone)
■ The amount of exercise taken
■ The types of fats consumed in the diet
■ Disease (such as hypothyroidism, growth hormone deficiency, diabetes, nephrotic syndrome, renal failure, obstructive jaundice, anorexia nervosa)
■ Alcohol abuse
■ Chemicals (see box, page 194)

blood vessel walls, thereby furring them up with fatty plaques. On the other hand, HDL cholesterol actively removes or 'cleans up' deposits of cholesterol on the blood vessel walls. Therefore, the higher the ratio of HDL-cholesterol to LDL-cholesterol, the lower the risk of heart disease. High levels of other blood fats, such as triglycerides, are also linked to heart disease.

Cholesterol – the chemical connection: The chemicals most strongly associated with a cholesterol-raising effect appear to be the organochlorine pesticides and pollutants, such as DDT, lindane, PCB and dioxins. It seems that the higher the body levels of these highly persistent and exceedingly common body contaminants, the higher the level of cholesterol and triglycerides in the blood. Not only is this cholesterol-raising effect found in people who work with these chemicals, but it is also seen in those who are merely exposed to higher levels of these toxins from their environment and diet.[143, 144, 145]

Many commonly used pesticides, such as the insecticide organophosphate, also appear to increase cholesterol levels by blocking the pathway by which cholesterol is converted into useful substances, such as hormones.[146]

Heavy metal exposure is also strongly implicated. For instance, metal workers exposed to higher levels of lead have

Chemicals that increase cholesterol levels

High cholesterol levels can be caused by the following chemicals:
- Pesticides (such as organochlorines, organophosphates and carbamates)
- Environmental pollutants (dioxins and PCBs)
- Toxic metals (such as lead, mercury, copper and cadmium)
- Chlorine
- Solvents (such as trichloroethylene and alcohol)
- Medications (such as oral contraceptives, thiazide diuretics, beta blockers, calcium channel blockers and corticosteroids)

been found to have higher levels of cholesterol.[101] Workers exposed to copper and cadmium also have abnormally high levels of blood fats.[147, 148] But not just metal workers are at risk, as people who are exposed to higher levels of mercury from their diet (for example from seafood) and from other sources such as amalgam fillings have also been found to have higher levels of bad cholesterol and lower levels of good cholesterol.[149]

Even those who drink chlorinated water appear to be at risk. A study in Wisconsin, USA, found that those living in communities that chlorinated their water had higher levels of blood cholesterol than those communities that did not.[150] Solvents such as alcohol and the widely used dry-cleaning agent and paint thinner trichloroethylene also appear to damage cholesterol metabolism.[151, 152]

Since reducing your body's exposure to the above chemicals can result in lower cholesterol levels, it makes sense to do all you can to achieve this. As optimum nutrition plays a vital role in detoxing, this should be tackled simultaneously.

Nutrients that lower blood lipids: Good nutrition is particularly important for those who have high levels of cholesterol, along with a balanced supplement programme (see Chapter 4). I will now highlight some nutrients that play a particularly important role in lowering high cholesterol levels.

As with many other disorders related to toxic chemicals, one of the recurring themes is a higher need for antioxidants. Antioxidants, such as vitamins C and E and co-enzyme Q10, tend to be deficient in those with high cholesterol levels. Supplements of these nutrients help lower levels of bad cholesterol and triglycerides while increasing the levels of good cholesterol.[153, 154, 155]

As mentioned previously, homocysteine is a protein which is known to significantly increase the risk of cardiovascular diseases and is also linked to higher levels of blood cholesterol. Homocysteine levels tend to increase when body levels of certain vitamins, such as folic acid, B6 and B12, are low. Therefore supplementation or higher levels of these nutrients not only successfully lowers the levels of homocysteine but also appears to lower levels of blood cholesterol.[156, 157] Vitamin B3 and B5 supplements can also actively lower cholesterol levels.

Other nutrients that help lower blood lipid levels include magnesium, zinc, selenium and chromium. This was clearly demonstrated in a study in which diabetics who were deficient in magnesium were given supplements for 12 weeks. Not only was there a significant fall in bad LDL cholesterol and triglycerides, but levels of the good HDL cholesterol rose.[158] Zinc supplements were found to produce beneficial increases in HDL levels in patients undergoing renal dialysis.[159] Selenium levels also appear to influence cholesterol levels, as a study showed that those with lower levels of selenium in their diets tend to have lower levels of good HDL cholesterol.[160] Chromium was found to protect the body from the lipid-raising effects of the heavy metal arsenic, a contaminant in the water supply in some countries. It also appears to be able to increase HDL levels in its own right.[161]

Other important lipid-lowering nutrients are the omega-3 oils, which are particularly powerful in reducing triglyceride levels while improving the cholesterol ratio.[154, 162]

Finally, soluble fibre supplements such as psyllium seed husks and pectin are well known for effectively and safely lowering levels of cholesterol, as they bind the cholesterol in bile as it passes through the gut, and carry it out of the body before it can be reabsorbed.[110] Eating foods high in natural soluble fibre will not only effectively lower the levels of cholesterol but also reduce the body burden of cholesterol-raising chemicals, found in particularly high concentrations in cholesterol. In this way you will effectively kill two birds with one stone. Other ways of lowering blood fat levels include:

- Cutting down on saturated fats in the diet.
- Increasing dietary levels of unsaturated fats in the form of oils, such as walnut, sunflower or olive oil.
- Increasing the proportion of vegetable and whole grain foods in the diet (vegetarians tend to have lower cholesterol levels).
- Eating garlic and soya protein.
- Cutting down on refined sugars (which lower levels of good HDL cholesterol).
- Drinking alcohol only in moderation.
- Cutting down on foods high in trans fatty acids (such as margarines – the hardening process causes these to form).
- Exercising more (which raises the levels of good cholesterol and lowers the level of bad cholesterol and triglycerides).
- Avoiding recreational drugs (which are known to raise blood levels of cholesterol).
- Giving up smoking (as tobacco lowers good HDL cholesterol levels along with its other harmful effects).
- Cutting down on real coffee (which is known to increase cholesterol levels).

Improving the health of your heart

In the Western world a staggering one out of every two people dies from heart disease, making it one of the commonest killers of the twenty-first century. Yet it was not always this way because just over 100 years ago, heart attacks were virtually unheard of. This extraordinary emergence of a disease over a few generations reflects a dramatic change in the underlying factors predisposing us to heart disease.

Owing to the huge numbers of people being affected by heart disease, many billions of pounds have to date been spent on research into the underlying causes – and yet there still appears to be a gaping hole in our knowledge base regarding the effect that many modern toxic chemicals have on heart disease. In light of their well-known toxic effect on the cardiovascular system and ever-growing presence in our lives, this is somewhat surprising.

What is heart disease? The heart is a pump, made up of specialised muscle. With each heartbeat, blood is pushed through the heart and around the body via blood vessels known as arteries, in order to carry nutrients and oxygen to all the body's tissues. The blood passes through these tissues delivering the nutrients and oxygen and taking away waste products. On its way back to the heart, transported in the veins, the blood passes through the kidneys, where most of these waste products are filtered out, formed into urine and sent to the bladder to be removed from the body. Once the blood has arrived back at the heart, it is directed into another set of arteries, this time leading into the lungs. Here the blood gets re-oxygenated, and more waste products, in the form of carbon dioxide, are removed. Then the blood is returned to the heart, and the cycle starts again.

The term 'heart disease' does not make clear that the main damage is to the coronary arteries that supply the tissues of the heart with nutrients and oxygen. Under certain conditions, a fatty substance, known as a plaque or atheroma, gets deposited on the lining of the artery. This process is known as atherosclerosis and is commonly referred to as 'furring up' or 'clogging' of the arteries.

This build-up leads to narrowing of the arteries. If a blood clot forms at this narrowing, the artery becomes blocked. In a

Ischaemic heart disease

A common disorder of heart function, ischaemic heart disease is caused by insufficient blood flow to the muscle tissue of the heart. The decreased blood flow may be due to narrowing of the coronary arteries (atherosclerosis) or to obstruction by a blood clot (coronary thrombosis). Severe interruption of the blood supply to part of the heart may result in the death of heart muscle.

coronary artery, this is known as a myocardial infarction. Severe problems arise as a consequence of this blockage. Once the blood supply to a part of the heart stops, all the tissues fed by the artery may die from lack of oxygen. The outcome depends on the coronary artery involved, the extent of the heart tissue affected and the length of time the tissue is deprived of oxygen. For instance, if the part of the heart that contains the specialised cells that generate the heartbeat is affected, there is a much greater risk of developing abnormal and potentially fatal heart rhythms. In severe cases it leads to a heart attack, which could trigger a cardiac arrest.

Some people are alerted to the danger by way of heart pain, known as angina. Angina is caused by a partial blockage in the coronary artery due to atherosclerosis. In this situation, enough blood gets through to keep the heart muscle tissue alive, but not enough to supply its total needs. This causes chest pain on exertion, in the cold and with stress. However, if angina is identified and dealt with appropriately, a potentially fatal heart attack can be avoided.

How is the heart susceptible to chemical toxicities? There appear to be two main ways in which toxic chemicals trigger heart problems. The first is mainly due to an immediate poisoning effect on the heart tissues. The second arises from the cumulative effect of longer-term exposure to toxic chemicals.

The parts of the heart most sensitive to direct chemical damage are the nerves, the highly specialised heart tissue (pacemaker) that controls the rate at which the heart beats, and the coronary arteries. Poisoning to the nerves and pacemaker can trigger the spectrum of abnormal heart rhythms, or arrhythmias. Chemical damage to the coronary arteries can cause them to go into spasm, thereby triggering angina or, if the reduction in blood flow is severe, even a heart attack.

Longer-term heart damage can be caused by a higher background level of chemically triggered factors predisposing to heart disease, such as diabetes (see page 170), high cholesterol or high blood pressure.

Which chemicals are known to damage the heart? It did not take much research to discover that many chemicals appear to possess a powerful ability to damage the heart. It is not only people who work with chemicals who are at risk, as many of these substances are now so widespread that they are already present in the population in levels high enough to cause significant damage to the heart.

Direct exposure to some of the more commonly detected pesticides on our foods, such as organophosphates, carbamates and organochlorines, greatly increases the risk of developing abnormal heart rhythms. This can be clearly seen in those who deliberately ingest such substances in order to harm themselves, or in those who are exposed to higher levels of pesticides owing to their lifestyles, diet and environment.[163, 164, 165] In addition, certain chemicals such as the organophosphates can actually cause heart muscle to break down.[166, 167]

Toxic metals, such as arsenic, lead and mercury, are also strongly implicated in triggering ischaemic heart disease and abnormal heart rhythms. They are also thought to play a part in heart failure, a condition in which the heart is unable to cope with its workload efficiently, usually due to defects or disease. The higher the level of these toxic metals in the body, the greater the risk of heart disease.[168] For example, the 15 per cent of the population with the highest levels of lead in their bodies (a group made up of both chemical workers and non-chemical workers) have a raised incidence of ischaemic heart disease and abnormally slow heart rhythms. So everyone is at

---

Chemicals linked to various forms of heart disease

■ Toxic metals (arsenic, lead, mercury)
■ Pesticides (organophosphates, carbamates, organochlorines)
■ Environmental pollutants (dioxins, PCBs)
■ Solvents (motor exhaust fumes)
■ Halogens (chlorine, fluoride)
■ Plastics (vinyl chloride)
■ Air pollution (sulphur dioxide)

risk from lead-induced heart damage, not just those working with lead.[169, 170, 171]

Halogens, such as chlorine and fluoride, also trigger abnormal heart rhythms. In one study, two children accidentally exposed to cleaning fluid containing fluoride had potentially fatal arrhythmias. If you consider that fluoride is a well-known poison, this is hardly surprising.[172, 173, 174] The simple action of drinking chlorinated tap water during pregnancy is also known to increase the risk of heart defects in the unborn baby.[175]

Other heart-toxic chemicals that ordinary citizens are exposed to in everyday life are the persistent environmental pollutants. There is a strong link between ischaemic heart disease and the level of chemicals such as PCBs and dioxins in the body.[98, 176, 177, 178] Higher rates of ischaemic heart disease are also found in populations with higher levels of air pollution comprising substances such as sulphur dioxide and solvents in motor exhaust fumes. Indeed, an increase in air pollution leads to an increase in the number of admissions to hospital for ischaemic heart disease and even heart attack, on the same and on the following day.[179, 180, 181]

Nutrients to strengthen the heart: There is currently a great deal of controversy about the usefulness of certain antioxidant nutrients in preventing heart disease. Some recent studies have claimed that these have little beneficial effect, while other research has found that they not only lower the risk of developing heart disease but are also effective in reducing problems in those with existing heart disease.[182] Many nutritional experts take the view that the former studies are basically flawed because they do not take into consideration the fact that antioxidants should not be used on their own, like drugs. To be effective they need to be used in combination with a good level of all the other nutrients known to be essential to heart health.

This view was also expressed in an editorial in the *Journal of the American Medical Association* (*JAMA*). They argued that owing to the known importance of vitamins in preventing chronic diseases such as heart disease, together with the known low levels of these nutrients in the general population, all adults should take vitamin supplements over the long term.[141, 183]

The nutrients highlighted as being both very low in the population and essential for good heart health were vitamins B6, B12 and folic acid. However, these are not the only nutrients that are known to benefit the heart. A lack of antioxidant nutrients such as vitamins A, C and E, selenium and co-enzyme Q10 is thought to play a critical role in one of the major risk factors for heart disease, namely atherosclerosis. Therefore these nutrients can play a leading role in protecting the heart against chemical damage.[184]

People who take co-enzyme Q10 after having a heart attack run a lower risk of developing further heart attacks or other deaths resulting from cardiac disease.[155]

Many other nutrients have a more accepted role in helping to prevent, or aiding recovery from, heart disease. The mineral magnesium is a good example. Treatment with magnesium reduces the rate of abnormal heart rhythms (particularly in those with heart failure). It can also increase the success rate following coronary angioplasty (a procedure in which coronary arteries are unblocked by means of a tiny balloon inserted into the blood vessel and inflated). Magnesium can dilate coronary arteries and prevent blood from clotting.[185, 186] This could also explain why magnesium supplementation can increase exercise tolerance and reduce exercise-induced chest pain in those with coronary artery disease.[187]

There is growing evidence that a good daily intake of omega-3 oils can decrease the risk of myocardial infarction and heart attack in patients with ischaemic heart disease.[188] Omega-3 is also known to help strengthen the heart muscle in those with heart failure,[189] counteract arrhythmia,[190] and, like the antioxidants, protect the heart and coronary vessels against chemical damage.[191] Other useful nutrients include the amino acids carnitine, which improves cardiac performance in those with coronary artery disease and cardiomyopathy (a disorder where the heart muscle is damaged), taurine, which can potentially reduce the development of atherosclerosis, and glutamine, which can help strengthen heart muscle in those suffering with heart failure.[192, 189, 193]

In summary, it seems sensible for those who have heart disease or who want to prevent it to lower their on-going exposure to chemicals, while taking soluble fibre and nutritional supplements to deal with existing levels of body pollutants. A balanced supplement programme, as suggested in Chapter 4, is recommended. Other measures for preventing heart disease include:

- Cutting down on saturated fats (particularly trans fatty acids in margarines).
- Reducing intake of refined carbohydrates (such as processed flour and sugars).
- Increasing the proportion of whole foods, such as fruits, vegetables, nuts and whole grains in the diet.
- Regular exercise.

Drug-free ways to lower high blood pressure

One day, 11 years ago, I had just started in my new research post at Oxford University when one of my old colleagues gave me a call, ostensibly to see how I was getting on. After the usual pleasantries, she casually mentioned that someone had told her that her blood pressure might be a bit high. They weren't sure exactly how high, since she was very overweight and the armband did not fit around her arm properly. After some extremely hard persuasion, due partly to her embarrassment about her excess weight, partly to her strong dislike of making any sort of fuss and probably from a fear of being ill, I managed to convince her to get it measured properly at her doctor's surgery that same morning. It wasn't long before I was contacted with the news that her blood pressure (at 220/135 mmHg) was way higher than the highest I had ever heard of previously. The World Health Organization defines high blood pressure as being consistently over 160/95 mmHg.

Despite being initially told that such a high pressure would have caused permanent damage and her life expectancy would be five years at the most, 11 years on, at the age of 65, she is still going strong. With a combination of supplements, detoxification and exercise she has now come off all the very powerful medications previously prescribed for her high blood pressure (which also gave her unwanted side-effects) and is over 38 kg (6 stone) lighter. The improvement has been so remarkable that her cardiologist still talks with amazement about the day when he first saw her all those years ago.

This demonstrates that medicinal drugs are only one of the many ways in which high blood pressure can be effectively reversed. As well as being more natural, these complementary ways tend to work because they treat the cause of raised blood pressure rather than the condition itself. But before I write more about these natural methods, I will start at the beginning by explaining what blood pressure is and what controls it.

What is blood pressure? Keeping a continual blood flow is uphill work. The heart pumps the blood around the body under some degree of pressure. The blood pressure is simply a measurement of the pressure at which the blood leaves the heart. If it is too low (hypotension) we will not get enough oxygen and nutrients to vital organs such as the brain, and we may faint (or in extreme cases go into shock). If too high (hypertension) then this can cause another set of problems such as increasing the risk of strokes or heart disease.

The blood pressure reading itself consists of two numbers, 'normal' blood pressure being somewhere around 120/80 (mmHg). The higher of the two numbers is known as the systolic blood pressure. It records the peak pressure in the arteries as the blood is initially forced out of the heart. The second reading, the diastolic blood pressure, reflects the pressure in the arteries between heartbeats when the system is in its most relaxed phase. It is the diastolic reading that is generally thought to be the more important of the two, as it gives an indication of the overall pressure continually present in the system.

What causes high blood pressure? The blood vessels are muscular tubes lined with a thin layer of membrane. If the vessels become blocked, narrowed or lose elasticity, following either a contraction or stiffening of the muscle in their wall or from a build-up of substances lining the blood vessels, this will reduce the amount of blood that can pass through. Thus, in order to keep the blood flow constant, the heart will have to pump the blood a little harder, thereby raising the blood pressure, in order to get the same amount of blood to the tissues.

There is no internationally agreed level above which everyone's blood pressure is considered high. Since existing levels are arbitrarily set, definitions of what constitutes a high blood pressure that requires treatment can vary according to the age of the individual (blood pressure increases with age) but also from country to country.

If blood pressure is deemed to be high, attempts are made to bring it down because of the increased risk of developing long-term health problems such as strokes. The type of treatment chosen depends very much on what appears to be causing the raised blood pressure in the first place. In around 5 per cent of cases a specific underlying cause can be found. In this situation, treating the underlying cause, if possible, or stopping the offending drugs usually resolves the situation. However, for the vast majority of people with high blood pressure, no such cause can be found. In this situation a diagnosis of 'essential hypertension' is made.

Known causes of high blood pressure

- Birth defects
- Being overweight
- Kidney disease
- Hormonal diseases
- Medications (such as oral contraceptives containing oestrogens, corticosteroids, non-steroidal anti-inflammatory drugs)
- Toxic chemicals (such as pesticides, the toxic metals lead, mercury, arsenic and cadmium, alcohol, solvents, plastics and halogens)

For some reason, mainstream medicine tends to disregard toxic chemicals as a cause of high blood pressure. Many toxic chemicals have powerful actions in raising blood pressure. But since no tests for these substances are made during a conventional medical check for the condition, their potential role in triggering high blood pressure is missed, and with it a real opportunity to tackle the problem effectively. The result is that in people with no 'obvious' cause of high blood pressure, their condition ends up being labelled as 'essential hypertension'.

How chemicals could bring about hypertension: There appear to be two main ways in which toxic chemicals cause high blood pressure. The first relates to their short-term ability to trigger contraction of the muscle layer in the blood vessels. The second is due to their longer-term actions in raising LDL cholesterol levels, thereby increasing the size and number of atheromatous plaques formed, which fur up the insides of the blood vessels. So where is the evidence that links chemical contamination to high blood pressure?

As mentioned previously, the higher the level of heavy metals detected in the body the greater the overall blood pressure. For instance, people exposed to higher levels of mercury at work, such as dentists, are at greater risk of developing hypertension. Children exposed to higher levels of mercury in the womb, from contaminated seafoods, for example, also have an increased chance of developing high blood pressure.[194, 195]

Pesticides appear to possess both short-acting and longer-term blood pressure-raising effects. For instance, raised blood pressure is found in those who have deliberately ingested organophosphates and carbamates, in order to harm themselves.[196, 197] It is also found in those who have been exposed to pesticides over longer periods of time due to their work.[198, 199]

Unfortunately, one of the most persistent groups of environmental pollutants now found in all of our bodies is strongly linked to higher blood pressure. This is the organochlorines family, and includes the now banned pesticide DDT and the industrial pollutants PCBs and dioxins. The higher the levels of these substances in our bodies, the greater the blood pressure tends to be.[200, 201, 202, 203, 204]

Alcohol and other industrial solvents (benzene and xylene) found in paint, car exhaust fumes, household cleaning solutions and perfume, can bring about high blood pressure.[205, 206] Other chemicals linked to high blood pressure are chlorine (in tap water), fluorocarbons, freon, carbon disulphide, asbestos, ozone and plastics.[207] Factory workers exposed to the plastic vinyl chloride over a number of years are known to have a markedly higher risk of developing hypertension. The higher the level of chemical in their bodies, the greater the risk of the disorder.[208] If you think about all the places you can find plastics and all these other chemicals in our modern world, it is no wonder that more and more people are developing high blood pressure.

Blood pressure-lowering nutrients: The food we eat also appears to play a major role in determining our blood pressure. This is because many nutrients play an essential role in enabling the normal blood pressure control mechanisms to work properly. A balanced supplement programme as suggested in Chapter 4 is recommended, but the following nutrients in particular are critical to the production of the natural substances that control blood vessel constriction and dilation:

- Vitamins A, C and E.
- Minerals magnesium, potassium, zinc, selenium, copper, calcium, chromium and manganese.
- Omega-3 oils.
- Co-enzyme Q10.

Deficiencies in any of these nutrients could lead to excessive constriction of the muscle in the blood vessel walls and hence high blood pressure.[209] However, out of all of the above minerals, magnesium is possibly the most important. Often called 'the relaxing mineral', magnesium is very effective in lowering both systolic and diastolic blood pressure by helping the muscle in the blood vessel walls to dilate. Deficiencies of this mineral are particularly common, however, so it's a very good idea to take a separate magnesium supplement since the levels available in regular multivitamin and mineral supplements are normally very low indeed.[210, 106, 211]

Muscle elasticity is also important in controlling the pressure throughout the body's network of arteries, as a loss of elasticity or a 'hardening of the arteries' (commonly associated with a lack of vitamin C and increasing age) means that the pressure has to increase in order to maintain an adequate blood flow throughout the system. This is yet another reason for taking extra vitamin C supplements.

Other nutrients that the body needs to lower blood pressure levels include vitamins B6, B12 and folic acid. Their importance can be gauged by the fact that even slightly lower than normal levels of these nutrients in the body can trigger high blood pressure. Fortunately, the system can be rebalanced by taking the appropriate supplements.[142] Since vitamin D deficiency can increase the risk of hypertension, this needs to be part of any supplement programme.[212] Lastly, the amino acid taurine has been shown to lower blood pressure.

Other ways to lower blood pressure

- Weight loss
- Exercise
- Yoga and relaxation techniques
- Reducing stress in everyday life
- Cutting down on salt intake and alcohol
- Stopping smoking
- Eating fewer saturated fats
- Drinking less caffeinated tea and coffee
- Eating garlic
- Eating more soluble fibre
- Tackling food allergies (these can contribute to hypertension in some people)
- Choosing low-fat dairy products
- Eating a diet high in fruit and vegetables

Considering the blood pressure-lowering effects that nutrients possess, it seems surprising that conventional medicine overlooks this safe and easy treatment.

Stroke prevention

Few things can be as frightening as feeling fine one minute and being struck down the next, without any warning, with a sudden loss of basic physical and mental skills. Yet this is the situation millions of people find themselves in every year after suffering a stroke. The nightmare does not end there for those who survive this disaster, as many are left with extensive physical and mental disabilities. Strokes are the most important cause of adult disability in the Western world.

One would imagine that owing to the sheer numbers involved, medical science would by now have found an effective way of preventing strokes or limiting the damage.

Nevertheless there does appear to be some light at the end of the tunnel as many conventionally trained specialists are beginning to realise that nutritional therapies have a great deal to offer. Not only can these therapies help treat and reduce the extent of the damage caused by strokes, but they can also help prevent strokes from happening in the first place. To discover why in many cases they can be so effective, we need to know more about the causes of strokes.

What is a stroke? A stroke is a non-specific term for the wide-ranging symptoms – such as paralysis, speech difficulties and loss of certain mental abilities – caused by brain tissue damage. In most cases (approximately 85 per cent) this brain damage follows a sudden interruption in the blood supply to a part of the brain because of a blockage in a blood vessel. This type of stroke is called a cerebral infarction. The other main cause of stroke results from a bleed into the brain from a ruptured blood vessel. This is known as a cerebral haemorrhage. The type and extent of symptoms experienced by an individual depend on the part of the brain that has been affected and the extent of the damage.

Cerebral infarctions are caused by diseased or severely narrowed blood vessels or a blood clot that blocks the blood supply to a part of the brain. Often blood clots form on diseased blood vessels. Cerebral haemorrhages tend to be caused when existing weaknesses in the brain's blood vessels are stressed to the point of rupturing. These weaknesses can be triggered by high blood pressure or by existing blood vessel disease.

Symptoms appear rapidly in the first few minutes and are normally fully developed after an hour or two. This timescale can be used to differentiate a full-blown stroke from a much lesser form of stroke, known as a TIA, or transient ischaemic attack. Despite causing similar initial symptoms, TIAs usually last only for a few minutes and the effects are gone within 24 hours. They tend to be caused when smaller clots briefly block brain blood vessels and/or when blood vessels in the brain constrict. TIAs are very important as they act as an early warning system. They alert the patient to the increased risk of developing a full stroke, and give the opportunity to have the problem fully investigated – so the appropriate preventive treatment can be started as soon as possible.

Stroke prevention: As it is very difficult to predict when a stroke may occur, prevention tends to involve identifying all the major factors known to increase the risks. By tackling these, it is thought possible to lower the overall risk of developing a stroke.

The main risk factors for stroke are:

- Excess weight.
- High blood pressure.
- Cigarette smoking.
- Stress.
- Diabetes.
- High blood lipids (cholesterol).
- Excess blood platelets (polycythaemia).
- High alcohol intake.
- Family history.
- Medications (such as oral contraceptives).

■ Blood clots (from cardiovascular disease).

■ Injury.

From the presence of risk factors such as cigarette smoking and medications you can see that there is already an acknowledged link between toxic chemicals and stroke. However, this link is strengthened by the fact that many of the other risk factors – such as high blood pressure, diabetes, excess weight and high blood lipids – are also strongly linked to toxic chemicals. But as the link between stroke and chemicals is not widely known, few will have been adequately informed about the importance of lowering their exposure to toxic chemicals. If you consider that strokes are the third most common cause of death, the sheer numbers involved would suggest that this should be an extremely worthwhile consideration for many, particularly those at high risk.

Chemicals and strokes: Many direct links between pesticides and strokes can be found. For instance, carbamates, chemicals commonly used as pesticides, not only trigger strokes but may also increase the degree of brain damage following a stroke.[213] Exposure to organophosphates, also commonly used as pesticides, can bring about symptoms almost identical to a stroke,[214] and workers exposed to organochlorine pesticides over the long term are at a higher risk of developing a stroke.[215] Lastly, there is a wealth of evidence that links a wide range of pesticides to many of the other major stroke risk factors, such as obesity, diabetes and hypertension.

Toxic metals are also linked to stroke. For instance, a study investigating the long-term risks of arsenic exposure (from contaminated water and other environmental sources) reveals that the higher the exposure, the greater the risk of developing a stroke.[168] Cigarette smoke, which contains several heavy metals such as cadmium, can also increase the stroke risk.[216] Heavy metals such as lead and mercury can play an important role in the development of stroke risk factors such as high blood pressure.

Air pollutants such as sulphur dioxide and carbon monoxide

appear to increase the stroke risk. One South Korean study revealed that high levels of air pollution caused an increase in the number of people suffering strokes.[217]

Managing strokes – the nutritional solution: Epidemiologic evidence, animal studies, angiographic and ultrasound studies in humans and a limited number of clinical trials are now suggesting that certain antioxidants, such as vitamins C and E and blueberries, may protect against developing a stroke.[218] This could be due to the fact that during a stroke the levels of antioxidants are rapidly depleted as they are used to mop up some of the damage caused by the stroke. This is why many believe that treatment with antioxidants may help prevent tissue damage and improve both the survival and neurological outcome.

Other nutrients of value include vitamins B3 and D, which if present in good levels appear to reduce the amount and extent of brain damage following a stroke. The mineral magnesium significantly reduces the extent of brain damage and dependence and increases the chances of survival if given within six hours of a stroke. This finding is reflected in animal experiments where magnesium is seen to reduce the amount of stroke-induced brain damage by a highly significant 25–61 per cent.[219, 220] Higher levels of vitamins B6, B12 and folic acid can also reduce the incidence of stroke, whereas lower levels of these nutrients are known to increase the risk of stroke. Many major studies have shown that people who take these nutrients as dietary supplements have a dramatically lower risk of developing a stroke or TIA compared to those who don't.[221, 218, 222, 223] The minerals copper and zinc are thought to protect against stroke-induced tissue damage.[224] The protective effect provided by zinc appears to be most effective as a preventive but can also be of value if given within hours of a stroke.[225]

Lastly, several major studies have shown omega-3 oils (found in walnuts, soya beans, rapeseed oil and fish) can significantly reduce the risk of getting a cerebral infarction stroke, although they have no apparent effect on the risk of getting a cerebral haemorrhage.[226, 227]

A balanced supplement programme as described in Chapter 4 is recommended, taking into account the above supplements in particular.

General and dietary advice for lowering your stroke risk: In addition to cutting down the exposure to toxic chemicals and taking supplements to ensure that sufficient levels of nutrients are being ingested, it is a good idea to make the following lifestyle changes in order to minimise other stroke risk factors:

- Maintain a healthy weight.
- Increase exercise levels (the risk of stroke in someone with a sedentary lifestyle is almost double compared to a more active person).
- Stop smoking.
- Change the diet to one higher in fresh fruit and vegetables (as these are rich in antioxidant chemicals called flavonoids).
- Eat more garlic (which thins the blood, reducing the risk of thrombosis).

12

Fighting Cancer

'Cancer Research UK are now recognising the considerable anti-cancer potential of medicinal mushrooms. This is also now being recognised in America as a novel area of complementary medicine and clinical trials will be organised in the next year.'

DR JOHN SMITH, EMERITUS PROFESSOR OF BIOCHEMISTRY,
STRATHCLYDE UNIVERSITY (AUGUST 2004)

Cancer - you can fight back

When I was a junior doctor, the worst job I ever had to do was to tell people that they had cancer. This unenviable task never got any easier with time, because for each and every one of the people affected the news always came as a devastating blow. They knew as well as I did that uttering those three words, 'You have cancer', was like passing sentence on a person for a crime they did not know they had committed and for which there was often no reprieve. In a flash, people fear the worst. Despite the many cancer success stories in the press, they instantly remember the people they have known or loved who succumbed to this unforgiving disease.

The good news is that far from being a hopeless situation, there appears to be a great deal we can now all do to fight back. In addition to the currently used 'conventional' treatments there is an ever-growing number of proven alternative and complementary methods which can open up fresh hope for those who are receptive to a new way of thinking. Further good news is that many of these new methods, such as taking vitamins and mineral supplements, and lowering exposure to chemicals, are highly effective in preventing cancer in the first place.

Many scientists are now exploring and researching radically new ways to strengthen the body's own natural mechanisms for suppressing cancer growth. One of the scientists taking this new approach is the renowned researcher Dr Gershom Zajicek of the HH Humphrey Centre of Experimental Medicine and Cancer research in Israel.[228] He believes that cancer begins as a metabolic deficiency caused by carcinogens (cancer-causing agents). He is of the opinion that in a healthy body, balance is maintained and cancer never develops, or if it does, it is kept in tight check by the homeostatic systems of the body.

Whether he is right or wrong, what is certainly true is that we are all continually exposing our bodies to a larger number of carcinogenic substances that are also known for their abilities to markedly disturb metabolism and promote nutrient deficiencies.

Around half of all chemicals tested cause cancer: Of all the different substances known to cause cancer, chemical carcinogens appear to play a very prominent role. The known list of cancer-causing chemicals is extremely long, and getting longer by the day. It includes a roll-call of the usual suspects such as pesticides, environmental pollutants, toxic metals, solvents, plastics, fluoride and many other types of man-made chemicals found in our everyday environment.

However, the real situation could be far worse than already suspected, as a US governmental oversight agency revealed, in 1987, that of the more than 50,000 chemicals in commercial use, only 284 had been tested on animals for their cancer-causing potential by the government in the preceding 10 years! Of these, 144 (about half) had been shown to cause cancer in animals. So, somewhat incredibly, the vast majority of industrial chemicals now in use have never been tested for their carcinogenic properties. One can only speculate what the results would be if such tests were to be carried out. Therefore, the assumption most of us make, that if something is for sale, everything in it should have already undergone a thorough battery of tests and be totally safe, is no longer valid – if indeed it ever was.

But not only do chemicals trigger a wide range of adult and childhood cancers – the most common being prostate, breast, brain, immune system (lymphomas and leukaemias), urinary tract, and liver – they can also stimulate cancer growth, make existing cancers much more aggressive and enhance their ability to spread throughout the body.

Furthermore, in a US government-sponsored safety and health document, produced by the CSEA Occupational Safety and Health department, scientists estimated that as many as 33 per cent of all cancers are related to workplace exposures to carcinogens (December, 1998). For example, painters and decorators, metal welders, hairdressers, dental workers, miners and builders are all exposed to numerous carcinogens from occupational exposure.

Considering that chemicals make up the majority of these carcinogens, and we are also exposed to these same toxins in our homes, the true extent to which chemicals are triggering cancer is likely to be much greater. With statistics like these, is it any wonder that so many people are getting cancer?

Turning the situation around: Many medics now advocate cancer treatments that incorporate nutritional and other proven techniques. There are now many specialist cancer centres that successfully use these methods. The Bristol Cancer Help Centre in the UK is an example of such a centre. It uses diet, nutritional supplements, counselling, relaxation techniques, exercise and

The Bristol Cancer Help Centre mission statement

Bristol Cancer Help Centre is the UK's leading holistic cancer charity that has pioneered the Bristol Approach to cancer care, for people with cancer and those close to them. This Approach works *hand-in-hand with medical treatment,* providing a unique combination of physical, emotional and spiritual support using complementary therapies and self-help techniques, and practical advice on nutrition. People can access the Bristol Approach through residential courses run by an experienced team of doctors, nurses and complementary therapists.

other methods to enhance the treatment and quality of life of those receiving conventional forms of cancer therapy.

Their whole philosophy is based around helping the body rid itself of cancer. Their therapies are designed to work with the body. Just because they don't make you feel ill, it doesn't mean that they are not helping you to fight cancer cells! Many studies have shown different nutrients to be highly effective not only at treating cancers, but also in preventing them.

Indeed, the cancer-suppressing actions of a whole range of different nutrients are often so marked that they are referred to by those specialising in conventional medicine as 'chemoprevention'.

Nutrients that block cancer growth: Antioxidants are one of the most important types of chemopreventative agents. Nutrients such as vitamins A, C and E, and minerals zinc and selenium, kill cancer cells and also slow down the rate of cancerous growth, which reduces the aggressiveness and extent to which cancer cells invade the rest of the body. Antioxidants can also prevent new cancers from forming in the first place.

Antioxidants offer protection from the wide range of cancer-causing chemicals we are regularly exposed to, as well as those used in chemotherapy. The benefits of using nutrients alongside chemotherapy or radiotherapy include reduced side-effects, and lower incidences of cancer recurring in those who have the highest levels of these nutrients in their diets and bodies.

A large number of other nutrients also possess anticancer qualities. These include vitamin D and the B group, which have powerful tumour-suppressing actions; minerals such as magnesium, which reduce the risk of death from cancer (for instance, the higher the level of magnesium in drinking water, the lower the risk of death from breast cancer); essential oils such as omega-3, which, in addition to reducing the risk of cancer, inhibit cancer growth and reduce cancer spread (metastases). Mushroom extracts (which are also very useful in reducing chemotherapy side-effects), plant and herbal extracts, such as lycopene, and soya products also have their own particular anti-cancer properties.

Nutrients with anticancer qualities

Antioxidants:
- Vitamins A, C, E
- Zinc
- Selenium

Non-antioxidants:
- Vitamins B, D
- Magnesium
- Omega-3 fats
- Lycopene
- Therapeutic mushroom extracts – such as shitake

When we get cancer, our need for nutrients to fight it is greatly increased, yet our intake tends to fall. This is due to a reduced food intake, inadequate digestion, malabsorption, vomiting, and increased nutrient demand as a consequence of cancer therapy. This has the effect of reducing the ability of cancer patients to fight back naturally, as their inbuilt cancer-fighting systems need a good supply of nutrients to work.

Soluble fibre is a great detoxing agent. Unlike the above nutrients, which help protect against the harmful effects of chemicals by feeding the body's natural detoxification systems, soluble fibres work by latching on to the toxic chemicals in the body and carrying them out. It is not surprising that people who eat more of these chemical-binding fibres tend to have a reduced risk of developing a wide range of cancers, and if they do contract cancer are able to suppress tumour growth and its spread throughout the body. This could explain why soluble fibres can protect the body from developing cancer, even during exposure to known carcinogenic chemicals.

Novel cancer treatments are currently being researched. One promising substance is therapeutic mushroom extracts, which can be used to reduce the effects of conventional cancer treatments and to help fight cancer in their own right. Certain therapeutic mushrooms have been successfully used in Asia for centuries and are now starting to be used in the West.

Complementary treatments which have been used to help tackle cancer

- Avoidance of chemicals (see Chapter 3).
- Detoxification (see Chapter 4).
- Nutritional therapy. Although the basic programme recommended in Chapter 4 is a great starting point, for best results have your vitamin, mineral and fatty acid status checked by blood tests. A good supplement programme, tailored to your individual requirements, will help to change your internal environment to make it more hostile to cancer (see Appendix B).
- Dietary changes. Poor nutrition increases the toxicity of chemicals, so you should choose whole, unadulterated foods. Reduce the amount of protein and fat from animal produce, and eat as much raw fruit and vegetables as possible. Avoid salt, sugar and stimulants.
- Exercise. This is a great way to boost the body's natural ability to kill cancer cells by strengthening the immune system. For general guidance, see page 57.
- Relaxation techniques. Techniques such as meditation, yoga and special breathing methods aid relaxation and help manage stress. They can be very effective in boosting the cancer-fighting immune system.

Maintaining a positive mental attitude: Lastly, I cannot overemphasise how important a positive attitude is in improving your chances of recovering. I recall the face of a young man in his 30s with very young children on being told he had cancer. His haunted look is still with me 10 years on. It was soon clear that he had lost the will to live, despite not having a very advanced form of the disease. He just gave up the fight there and then. Two weeks later he was dead.

On the other hand, I have seen people with extensive disease whose sheer battling spirit and determination helped them survive far longer than had been expected. These fighters appeared to be better at surviving as they simply refused to give in. They were the ones who explored all the available options and changed their lifestyles accordingly.

Rather than being cancer patients, they were people who by the way also had cancer. They knew that life doesn't have to end with the diagnosis. It just marked the beginning of a different period of their lives.

Beating breast cancer

Readers of my first book will realise that my whole interest in the field of environmental medicine was triggered when I stumbled across a link between toxic chemicals and breast cancer. This life-changing discovery was in a newspaper article. I discovered that synthetic chemicals were already in the general environment in levels high enough to lower the fertility of a great number of animal species, seemingly due to the ability of these substances to mimic the action of female hormones. These hormone mimics are commonly referred to as xenoestrogens – 'xen' meaning foreign and oestrogen being the hormone they mimic.

Initially, the very existence of these chemicals came as a complete revelation to me, probably because the mainstream branch of medicine on which I had previously worked almost completely ignores their presence. However, once understood, it enabled me to provide an answer to a really important question that had been nagging at me ever since I was at Oxford. The question being – what is underlying the current breast cancer epidemic?

Breast cancer and the environment: Breast cancer is now the commonest cause of cancer death in women worldwide and the numbers show no signs of slowing down. We are facing a cata-strophic global epidemic. Not only would finding a cause help prevent millions from getting this cancer in the future, but it would also potentially help those millions already affected with the disease. This same question has in fact been puzzling scientists for years.

Despite the known link between some cases of breast cancer and the genetic inheritance, the rapid explosion in numbers suggests that other factors, especially environmental ones, are at work here. This fits in with other observations. For example, women migrating from a low-risk to a high-risk area eventually acquire the same higher risk of the new area. Indeed when one scientist, Professor William Rea, tried to estimate to what extent environmental factors play a part in the current epidemic, he came up with the astonishingly large figure of over 95 per cent of cases.

The good news is that, unlike genes, which are handed out to us at conception, we can alter and improve our environment – once we know what to avoid. One of the major groups of chemicals thought to be behind the breast cancer epidemic are the xenoestrogens. To appreciate why, it helps to have an overview of the strong relationship between the hormones these chemicals mimic, namely the oestrogens, and breast cancer.

Oestrogen – the Jekyll and Hyde hormone: Oestrogens are the hormones that make women different from men and play a fundamental role in controlling all aspects of female fertility. So, it's disconcerting to discover that they have been classified as known human carcinogens. Nonetheless, this darker side goes some way towards explaining the increasingly numerous reports finding that the combined oral contraceptive pill and hormone replacement therapy carry an increased risk of breast cancer.

This cancer-provoking effect appears to arise from the natural ability of oestrogens to switch on breast cell growth and turnover. Both natural and synthetic oestrogens trigger these events after 'docking' on to highly specialised receptor sites in breast cells. The action of 'docking on' turns on the cellular switch that triggers cell division. Then, almost as soon as the cell is switched on, this mechanism is turned off, because the oestrogen is grabbed by a specialised protein that binds to it tightly, preventing it from getting free and stimulating more tissues.

Excessive stimulation of these receptor sites from higher levels of either natural or synthetic oestrogens is thought to be one of the main factors behind normal cells turning cancerous. It also is likely that these substances make existing cancer cells more aggressive.

Drowning in a sea of xenoestrogens: Since oestrogens can trigger breast cancer, it seems logical that chemicals that can mimic the actions of oestrogens should also be able to trigger breast cancer. While the strength of the breast cell stimulation triggered by xenoestrogens is generally much weaker than that caused by natural hormones, their fat-loving nature, in combination with the high percentage of fat tissue in breasts, means that xenoestrogens accumulate in breast tissue at levels hundreds of times greater than the hormones they mimic.

In addition, our bodies appear unable to remove many xenoestrogens from breast cells once they have docked on, owing to their widely varying forms. The upshot is that breast cells are being falsely stimulated 24 hours a day.[229]

A vast number of chemicals are now known to mimic the effect of natural oestrogens. Indeed, owing to the extent to which xenoestrogens have crept into virtually every aspect of our lives, our modern environment has been likened by scientists to 'living in a sea of oestrogens'.

'Oestrogenic' origins of plastic: You may think that this ability of chemicals to mimic oestrogens is largely accidental, but in some instances this could not be further from the truth. Take for example the plastic known as Bisphenol A (see Appendix A.6). Its adaptability has made it one of the most common plastics used today. It can be found in a whole range of products, from the linings of food tins to dental fillings and baby feeding bottles.

However, few realise that this 'plastic' was first developed in the 1930s as a potential synthetic form of oestrogen. A paper published in *Nature* in 1936 announced research to that effect.[230] So, far from accidentally possessing oestrogen-mimicking properties, it seems that this plastic was specifically created for that purpose!

Chlorine – breast poison on tap? Another chemical that turns compounds into xenoestrogens is the element chlorine. Previously used as a chemical warfare agent in the First World War, chlorine can now be found in an extremely large number of synthetic chemicals, many of which have been found to promote breast cancer. At the simplest level, those who drink chlorinated water are at a higher risk of developing breast cancer. It seems that chlorine reacts with some of the other substances in the water to form trihalomethanes, compounds linked to breast cancer. This cancer-inducing effect has been demonstrated in a study of women who drank chlorinated tap water in Louisiana, USA.[231]

Other chlorine-containing chemicals known to cause breast cancer are the organochlorines (see Appendix A.1). These notorious, highly toxic and persistent groups of chemicals include the pesticides DDT and lindane, as well as the environmental pollutants PCBs and dioxins. Much of the research into chemicals and breast cancer includes studies that show breast cancer patients to have higher levels of these chemicals in their breast tissue and blood.

Other chemicals that cause breast cancer: Many other chemicals have the ability to trigger breast cancer. Although the exact mechanisms are as yet unknown, one way could be by increasing levels of cancer-inducing free radicals. Another could be by damaging DNA.

The logical next step is to lower our exposure to such chemicals. But before we can expel them from our bodies or learn how to avoid them, we first need to know which chemicals to target.

Substances linked to breast cancer

- Medications (such as synthetic oestrogens used in hormone replacement and the contraceptive pill)
- Pesticides (such as organophosphates and synthetic pyrethroids)
- Organochlorines (such as DDT, lindane, dieldrin and PCBs)
- Alcohols
- Solvents (chlorinated)
- Constituents of plastics (Bisphenol A, chloride)
- Toxic metals (such tributyl tin, cadmium, antimony, barium, chromium, lithium and lead acetate)
- Detergents
- Chemicals containing chlorine

Fighting back: As with most forms of cancer, it seems sensible to tackle the levels of cancer-inducing chemicals, as well as ensuring a good level of nutrition. Starting with the strong link between breast cancer, xenoestrogens and other chemicals, it would seem sensible not only to lower the levels of these chemicals in the body by detoxing (see Chapter 4), but also to avoid them where possible (see Chapter 3).

The second line of defence is to strengthen the body's ability to fight breast cancer by ensuring it gets sufficient levels of nutrition. Many studies now show that a whole range of nutrients and supplements are very effective in suppressing breast cancer formation and growth. These include the nutrients previously mentioned on pages 216–17, such as vitamins, minerals (particularly those with antioxidant properties) and essential fatty acids (particularly omega-3 oils) (see also page 218 for a general list of cancer treatments).

So, far from passively accepting our lot, there really is a great deal we can and should be doing to reduce the odds of getting cancer in the first place and, if we have got it, to fight back.

Suppressing prostate cancer

If breast cancer is the most important hormone-linked cancer in women, prostate cancer is the male counterpart. Despite superficially being very different, these two diseases have much more in common than first meets the eye.

Like breast cancer, prostate cancer is already extremely widespread. Indeed it currently holds the record of being the most common malignancy found in US males, and it is also the fourth most common cancer in the world. Although the number of women with breast cancer is rising by a very significant 1.5 per cent per annum, the number of new cases of American men diagnosed with prostate cancer between 1983 and 1989 rose by a much greater 6.4 per cent.[232]

In fact, the older a man is, the more likely he is to develop it. Statistics based on autopsies of men who have died from other causes reveal that, somewhat incredibly, 40 per cent of men over the age of 50 have prostate cancer. The risk increases as the decades pass, so, by the age of 80, a colossal 70 per cent of men have it. For men in their 90s, it's a near certainty.[233]

Prostate cancer is relatively harmless in most men: Despite the high figures of those affected by prostate cancer, up to 90 per cent of men with this disease never develop symptoms or become ill with it. This is because prostate cancer tends to be very slow growing, and is also very slow to spread. One study has shown that 86 per cent of patients with prostate cancer survive more than 10 years after diagnosis.[234] Furthermore, in two-thirds of cases, the cancer did not spread at all. So the chances are that if you are over 70, you are far more likely to die with prostate cancer than of it.[235]

Many men appear to be very good at keeping their disease under control. But even if you are one of those whose cancer has already started to spread, this unique ability to suppress cancerous growth can still help you. The insight into how many men manage to suppress this disease can also help prevent new cancers from arising. So what gives these men such special powers?

After investigating this phenomenon, two explanations stand out from the pile of research that has taken place over the last few decades. It seems that whether you become a victim or conqueror of this disease is largely determined first by your exposure to toxic chemicals, and second by what you eat.

Artificial chemicals make prostate cancer cells turn aggressive: Prostate cancer is one of the many cancers known to be powerfully triggered by a large number of chemicals currently found in our environment, such as pesticides, pollutants, heavy metals, plastics and solvents.[236] The levels of chemicals needed to trigger prostate cancer are not only encountered in those working with these substances on a day-to-day basis but, judging by the number of men who already have this disease, it seems that the 'chemicalisation' of our everyday lives has put virtually every single man at risk.

How passive cells turn aggressive

Scientists from the Medical College of Wisconsin, USA, presented their findings at the 90th meeting of the American Association for Cancer Research, held in Philadelphia on 10–14 April 1999. They noted that aggressive prostate cancer cells appeared to be different in their genetic makeup from dormant cells, and that environmental pollutants such as toxic metals (particularly cadmium), cigarette smoke, pesticides, or car and truck emissions could bring about this transformation, turning non-aggressive prostate cancer cells into killer cells. Furthermore, they found that exposure to these toxic pollutants could trigger aggressive cells to attack and invade the surrounding tissue, and thus spread more rapidly through the body.

As well as triggering the onset of prostate cancer, chemical toxins are believed to act on already-established cancers to accelerate their growth, converting previously slow-growing cancers into killer cancers.

Good nutrition is the natural enemy of prostate cancer: The second most important natural defence mechanism against prostate cancer is our diet. Antioxidants include some of the most effective nutrients used in suppressing and preventing prostate cancer. They include a range of compounds such as the vitamins A and E, the minerals selenium and zinc, as well as the phytonutrient (plant chemical) lycopene, which is responsible for the red colour in fruits and vegetables, particularly tomatoes. Many studies now confirm that the higher the levels of many of these nutrients in the body, the lower the risk of developing prostate cancer, or if it does develop, the slower the rate of tumour growth.[237, 238, 239] The best effects are seen with a combination of these nutrients used.

Other nutrients with anticancer powers include vitamin D which is particularly effective at inhibiting the growth of prostate cancer cells,[240] omega-3 oils, which also slow down cancer growth, and soya products, owing to their high levels of isoflavonoids (or phyto-oestrogens).

Indeed many of these basic nutrients appear to be so toxic to most prostate cancer cells, they are increasingly used to treat prostate cancer under the banner of 'chemo-preventative' agents. Their use is thought by many to be more successful in some cases than certain conventional forms of treatment. As well as these specific prostate cancer treatments, see page 218 for a general list of cancer treatments.

Immune system cancers – lymphoma and leukaemia

Over the last few decades, the number of people with immune system cancers, such as lymphomas and leukaemias, has been steadily increasing. But the real situation was only thrown into the spotlight when Jacqueline Kennedy Onassis developed an increasingly common form of cancer, known as non-Hodgkin's lymphoma (NHL). Suddenly people started to sit up and take notice.

The rise of this cancer has been pretty marked, with the number of people developing it over the last 20 years rising by a massive 80 per cent, and showing no signs of slowing. Indeed, with every passing year, the number of people developing it increases by approximately 3 per cent, making it one of the fastest-growing cancers in the world.[241] This complete turn-around in a once-rare tumour means that it is now the fifth most common cancer in the USA. But before we look at why this particular form of cancer is rocketing, it helps to know a bit more about immune system cancers.

What are immune system cancers? The main forms of immune system cancers are leukaemia, Hodgkin's lymphoma, non-Hodgkin's lymphoma and multiple myeloma. While all of them have increased in incidence over the years, the most dramatic increase has been with non-Hodgkin's disease.

Despite having different names and characteristics, all these cancers originate from cells in the immune system, especially the lymphocytes, or white blood cells. These white cells play an essential role in protecting the body from all the bugs and foreign bodies that we are exposed to. These cells often collect in the lymph nodes, which are kidney bean-shaped nodules scattered throughout the body. White cells travel around the body in the blood and lymph vessels.

Some white cells produce vast quantities of proteins known as antibodies which label the invader for destruction. Other cells are designed to destroy micro-organisms on contact. The type of cancer, and therefore the symptoms and ultimate prognosis, depends on which type of cell becomes cancerous. For instance, multiple myeloma occurs when mature antibody-producing cells become cancerous, multiply and start churning out excessively large quantities of one type of antibody. These cells build up in the bone and other tissues and can be detected in large quantities in the blood. Leukaemia occurs when certain types of white blood cell are produced in large numbers in the bone marrow and found in excessive quantities in the bloodstream. And lymphomas occur when immune cells in lymph nodes turn cancerous and multiply uncontrollably. This results in an abnormally large lymph node.

What is behind the increase in immune system cancers? To discover what appears to be behind this increase in immune system cancers, we must look at the type of people developing these problems. A large number are associated with certain occupations. As many of these jobs involve exposure to a higher level of chemicals, this is high up on the list of possible triggers for immune system cancers.

Occupations linked to immune system cancers

- Farmers
- Drivers
- Hairdressers
- Pesticide operatives
- Cooks
- Waiters
- Bartenders
- Caretakers
- Cleaners
- Textile workers
- Machinery fitters for metal processors
- Rubber workers
- Painters
- Tailors
- Electrical workers
- Plumbers

Factors that trigger the development of immune system cancers

- Pesticides, such as fly sprays, cockroach repellents or weed killers (children who live in houses treated with indoor pesticides have a higher rate of leukaemia)
- Environmental pollutants (artificial chemicals which now contaminate our food, water and air)
- Plastics (vinyl chloride, synthetic fabrics and phthalates)
- Traffic-related air pollution (such as petroleum, petroleum products, engine exhausts)
- Solvents (benzene)
- Infections (zoonotic microbes, viruses)
- Chemicals in household products, such as hair dye (hair dyes have been linked to non-Hodgkin's lymphoma, and hairdressers are more prone to Hodgkin's disease), cosmetics (cosmetologists have a higher incidence of Hodgkin's lymphoma), products that contain PVC and other plastics, and chlorinated tap water
- Medications (immunosuppressive drugs, treatments for rheumatoid arthritis, HIV drugs)
- Genetic predisposition
- Certain medical conditions (such as HIV)
- Energy sources (electricity and radiation)

If we look a bit more deeply into this, we will see this suspicion confirmed, as a large number of chemicals appear to trigger immune system cancers. But it is not just work exposure that appears to predispose people to these cancers, because any form of exposure in our lives, such as treating the house with pesticides, can result in a higher risk of cancer.[242]

My husband lost his much-adored mother from an immune system cancer when she was still very young. She was a housewife and a mother, and had never previously worked with chemicals. So don't think that just because you don't work with chemicals you are not at risk. Considering the increase of the following mentioned substances in our everyday lives, is it any wonder that these cancers are on the increase?

Nutritional demands put on the body by these diseases: People who eat inadequate levels of nutrients put themselves at a greater risk of developing immune system cancers. Also poor nutrition in people who have these forms of cancer could potentially be fatal. This is because these forms of cancer increase the demand for certain nutrients, particularly vitamins. If they are not met by an increased intake, some people develop life-threatening vitamin deficiencies. The risk of this is greater if they are treated with conventional therapies, as these increase the body's needs for certain nutrients.[243, 244]

So whether you have one of these illnesses and want to fight cancer naturally and ease some of the symptoms you may be experiencing, or will shortly be undergoing chemotherapy and want to minimise treatment side-effects, or want to do what you can to prevent getting one of these cancers in the first place, it seems like a sensible idea to ensure that your body gets all the nutrients it needs.

In addition to reducing your exposure to toxic chemicals and embarking on a detox programme (see Chapter 4), the following treatments could prove useful:

- Heat therapy. Raising the whole body temperature in combination with taking the bioflavonoid quercertin has been found to be very successful in treating, and in some cases curing, people with lymphoma.
- Increase your intake of fruit and vegetables, as an alkaline diet aids detoxification. High consumptions of cruciferous (cabbage family) and carotene-rich vegetables and all types of fruit also have a protective effect. Eating organically where possible will help to reduce your exposure to toxic chemicals, while increasing the amounts of nutrients that you take in.
- Reduce your intake of red meat, as a higher incidence of non-Hodgkin's lymphoma (NHL) was found in those who had a high intake of pork, beef or lamb. They had doubled the risk of developing NHL compared with those who consumed these meats less than once a week. In addition, the higher the intake of animal fat in general the higher the risk of NHL.

■ Reduce the level of trans fats in the diet, for example, from margarine (only margarines labelled as trans fat free are acceptable). A high level of trans fats was found to increase risk of NHL by two and a half times.[245]

13

Chemical Sensitivities
MULTIPLE CHEMICAL SENSITIVITY

'Today we are witnessing another medical anomaly – a unique pattern of illness involving chemically exposed people who subsequently report multi-system symptoms and new-onset chemical and food intolerances. These intolerances may be the hallmark for a new disease process, just as fever is a hallmark for infection.'

DR MILLER, DEPARTMENT OF FAMILY PRACTICE, UNIVERSITY OF TEXAS
HEALTH SCIENCE CENTER, SAN ANTONIO, USA

Poisoned by the 21st century

Multiple Chemical Sensitivity (MCS), also known as environmental illness, is now one of the most common but least understood illnesses in the developed world. Despite not being recognised by the majority of medical doctors, a recent study carried out in California by physicians specialising in environmental medicine revealed that 6 per cent of the public had been diagnosed with MCS by their physicians, and a whopping 15.9 per cent reported being 'allergic to or made sick by a number of everyday chemicals'.[246]

Considering that approximately 40 per cent of those with MCS had to consult 10 or more medical practitioners before being diagnosed, it not only exposes the complete failure of the current medical system to help people with this problem, but also shows the lengths that many sufferers are driven to, in order to get proper treatment.[247]

It seems that people with MCS have to be extremely persist-ent and need a thick skin. While they are trying to get their condition diagnosed, many have to run the gamut of doctors who actively try to persuade them that their problems are 'all in the mind' and that chemicals have no role in triggering their symptoms. As one paper states, 'The greatest challenge in treatment is to overcome the patient's disabling belief in a toxi-cogenic explanation for his or her symptoms'.[248]

So what is multiple chemical sensitivity? Despite the 'it's all in the mind' brigade, MCS has established itself as a very genuine condition in significant parts of the medical community. These specialists understand the effects that chemical toxins can have on our health, and have come up with the following definition outlining this new illness, which tends to affect ordinary people as well as industrial workers, communities with contaminated air or water supplies and others with unique exposure to particular chemicals.

MCS is a condition in which previous exposure to a signifi-cant level of solvents, pesticides or other chemicals appears to render people hypersensitive to a wide range of unrelated and previously tolerated chemicals, at very low levels, which do not affect the general population at large. Following exposure to one or more of these chemicals, even seemingly innocuous and unre-lated substances such as perfume bring about an almost immediate reaction, resulting in the rapid onset of a collection of widespread symptoms affecting many organ systems.

Symptoms range from headaches and depression to breathing difficulties, flu-like symptoms, ear, nose and throat disturbances, gastrointestinal problems, musculo-skeletal problems and even heart and circulatory disorders.

Indeed, Professor William Rea, author of the four-volume series *Chemical Sensitivities*, who has treated more than 20,000 environmentally ill patients, believes that as chemicals can affect virtually every part of our bodies, we may manifest any symptom in the textbook of medicine.

Many are forced to change lifestyles just to avoid these

substances. The symptoms can be so extreme that some sufferers have to move home to live in less-contaminated surroundings. The extent of these often life-threatening health problems helps us understand why many extremely sick people are driven to consult 10 or more doctors in order to get help.

Gulf War syndrome – another MCS? Unexplained symptoms reported by veterans of the first Gulf War with Iraq, in 1991, have caused heated international debate for many years. The symptoms reported include fatigue, skin rash, muscle and joint pain, headaches, loss of memory, shortness of breath, gastro-intestinal and respiratory symptoms, and extreme sensitivity to commonly occurring chemicals.

Interestingly, the key to the puzzle of Gulf War syndrome (GWS) may be the particular combination of the numerous toxic chemicals that these soldiers were exposed to as a result of their posting. It has been hypothesised by researchers at Duke University, Durham, USA that the combination of pesticides, such as organophosphates and carbamates, along with the solvents and toxic metals and other nasties in the vaccinations they were given, may have brought about more severe nerve damage than any one of these substances could have caused individually.[249, 250]

This chemical cocktail may have acted as the initial trigger for MCS and could explain why veterans of the first Gulf War now have a significantly higher prevalence of symptoms suggestive of MCS than equivalent non-Gulf War military personnel.[251]

Many scientists now believe there to be a robust association between Gulf War syndrome and MCS. However, in the event that this were to be proven, the respective governments would potentially be liable for any damage caused to the soldiers by exposing them to a whole raft of toxic chemicals. So, not too surprisingly, this diagnosis appears to have been fought every step of the way.

MCS – a political hot potato? Unfortunately for the many millions of people thought to be debilitated by MCS, the issue involves some of the most powerful industries in the world with enormous vested interests in keeping the lid tightly on this problem.

Question: When is a disease affecting approximately 6 per cent of the population not a real disease?
Answer: When huge financial vested interests are at stake.

Just the thought of legal action from potentially millions of people damaged by everyday chemicals sends shock waves throughout the industries responsible. So, despite copious evidence revealing MCS to be a genuine disease triggered by chemicals, the efforts made by many in brushing this whole issue under the carpet have been vigorous. No wonder an international workshop on MCS held in Berlin in 1996, sponsored by major chemical companies, concluded that MCS should be treated as a psychological problem. These proposals were later rejected by many top scientists and international bodies such as the World Health Organization, highlighting the gulf between industry and independent scientific evidence on this issue.

New theory of chemically induced disease: Dr Miller, from the Department of Family Practice, University of Texas Health Science Center at San Antonio, USA is one of the growing number of scientists to champion the ground-breaking concept that we appear to be on the threshold of a new theory of disease, triggered by toxic chemicals.

So MCS might be one of these new diseases, and this new disease process might be the key to explaining the emergence of a new type of chemically related disorder, such as Gulf War syndrome, chronic fatigue syndrome (see page 240) and attention deficit hyperactivity disorder (see page 263). Their common origin not only explains the similarity of symptoms in these conditions but also why many people affected by one of these illnesses, such as MCS, are also much more likely to have another, such as chronic fatigue syndrome.[252]

Disbelieving doctors

Patients with MCS don't simply have an industry with enormous vested interests to contend with, they also have to fight their corner against a doubting medical profession. Since few doctors were taught about the toxic behaviour of certain chemicals at medical school, many are loath to acknowledge the existence of this disease, even in the face of overwhelming evidence. Maybe this is because it is easier to dismiss the condition than have to admit to their lack of knowledge or learn a whole new set of treatment rules, which admittedly takes some time to do. It also has to be said that toxic chemicals were not around in such variety and quantity when many of these doctors were at medical school. However, the world has now changed – and with it people's health.

Treatments for MCS: MCS is usually diagnosed by an experienced doctor specialising in environmental medicine or clinical ecology, following a discussion of the patient's medical history, physical examination, tests for immune functioning and toxins, and possibly neuro-imaging. There are a number of treatments available to the MCS sufferer.

For example, avoidance of all forms of chemicals, not only in foods and drinks but also in the environment, is one of the cornerstones of treatment (see Chapter 3). This includes not only the chemicals that trigger the sudden attacks but also the entire range of chemicals. They all put pressure on the already beleaguered detoxification system. As people with MCS tend to have higher levels of fat-soluble toxins (such as organochlorine pesticides and solvents) than non-affected people, detoxification is essential. Only by reducing the existing body burden of chemicals can the body deal with future ones (see Chapter 4).

To help power these detox reactions, the body needs a very good supply of nutrients such as vitamin and mineral supplements, in combination with antioxidants, alkalising salts and amino acids. This is because chemical damage both inhibits nutrient absorption and brings about an increased need for nutrients. In fact, nutrient deficiency is usually the rule in MCS.

Other methods useful in managing chemical sensitivities include:

- Dietary management. The diet must be carefully managed to exclude foods that trigger reactions. It is also preferable for the patient to base their daily diet on organic produce.
- Exercise. This is a great way to boost the body's ability to detoxify.
- Specialist treatment centres. Owing to the potentially serious nature of this condition, those with extreme sensitivities should be treated under the supervision of a medically qualified person specialising in this field. In the UK, experts can be found at Breakspear Hospital, Hemel Hempstead, Herts, or in the USA, at the Environmental Health Center in Dallas, Texas.

Trigger factors for MCS symptoms

Reactions in MCS are triggered by a vast array of everyday chemicals from perfume to diesel exhaust. The common ingredients in most of these chemical products are hydrocarbon-based volatile organic chemicals (VOCs, see Glossary page 343). Phenols (containing the organic solvent benzene) are commonly implicated. With everyday cosmetic and household chemical products, it is generally the addition of a perfume that makes them bad news for MCS sufferers. Typically a sufferer will notice a sensitivity to one or two things to start with, perfume and cigarette smoke for example, and then will rapidly become sensitised to more and more chemical sources over a relatively short period of time.

Common chemical triggers in MCS:
- perfume or perfumed products
- petrol
- diesel exhaust
- cleaning agents such as detergents
- cosmetics such as nail polish
- paint and solvents
- new carpet
- adhesives
- food additives and preservatives

It is difficult to avoid all of these substances. Whilst most people can adapt their living area to be less polluted by using more environmentally friendly products, they have to restrict their movements outside their houses to open areas where they can rapidly get away from people wearing perfumes or aftershaves before they become ill.

Typical MCS symptoms: Although the following symptoms are very common, you will know they are chemically related if they regularly occur immediately after being exposed to a relatively small amount of chemicals, such as a whiff of perfume or a puff of cigarette smoke. They can also be disproportionately extreme. One patient I know experiences a severe asthma attack if he smells aftershave on someone standing near him.

Mental symptoms:
- Irritability
- Mood swings
- Inability to concentrate or think clearly
- Poor memory
- Fatigue
- Dizziness
- Mental exhaustion (also called 'brain fog')
- Headache
- Lightheadedness
- Drowsiness

Gastrointestinal symptoms:
- Diarrhoea
- Cramps
- Upset stomach

Other symptoms:
- Sneezing
- Runny or stuffy nose
- Wheezing
- Itching eyes and nose
- Chest pain
- Muscle pain
- Tingling of the fingers and toes
- Poor muscle coordination

14

Musculo-skeletal Health

'The UK definition of chronic fatigue syndrome (CFS) was developed by a panel of physicians who were primarily psychiatrists, with few if any clinicians who had ever looked at an epidemic of ME.'

DR BYRON MARSHALL HYDE MD, NIGHTINGALE RESEARCH FOUNDATION

Chemical-induced musculo-skeletal damage

When researching my first book, *The Detox Diet*, which examines the effects chemicals have on our weight, I have to admit that I was absolutely staggered by the extent to which the majority of toxic chemicals appear to be able to damage virtually every part of our musculo-skeletal system. But what really made me sit up and take notice was the fact that I now had my first real insight into what was behind the hitherto little understood disease of chronic fatigue syndrome, otherwise known as ME.

Whilst Chapter 6 explained how avoiding chemicals and improving your nutrition could maximise your fitness potential and musculo-skeletal system, this chapter explains how chemicals appear to be behind a number of musculo-skeletal diseases. To find out how you can improve your health if you currently suffer from chronic fatigue syndrome, arthritis, or one of the many connective tissue disorders linked to our increased exposure to chemicals – read on!

Free yourself from chronic fatigue

For some people, things have gone much further than just being 'tired all the time'. They get so tired that they can hardly get out of bed, let alone go to work. For them, lack of energy has gone well past the stage of being just a nuisance. It now dominates all aspects of their lives. It can turn a previously active existence into a living nightmare.

This condition is now commonly referred to as chronic fatigue syndrome, but it is also known under many other names, such as ME (myalgic encephalomyelitis), post-viral fatigue syndrome, fibromyalgia (muscle pain), CEBV (chronic Epstein-Barr virus), and 'yuppie flu'. No age group is excluded, but it appears mainly to target people between the ages of 20 and 40. Conservative estimates of numbers affected by this extremely debilitating disease stand at 1.4 per cent.[253]

It is a complex illness characterised by incapacitating fatigue (experienced as exhaustion and extremely poor stamina), neurological problems, and a constellation of other diverse symptoms that can include poor sleeping patterns, recurrent sore throat, painful and aching muscles, painful joints, headaches and excessive post-exercise fatigue. These symptoms tend to wax and wane, but are very often severely debilitating and can last for several months or even years on end.

Despite recently being recognised by the World Health Organization as a disease in its own right affecting large numbers of people, many of its victims are still battling for the disease to be accepted as a true entity rather than being thought of as a product of hysteria – a view still held by a large section of the medical profession. There may be no visible signs of illness – but no doctor would say that a person with a headache was 'hysterical', even though there are no visible signs of a headache.

The widespread resistance to CFS being accepted as a 'real' condition is probably due to a relative lack of knowledge about both its causes and treatment. However, a certain amount of work into identifying the causes of CFS has actually been carried out, leading to the following theories.

Substances that lower mitochondrial energy production
■ Pesticides such as organophosphates, organochlorines, pentachlorophenol and many others.[254, 255, 256]
■ Herbicides, such as 2,4-D.[257]
■ Persistent environmental contaminants, such as PCBs and dioxins.[258]
■ Solvents.[259]
■ Toxic metals.[41]
■ Plastics.[260]
■ Drugs, such as antibiotics,[261] non-steroidal anti-inflammatories[262] and anti-parasite drugs.[263]
■ Fluoride.[264]

CFS – the latest theories: It seems that most people researching this subject are divided into two main camps. The first is made up of those who blame a persistent virus, and not the immune system for allowing the virus access in the first place. The second includes those who see CFS as a disease activated by many different triggers, one of which can be a virus, but only in combination with other factors.[265]

These other trigger factors are thought to include fungal (candidiasis) and bacterial infections, in addition to viral ones, mineral and vitamin deficiencies, and finally allergies or sensitivities to foods, pollutants, animal and plant products, and chemicals.

As you can imagine, I am very much in the latter camp, from the very moment of discovering that the majority of chemicals currently residing in the body can severely incapacitate our vital energy-producing mitochondria. For a long time now I have been eager to write about what this really means to CFS sufferers. This need has increased with time as the more I learn, the more I am convinced that toxic chemicals are not just responsible for lowering energy levels, but could be playing a key role in triggering this life-shattering syndrome.

How CFS is diagnosed: Most cases of CFS are diagnosed by discussing the patient's medical history and by performing a full physical examination. In general, to be diagnosed with chronic fatigue syndrome, a patient must satisfy two criteria. He or she must:

- Have severe chronic fatigue of six months' or longer duration in the absence of other medical conditions that might cause this symptom.
- Concurrently have four or more of the following symptoms: substantial impairment in short-term memory or concentration, sore throat, tender lymph nodes, muscle pain, multi-joint pain without swelling or redness, headaches of a new type, pattern or severity, unrefreshing sleep, and post-exertional malaise lasting more than 24 hours.

Sufferers may also be tested for any of the large number of abnormalities commonly associated with this condition. The problem with the following tests is that none of them is found among the battery of conventional procedures ordered by most general practitioners. Most of these tests are either research-based techniques, or are too expensive or invasive, or only tend

The following signs, as revealed by the tests listed, may indicate chronic fatigue syndrome:

- Fewer and more damaged mitochondria (revealed by muscle biopsy).
- Markedly lower levels of energy production and a greater build-up of waste products following exercise (revealed by magnetic resonance spectroscopy – a research technique I used to study muscle metabolism at Oxford).
- Increased presence of infectious organisms, possibly due to a weaker defence/immune system (revealed by blood tests).
- Lower levels of energy-releasing and other important energy-controlling hormones (revealed by blood tests).
- Higher levels of toxic chemicals in body tissues, particularly organochlorines (revealed by toxicity tests).
- Widespread immune-system damage, mixed pattern, as some parts are suppressed while others are in overdrive (based on general symptoms).

to be ordered and understood by physicians who specialise in the field of environmental medicine (see Appendix D for details of doctors who are specialists in this area). So even if you have CFS, it won't necessarily be recognised.

So, far from being all in the mind, CFS appears to be associated with a significant number of physical defects. Energy-producing systems are grossly impaired, giving chronic fatigue syndrome its name, and many other systems also appear to be affected. This widespread damage could readily account for the other numerous and seemingly disconnected symptoms commonly accompanying CFS.

The evidence pointing towards chemicals underlying CFS: To date, chemical exposure is the only single factor known to bring about all of the above detectable disorders and symptoms associated with chronic fatigue syndrome. No other single cause has yet been found to achieve this widespread degree of destruction, which strengthens my belief that chemicals are playing a major role in the current CFS epidemic.

More corroborating evidence can be gleaned from the fact that CFS is a fairly recently identified disease whose emergence has coincided with our greater exposure to everyday toxic chemicals. While this does not prove that the two are linked, the fact that these chemicals are now in our bodies at levels that appear to be producing all the signs and symptoms of CFS gives extra credibility to this hypothesis.

We also know that fatigue syndromes are particularly common in workers who are exposed to pesticides, insecticides and other chemicals. For example, veterans of the first Gulf War exposed to these chemicals have much higher rates of CFS than non-exposed veterans.[266] In addition, a recent study of sheep farmers revealed that the greater their exposure to organophosphates used in sheep dip, the greater their risk of developing all the symptoms of CFS.[267]

These links get stronger as up to half of all those with CFS have been found to have multiple chemical sensitivities, as described in Chapter 13.[268] The reverse also holds true, as up to

40 per cent of those with chemical sensitivities show all the symptoms of chronic fatigue syndrome.[252] Indeed, it can often be very difficult to distinguish between these two disorders, and to distinguish CFS from a number of other chemically related disorders, such as multiple sclerosis and the autoimmune disease systemic lupus erythematosus (SLE).[269]

So, on the basis of all this evidence, it seems that CFS should be placed alongside the growing list of environmentally triggered illnesses to which our modern day lives appear to have predisposed us.

Treatment for CFS: While this all makes perfect sense in theory, the question is – can we do anything about it? I strongly believe the answer is yes. Many people find that the combination of detoxing and a proper intake of nutrients can make the world of difference to their lives (see page 2).

There are many treatments currently being used for those with CFS. Although none of the treatments is considered consistently satisfactory, some are thought to be helpful. They include physiotherapy, exercise programmes, acupuncture, small doses of antidepressants and psychotherapy.[269]

However, none of them tackles the problem of toxic chemicals. So, here are my suggestions for those who want to lower their exposure to energy-draining toxins, alongside other treatments currently used for CFS.

Avoid all concentrated forms of toxic chemicals (see Chapter 3). Eat organic food, use organic toiletries and environmentally friendly household products as much as possible. Detoxification is also of benefit in lowering the body's chemical burden (see Chapter 4) but fasting should be avoided (unless under strict medical supervision) as this could mobilise toxins too rapidly from the body's fat stores, making the problem worse.

Nutritional supplements play an essential role. Many people with CFS are found to be deficient in one or more of the following nutrients:

- B group of vitamins (particularly B6, B12 and folic acid).
- Vitamin C (this highly effective nutrient has previously been widely used as an infusion to successfully treat CFS).
- Vitamin E (lower body levels of this vitamin are associated with increased fatigue symptoms).
- Magnesium (reportedly successful in treating CFS fatigue symptoms, particularly when given as an infusion).
- Zinc.
- Chromium.
- MSM-sulphur (to help remove existing stores of the energy-draining toxic metal mercury).
- Tyrosine (an amino acid building block for two vital energy-enhancing hormones).
- L-tryptophan.
- L-carnitine (helps boost mitochondrial energy production and reduces fatigue and other symptoms in those with CFS).
- Co-enzyme Q10.
- Essential fatty acids (omega 3, from fish oils and flax seed oil, is particularly effective in CFS. One study showed that essential fatty acid supplementation improved symptoms in 90 per cent of those with CFS within three months).[271]
- Pancreatic enzymes.[271]

Other nutrients found to be of benefit to CFS patients include vitamin D, iron, glutathione, N-acetylcysteine (an amino acid, sometimes abbreviated to NAC, which is a potent antioxidant and great detoxer, and sold as a supplement by Solgar), alpha-lipoic acid, Ginkgo biloba and (bilberry) *Vaccinium myrtillus*.[270]

Diet is also important in those with CFS. Some practitioners recommend cutting down on all simple sugars and refined foods, and concentrating on whole, unprocessed foods. Coffee and tea should be replaced by herb and fruit teas and plenty of spring or filtered water. Dairy products can be a common problem for those with CFS, as can wheat.

Nearly 50 per cent of patients with CFS appear to be infected with *Candida albicans*. If this diagnosis is confirmed, you could find a practitioner who would suggest an anti-candida diet. There are other forms of candida treatment available, including time-released caprylic acid, herbal formulations and grapefruit seed extract.

One study showed that 28 per cent of CFS patients were infected with the intestinal parasite *Giardia lamblia*.[265] If detected in multiple stool tests it can be treated with herbs (such as *Artemisia annua*) as well as by the rather more toxic antibiotic, metronidazole.

Finally, other treatments found helpful in CFS include acupuncture, massage with essential oils, homeopathy, deep relaxation and meditation.

Arthritis – natural ways to enhance your mobility

The ability to move from one place to another with ease is one of our very greatest assets. There is a growing number of people whose whole lives are centred around minimising their muscle and joint pain. As painful muscles or joints can transform the simple act of walking a few yards into a major life event, it is easy to understand why priorities change. The number of US adults affected by osteo- and rheumatoid arthritis, and other rheumatic conditions, has already passed the 70 million mark, and is set to double by 2030.

So, to optimise our chances of keeping mobile and looking good throughout our lives – as it's hard to look attractive when you are in constant pain – we need to keep as fit and healthy as the constraints of modern day lives allow. In order to do this we have to take care of the whole of our body to either reduce our own personal odds of getting one of these potentially debilitating musculo-skeletal conditions, or to minimise symptoms if we have already been affected.

Environmental wear and tear: We need to understand more about why the number of people with arthritis and other rheumatic conditions is rising. Conventional wisdom states that this is due to our ageing population. To an extent, this is true as the greater the wear and tear the body is subjected to, the higher the risk of developing osteoarthritis. So it seems logical that the older one is, the more susceptible to this form of arthritis one will become. As the average age of our population increases, it is reasonable to assume that the overall incidence of osteoarthritis should follow suit.

However, not all forms of arthritis showing an upsurge in recent years are so strongly linked to an ageing population, since the other important musculo-skeletal diseases – especially inflammatory conditions such as rheumatoid arthritis (RA), psoriatic arthritis, inflammatory spondylitis, systemic lupus erythematosus (SLE), scleroderma and systemic sclerosis (SS) – tend to be found in a much younger sector of the population. They generally strike victims between 20 and 40 years of age.

Although, like osteoarthritis, they can affect our joints, the way in which they do this differs significantly. Rather than resulting from ordinary wear and tear, these conditions wreak their damage through inflammation caused by an abnormally over-heated natural defence system, thought to be triggered by environmental damage (see Chapter 7).

Life-long fight: There is a fight going on in the bodies of those with these diseases. On one side is the immune system – and on the other certain components of body tissues. If the immune system is in good working order, it can easily distinguish its own tissues from foreign ones. However, problems occur if the system regards some of its own tissues as foreign invaders. This has disastrous consequences as the immune system throws its full destructive might against the body's own tissues.

The upshot of all this is that this battle can only be 'won' through the total destruction of the tissues targeted. Unfortunately, once this erroneous battle is started, there is little we can do to totally reverse it or stop it completely. The more our defence system tries to fight the 'invaders' the more ill we will become, and the worse our symptoms will get.

The type of tissue targeted determines the disease: The type of disease one gets and the accompanying symptoms experienced depend upon the tissues targeted for destruction. For instance, in rheumatoid arthritis, the main tissues targeted are the inner membrane lining the joints and sometimes joint cartilage. So it is not surprising that the main features of this disease are joint pain, swelling and inflammation.

For each of the other main connective tissue diseases, such as SLE (otherwise known as lupus), Sjögrens, systemic sclerosis and scleroderma, the body appears to react against particular types of tissue proteins. This can be found from blood tests, by identifying the auto-antibodies responsible.

Diagnosis also depends on the clinical features that a person might display. While it is relatively easy to diagnose RA in someone with typical joint symptoms alone, some people are unfortunate enough to get symptoms commonly found in several of the connective tissue diseases. This overlap is actually quite common. Those unfortunate enough to be affected by a hotchpotch of symptoms and multiple types of auto-antibodies end up with a broader diagnosis of 'mixed connective tissue disorder'.

Are chemicals pressing our self-destruct button? An understanding of why we develop these autoimmune disorders is vital if we are to have any chance of successfully dealing with them. Conventional medicine treats this problem, in effect, by trying to throw a bucket of cold water over the whole fight, to calm it down. It does this by using highly toxic drugs that suppress the immune system's ability to fight any invader, not just our own tissues. However, this method not only fails to tackle the cause of the problem, it also threatens our ability to deal with real invaders, such as harmful bacteria, when they come along.

A group of physicians specialising in occupational and environmental medicine has been tackling this problem for years. Initial observations alerted them to the fact that those working with or exposed to a wide range of toxic chemicals tended to be more susceptible to developing autoimmune connective tissue diseases. For instance, people who were exposed to the highest levels of mercury from their dental fillings were more likely to develop one of these diseases than those with fewer or no fillings.[272]

It seems that toxic chemicals increase the rate at which the body creates auto-antibodies.[273] This tendency of chemicals to start off a disastrous self-destruction process appears to be aided and abetted by a combination of genetic vulnerability and a poor nutritional status, as low body levels of vitamins and minerals, particularly magnesium, can trigger production of auto-antibodies.[274]

This ground-breaking research not only gives us more of an idea as to what is causing these diseases in the first place, but it also opens up numerous safe and highly effective ways that we can exploit these diseases, without poisoning our bodies with other highly toxic drugs that suppress the immune system.

Chemicals linked to rheumatoid arthritis and other connective tissue disorders: If chemicals are playing a major role in triggering these conditions in the first place, their removal could put the brakes on disease progression. So what are the likely culprits?

To date, the list of chemicals that appear to trigger different forms of arthritis and connective tissue disorders is very extensive and growing. They include substances from toxic metals used in dental fillings to solvents used in the dry-cleaning industry.[273, 78, 275, 276, 277] Indeed there are now thought to be more than 80 'therapeutic' drugs that can cause SLE (lupus).[278]

The following chemicals have all been associated with at least one of the autoimmune connective tissue diseases and in some cases all of them.

- Toxic metals (such as mercury, cadmium, arsenic, lead, antimony, tin, cobalt and gold).
- Silica and silicone breast implants.
- Oestrogenic substances and xenoestrogens.
- Pesticides (such as DDT and organophosphates).
- Environmental pollutants (such as PCBs and dioxins).

Renoir, Rubens and rheumatoid arthritis

Three famous artists, Rubens, Renoir and Dufy, are thought to have been early casualties of this particular form of chemical damage, possibly due to their love of bright and clear colours (Pedersen LM, 1988). They all suffered from rheumatoid arthritis, a disease triggered by exposure to heavy metals. In those days, the brighter and clearer colour paints tended to be made from heavy metals such as mercury, cadmium, arsenic, lead, antimony, tin, cobalt, manganese and chromium, whereas the earth colours tended to contain less toxic ingredients, such as iron and carbon compounds.

Analysis of the areas of various colours in randomly selected paintings by these artists compared to 'control' artists (contemporary painters without rheumatic disease) suggests that Rubens and Renoir used significantly more bright and clear colours based on toxic heavy metals and fewer earth colours. While their preference and increased use of these more vivid colours obviously helped them to enjoy extraordinary artistic success, it now seems that it could have come at a high price to their health.

Artists today are not so exposed, but heavy metal contamination in food and drinking water exists. So experience from the occupational exposure of old masters is still highly relevant.

- Solvents (such as vinyl chloride, epoxy resins, alcohol, benzene and trichloroethylene).
- Contaminated rapeseed oil.
- Diesel exhaust particles.
- Medications (including oestrogen, antibiotics, bleomycin and pentazocine).
- Cocaine.
- Hair dyes.
- UV light.

Connective tissue disorders: An early interest in the body and movement prompted me to study rheumatology for a few months at Yale University some 15 years ago. As this department was particularly strong in treating those with connective tissue disorders, I was fortunate to have closer access to those affected by this then relatively rare group of diseases. Little was I to realise the impact this experience would have on my life.

A couple of years later, my mother started to suffer from a variety of bizarre and seemingly unconnected symptoms. These consisted of muscle aches and pains, dry eyes, odd tingling sensations under her skin, in the pit of her stomach and in her face, heat sensitivity in her limbs, stabbing pains in her face, head, hands and feet, and an inability to perspire, causing heatstroke in warm weather. At least half a dozen professors specialising in different fields failed to diagnose her condition. Eventually she gave up hope of ever discovering what was wrong with her. Increasingly fearful of being permanently labelled a hypochondriac or, worse still to her, a malingerer, she opened her heart to me. Although she had been investigated for most major problems, no one had looked into the possibility of a connective tissue disorder.

A couple of months later, following a letter to her doctor requesting a referral, she saw Professor Isenberg, an international specialist in connective tissue disorders. He diagnosed Sjögren's syndrome, a disorder affecting the connective tissues, which effectively bind the body together, characterised by a lack of tears and saliva. He also gave her something she found much more valuable – a name for her condition. This label was her 'proof' to the world and herself that she really had problems and was not going mad!

Since that time, she has reduced her exposure to toxic chemicals, has had all her mercury amalgam fillings removed and is taking regular nutritional supplements. Although her symptoms have not gone away, she finds it easier to live with her problems, which are now little more than an inconvenience. Fortunately, it also seems that on this new regime the speed at which the disease is progressing appears to have slowed right down.

Treatment of osteoarthritis, rheumatoid arthritis and other rheumatic and connective tissue disorders: Although osteoarthritis differs in many ways from rheumatoid arthritis, different forms of arthritis still have many things in common, such as joint inflammation and higher levels of free radicals. Because of this, many of the treatments useful for those affected by osteoarthritis are also beneficial to those with rheumatoid arthritis and other rheumatic and connective tissue disorders.

In these conditions there is a life-long need for treatment, so, if at all possible, it is best to use the most natural and least toxic methods available to you. The following treatments are based on suppressing inflammation naturally by improving the functioning of the immune system. Fortunately, many studies have shown that this is possible in many cases.[279]

The first involves the avoidance of all forms of chemicals, particularly those known to irritate the immune system. Any unnecessary medicines should also be avoided. Detoxification is another key tool for slowing down disease progression (see Chapter 4).

Nutrient supplementation appears to help in all the above-mentioned types of arthritis, rheumatic conditions and connective tissue diseases. Not only can supplements help prevent the onset of disease, but they have been shown to alleviate symptoms, such as pain and stiffness, decrease disease progression and reduce the reliance on, or combat the side-effects of, non-steroidal anti-inflammatories and other medications.

Beneficial substances include:

- Omega-3 oils, particularly from fish and flax seed.
- Evening primrose oil.
- Antioxidant nutrients, particularly vitamins A, C and E, which are important for cartilage formation.
- Selenium, zinc and glutathione, which all help to reduce swelling and pain.
- B group of vitamins (blood levels of B6 and B12 tend to be particularly low in rheumatoid arthritis sufferers, and those low in B2 and B3 have more disease symptoms).
- MSM-sulphur – this helps people with joints that are injured, arthritic, stiff or painful.

Vitamin D may be beneficial for arthritis. In Sjögren's syndrome and other forms of arthritis, vitamin and mineral deficiencies, such as iron, B12 and folic acid, are common. Boron is thought to aid calcium metabolism. Glucosamine sulphate, a building block needed for the repair of bone cartilage, can be of value.[280]

Dietary management is often helpful since many clinical ecologists believe that rheumatoid arthritis is primarily an allergy to certain foods, as well as toxic chemicals. Some people with rheumatoid arthritis and SLE who were placed on food allergy elimination diets have reported an improvement in their symptoms. Arthritis can be exacerbated by foods, such as dairy products, soya, meat, fruit, vinegar and other acids, peppers, hot spices, chocolate, dry roasted peanuts, alcohol and soft drinks, wheat, gluten and members of the nightshade family, such as potatoes, peppers, aubergines, tomatoes and tobacco. As this could affect nutrient intake, elimination diets should only be done under the supervision of a specialist.[281]

The herb boswellia appears to have anti-inflammatory actions in arthritis. The Chinese medicine, *Tripterygium wilfordii* Hook F (TwHF), has been used for SLE.[282]

15

Childhood Disorders

'Among the 3,000 chemicals produced in highest volume (over one million pounds per year), only 12 have been adequately tested for their effects on the developing brain. This is a matter of great concern because this means the foetus and child are exposed to untold numbers, quantities and combinations of substances whose safety has never been established.'

J STEIN, 2002

Are current levels of chemical exposure creating a future health timebomb?

The effects of environmental toxins on adults are bad enough, but the thought of the even more severe effects they are having on our children truly horrifies me. Although these next few pages only scratch the surface of this vast subject, my aim here is to give just a taste, so that you can grasp the immense health problems that chemicals are already bringing to the human race.

One major problem stems from the fact that children are adversely affected by much smaller levels of chemicals than those considered 'safe' for adults. As most existing 'safety' limits for chemicals have usually only considered the needs of adults, this has meant that the unique needs of our children have been virtually ignored.

Children are not simply 'little adults'. They lack a mature detoxification system that can process and expel many of the chemicals they are now exposed to. Furthermore, because most of their body systems are still developing, the chemical poisoning

Diseases linked to childhood exposure to chemicals

- Developmental disorders (such as ADHD, autism and dyslexia)
- Immune system disorders (such as suppressed immunity, overactive immune system, autoimmune diseases, asthma, eczema and hay fever)
- Brain and nervous system diseases (such as memory loss, Parkinson's disease, depression and multiple sclerosis)
- Cardiovascular diseases (such as high cholesterol, high blood pressure, heart disease and stroke)
- Gut problems (such as food intolerances, inflammatory bowel disease, irritable bowel syndrome)
- Hormonal and metabolic imbalances (such as diabetes, thyroid disease, infertility and weight disturbances)
- Cancer
- Multiple chemical sensitivities
- Musculo-skeletal disorders (such as arthritis and chronic fatigue syndrome)

of these systems can cause immediate damage and also increase the overall risk of developing a wide range of chemically related diseases in later life.

Early exposure: The massive production and release of synthetic chemicals into our world means that we are now exposed to thousands of health-damaging substances before we are even conceived. Chemical contaminants in both the parents' bodies are known to influence the health of the egg and sperm in ways linked to a higher rate of infertility and miscarriage and a greater level of subsequent health problems in the offspring.

Once the foetus is growing, it continues to be polluted not only with the chemicals that had already accumulated in its mother's body, but also by the ones she is exposed to on a daily basis from the food she eats, the water she drinks and the air she breathes in – with potentially devastating consequences. It does not take much to make an impact. For instance, mothers who eat normal amounts of certain types of fish (which, depending on the source, can be one of the most polluted foods on our menus) tend to have babies with a lower average IQ than those born to non-fish eaters.[283]

Scandal of the anthrax babies

Deaths, stillbirths, miscarriages, physical defects and sickness are all being blamed on anthrax jabs given to British soldiers who went to Iraq. In the case of 33 Field Hospital – an army unit of 105 men and women who served in the Gulf in 2003 – not one pregnancy has been trouble-free since the war. In every case, one of the parents was given anthrax jabs.

One father who was given the anthrax vaccine and whose wife conceived shortly afterwards, subsequently lost his five-week-old baby, born 10 weeks premature with growth problems and limb defects. In the other pregnancies there was one stillbirth, two miscarriages, a forced termination (due to major developmental abnormalities) and two premature births.

Professor Malcolm Hooper, a member of the Ministry of Defence's Independent Vaccines Panel, said: 'This situation looks like a cluster and I am sure it is linked to the anthrax vaccine. This is hugely significant and should not be ignored'.

Once the child is born, it is then subjected to higher levels of fat-soluble pollutants in the mother's milk. However, this IQ-lowering effect seems to be mainly caused by exposure to these toxins while the baby is in utero, and not from subsequent exposure to these toxins from breast milk. While this should not discourage mothers from breastfeeding – as it has never stopped me – it seems a sensible precaution to minimise the potential toxin transfer to the baby in breast milk. For instance, she should not go on a food-restrictive diet while pregnant or breastfeeding, as this increases the mobilisation of fat-borne toxins from the mother's fat stores and raises the level of chemicals in her breast milk. She should also avoid using pesticides, and eat less polluted or 'cleaner' foods, such as organic products.

Bottle-feeding carries its own risks. In addition to any existing chemicals found in formula baby milk, more can be added from the plastics in the baby bottle. Most feeding bottles contain bisphenol, a fat-soluble chemical originally designed to mimic oestrogen. When the milk is in contact with the plastic for any length of time, these fat-soluble bisphenols leach into the milk. This whole process speeds up if the milk is heated up in the bottle, as higher levels of this gender-bending chemical will contaminate the milk. The older the bottle, the greater the degree of leaching.

One study revealed that mothers who ate at least 11.8 kg of fish from Lake Michigan – a lake known to be polluted – over a six-year period before they became pregnant, tended to have babies with an average IQ lower than those born to non-fish eaters. When examined in more detail, it emerged that this IQ-lowering effect, due to the chemical PCB, was seen in only the most heavily exposed children, being the top 11 per cent most contaminated mothers from the fish-eater group. However, interestingly, they also found that the top 3–5 per cent of mothers in the general population (who did not eat Lake Michigan fish) not only had similarly high levels of contamination (mainly from other animal-based dietary sources) but their children also had lower IQs.

So, it seems sensible for all future parents to limit the amount of foods likely to contain these IQ-lowering contaminants, such as farmed salmon and trout and other animal fats, as they tend to contain more PCBs (see Appendix A.1, page 281).

The nutritional habits of toddlers also increases the damage that chemicals can wreak on their future health. They eat and drink proportionately more food and water than do adults. Their behaviours, such as crawling on pesticide-treated carpets, means that they tend to absorb comparatively more chemicals through their skin than do adults. Lastly, the fact that most young children tend to spend much of their time indoors, and that most of the total daily exposure to airborne pesticides comes from air inside the home, means that children are exposed to relatively higher levels of chemicals from their environments than many adults.

Tackling childhood health: This helps to explain why more twenty-first century children appear to be falling ill, and why the age at which children are getting certain diseases is falling. At the heart of the problem are the following three factors: the increased exposure that children now get to toxic chemicals, reduced ability to deal with chemicals due to their immature detoxification system, and an often limited nutritional intake. So what can we do about this?

Ideally, to protect our children we need to start lowering their exposure to chemicals at the earliest possible stage. This means that prospective parents should embark on a detox programme even before they try to conceive (see Chapter 3). During pregnancy, the mother should reduce her exposure to all forms of chemicals, particularly during the first three months. After the baby is born, parents need to ensure at all times that sensible efforts are made to reduce all forms of chemical exposure. These efforts include avoiding concentrated forms of chemicals, such as pesticide sprays, taking care to wash and peel fruit and vegetables, eating more organic foods, filtering water – in other words, taking the same precautions with their children that I have recommended for adults.

Childhood vaccination - straight to the point

Now for the thorny subject of vaccinations. If you have read all of the book up to this point, you will have some insight into my growing worries over vaccination. My extensive research into the chemicals used in vaccines, together with my own personal experiences of vaccine-induced health damage, has led to my decision not to let my last two children be vaccinated at all. And to date they appear to have suffered comparatively few of the childhood health problems that have been experienced by my older two. To make sure that my excellent local (and very understanding) doctors are not penalised financially by my personal choice (as UK doctors are only paid for vaccines once a certain percentage of children are vaccinated), I have recorded my decision in my children's health records.

Since most children today get up to 28 immunisations, many parents are starting to ask a fundamental question: 'Which is the greater risk: getting and being injured by the disease, or being injured by the vaccine that purports to protect against it?'

For example, serious adverse events in US children after receiving the hepatitis B vaccine, including 48 deaths, are

Measles deaths

US Government figures reveal falls in measles deaths were mainly due to improvements in living standards, not vaccines.

The rate of death attributed to measles in Massachusetts between 1860 and 1970 had dropped long before the measles vaccine was introduced in 1963, according to government data. Decreased mortality in the nineteenth century is primarily attributed to improved basic hygienic measures, including purification of water, efficient sewage disposal, and improved food hygiene.

In their attempts to get people to accept vaccines for diseases such as measles, vaccine manufacturers, healthcare providers and public health officials usually neglect to mention that the number of deaths caused by measles was declining long before the vaccine was mandated.

reported three times as frequently as actual cases of hepatitis B in children under the age of 14. Indeed, many of the vaccines are used against diseases which nowadays simply don't exist. For instance, the only polio cases in the United States since 1991 have been those caused by the oral polio vaccine, whose use was discouraged only just recently! And even when they do exist, our better living standards have converted diseases such as measles from potential killers – as they can be in Third World countries – to mostly harmless childhood illnesses.

How the Childhood Vaccination Programme could be damaging children's health: Ever since mass vaccination of infants began in the last century, reports of serious brain, cardiovascular, metabolic and other injuries started filling pages of medical journals. For example, an article in the respected journal *Science News* on 22 November 1997, called 'The Dark Side of Immunizations', reviewed reports from several countries showing that vaccinated children, in addition to having a lower IQ, also have a higher incidence of behavioural problems, asthma and diabetes than unvaccinated children.

There is also evidence which points to childhood vaccinations being far more risky than adult vaccinations. Firstly we know that children, due to their relatively immature detoxification systems, are likely to be the most vulnerable to possible vaccine-induced chemical damage. Secondly, levels of chemicals which cause damage to children are far smaller than those known to damage an adult. And thirdly, because children's systems are still developing, chemical damage can cause additional health problems in our young such as developmental delays and diseases such as autism. This, together with the fact that these days our children have already been exposed to far more chemicals in the womb than their parents ever were, could help account for the unprecedented number of childhood vaccine-related illnesses now being seen.

The difficulty of breaking the 'vaccines are only good' myth: To understand how this situation came to pass we need to go back to the origins of vaccines. Vaccines were originally introduced following the observations of country physician Dr Jenner that

Some of the many outcomes of vaccination

Sudden infant death (cot death)	Learning disorders
Death	Gut malabsorption diseases
Brain damage	Eczema
Multiple sclerosis	Asthma
Autism	Hay fever
ADHD	Autoimmune diseases
Dyslexia	Diabetes

'Unnecessary' vaccines appear to be damaging animal health

Veterinarians [in the USA] are warning dog and cat owners that millions of dollars are being dished out for unnecessary and often dangerous vaccines. An open letter was written warning pet owners that several vaccines given to their pets on an annual basis actually lasted much longer than a year. It was also noted that vaccinations for conditions such as distemper, cat flu and parva virus could last sometimes up to a lifetime. So many of the annual booster jabs were actually unnecessary. This open letter also revealed the increased risk of 'adverse post-vaccination events' including problems such as autoimmune disorders, transient infections and a risk of cancer in cats. (BBC News, April 2004) milkmaids who had been infected by cowpox appeared to be resistant against contracting the more fatal smallpox. Ever since, this romantic medical breakthrough has resulted in virtually the entire medical community holding the concept of vaccinations tightly to its collective bosom.

However, things have changed from those early days in a way in which Jenner could never have predicted. Vaccines are now – unlike in his day – regularly loaded with some of the most toxic brain-damaging chemicals known to mankind.

The problem appears to arise from the fact that most doctors are simply not told about these additives. And even if they are, because they are not taught about the effects that these chemicals can have on human health, they fail to grasp their significance and the potential role they could be playing in triggering disease.

However, the decision on whether to vaccinate or not is totally up to the individual. Parents need to read up about this subject and draw their own conclusions. If you still want to go ahead and get your child vaccinated, at the very least make sure the vaccines used are mercury-free. While mercury has stopped being used as a preservative in routine childhood vaccinations (unlike aluminium which is still present), it continues to be found in many non-routine vaccines.

Nutrition for children

Nutrients play an important role in preventing chemically related damage and optimising our health. However, the combination of less-nutritious, increasingly processed food, together with a less-varied diet, means that the vast majority of children, from babyhood upwards, are no longer getting the nutrients they need to grow and develop properly – let alone defend their bodies against the onslaught of toxic chemicals. The good news is that this situation is easily remedied by making sure you give the nutrients they need in the form of supplements (see page 114).

So, in order for our future generations to survive and thrive in the twenty-first century, we all need to do our bit as parents

Nutrients in pregnancy and reduced cancer risk

Taking nutrient supplements in pregnancy can help reduce your child's risk of cancer. One study has shown that when mothers take a combination of vitamins and minerals throughout pregnancy, their offspring are 30–40 per cent less likely to develop a common form of brain tumour. This is consistent with findings for other childhood cancers.[284]

to protect our children from the accompanying hazards. Whilst the number of childhood disorders linked to exposure to toxic chemicals is extensive, I have decided to concentrate on the following increasingly common behavioural and learning problems, which tend to start in childhood, namely:

- Attention deficit hyperactivity disorder (ADHD).
- Autism.
- Learning difficulties.

By taking care to reduce harmful toxins and by ensuring optimal nutrition, you have the unique ability to give your children the best start in life that a parent can now give, which is good health. Whether your child is a toddler or a teenager, it's never too late to improve his or her health.

Natural ways of dealing with attention deficit hyperactivity disorder

One of the biggest problems faced by parents in recent years is the exponential growth in the number of 'problem' children with extreme and disruptive behaviour. The best recognised of the behavioural problems is attention deficit hyperactivity disorder (ADHD). This once extremely rare problem, which was first identified only 100 years ago, has become so widespread that it is now the most common brain-development disorder of childhood.

Your child may have ADHD if he or she has a mixture of the following problems:

- Cannot sit still, and fidgets excessively.
- Has difficulty concentrating on what they are doing.
- Has unpredictable, impulsive and often destructive behaviour.
- Has a difficult time settling down to sleep.
- Cannot adapt to new situations.
- Tends to be anxious and forgetful.
- Does not appear to listen when spoken to directly.
- Over-reacts to new stimuli.
- Talks excessively.
- Is always on the go.

As you can imagine, some of these behavioural problems could make life very difficult for other members of the family. Problems at school could add to the pressure on parents to get their child to conform.

Therefore it may come as no surprise that sales of Ritalin, the highly controversial drug used to sedate children with ADHD, have rocketed. With current estimates of children affected by ADHD ranging from 2–18 per cent, Ritalin is now one of the most prescribed children's drugs in the USA, with more than six million prescriptions a year and approaching $550 million in annual sales.[285] However, rising concerns about this drug's links with liver cancer, severe depression, addiction, psychosis and heart disorders have meant that Ritalin attracts more lawsuits than virtually any other drug in existence.[286] As a result, parents are now caught between wanting a better-behaved child and worries about the adverse reactions arising from its use.

The good news for parents of children with ADHD is that an increasing number of people are finding that symptoms of ADHD can be cut dramatically by using safe complementary or alternative treatments. This is not just wishful thinking, as these dramatic benefits have now been proved in a growing number of academic studies. But before I explain how they produce their 'magic', we need to know more about ADHD and what causes it.

About ADHD: ADHD is thought to affect two to three million children in the USA. Some children appear to have a greater problem with hyperactivity-type symptoms, others with poor concentration, and the rest have a combination of both. Although these symptoms tend to lessen during adolescence, a minority carry on to be afflicted by the same symptoms into mid-adulthood. In many cases ADHD in adult life is also associated with anxiety, mood and other disruptive disorders, as well as substance abuse. Poor concentration on its own is referred to as attention deficit disorder (ADD).

At the heart of these symptoms appears to be a marked inability of the brain to produce enough of the neurotransmitters (brain messenger molecules) known as catecholamines. These are critical in energising the body, initiating movement and improving concentration, among other things. Low levels of catecholamines result in hyperactivity and inattention. Ritalin, which encourages the release of catecholamines, appears to calm previously disruptive children.

Recent imaging studies have revealed that certain parts of the brains of ADHD children tend to be smaller than those of normal children, while other parts appear to be larger.[287] Those affected by ADHD also appear to have reduced blood flow to the brain. This is of great concern as something out there appears to be powerful enough to change not only the way the brain works but also its very structure. So what could be doing this? You guessed it – toxic chemicals.

Chemicals and ADHD: While genetics appears to play some role in triggering ADHD, the sheer increase in the number of those developing this condition would suggest that the factors responsible can only reflect recent changes in our diet and environment. Since an estimated 25 per cent of the industrial chemicals in our environment are known neurotoxins – that is, they are known to poison nerve and brain cells – these would seem to be the obvious major source of the problem.

If you delve a little deeper you will see that not only are chemicals powerfully able to change the shape of developing brains, but the vast majority of them can damage and reduce the level of catecholamines produced by brain cells. Indeed, some toxic chemicals are so good at creating ADHD-like symptoms, they are even used to produce animal models of the disease for research purposes.[288] It is therefore easy to understand how the ever-increasing exposure of our children to these known neurodevelopmental chemical toxins could be playing a major role in the ADHD epidemic.

Unfortunately, some of the chemicals most strongly linked to ADHD are those commonly found in the body of every prospective parent. Consequently, babies are exposed to these toxins from the moment of conception. For instance, the toxic metals toxins lead and mercury, and the environmental pollutants PCBs and DDT – all associated with ADHD – are already found in many people at levels known to damage brain development in unborn babies.[195, 289]

It is known that the developing brain is exquisitely sensitive to mercury. One study showed that the more mercury-contaminated foods a pregnant woman consumed, the worse the attention, language and memory problems seen in her child by the age of seven.[195] Lead also appears to be strongly linked to

Factors associated with ADHD

- Genetic factors
- Premature delivery
- Exposure to neurodevelopmental toxins (including toxic metals, such as mercury and lead, organochlorine pesticides and pollutants, such as PCBs, DDT and DDE, and pesticides, such as organophosphates and carbamates)
- Maternal smoking during pregnancy
- Adverse responses to food additives (such as preservatives and colourings)
- Food intolerances and 'allergenic' foods
- Refined sugars
- Nutritional deficiencies (vitamins, minerals and fatty acids)
- Sensitivities to environmental chemicals and fungi
- Thyroid diseases (which can also be triggered by toxic chemicals)

ADHD, as the higher the level of lead in a child's blood or hair, the more likely they were to get ADHD symptoms.[290]

Since the widely distributed organochlorine contaminants known as PCBs can powerfully and permanently lower the level of catecholamines produced in the brain, it is no surprise that the number of children developing ADHD is on the increase. Indeed, mothers who have higher body levels of other catecholamine-depleting toxins such as the organochloride pesticide DDT and its metabolite (breakdown product) DDE are more likely to have children affected by ADHD.[291]

Childhood exposure to other chemicals such as the pesticides commonly found in the diet is also known to cause behavioural problems such as poor attention, IQ and memory.[292] But perhaps the best-known connections between hyperactivity and chemicals are seen with food additives such as colourings and flavourings. Many studies have now demonstrated that children with ADHD show dramatic improvements after food additives are lowered in the diet.[292] So, although ADHD is known to be a complex disorder triggered by a number of different factors, it seems that lowering exposure to chemicals (see Chapter 3) in combination with removing existing ones from the body by way of a good detox programme (see Chapter 4) could provide an effective drug-free way of tackling symptoms naturally.

Nutrients and ADHD: Using nutrients to treat children with ADHD has in many cases been phenomenally effective. This is because virtually all the children with ADHD are deficient in at least one of the many essential nutrients needed for the brain to work properly. In fact the greater the degree of nutrient deficiency the worse the symptoms tend to be. For instance, a staggering 95 per cent of children affected by ADHD are known to be deficient in magnesium. The good news is that parents of children with ADHD who had magnesium and other nutrient deficiencies found that supplementation proved very helpful in alleviating many of their symptoms.[293]

Magnesium supplements should be taken separately (100 mg for younger children and 200 mg for older children) as virtually all multivitamin and mineral formulations contain insufficient levels of this nutrient.

This pattern of widespread nutritional deficiencies associated with those affected by ADHD symptoms includes the following nutrients, in addition to magnesium.

- B group of vitamins.
- Iron.
- Zinc.
- Calcium.
- Copper.
- Omega-3 oils (very important).
- The essential phospholipid, phosphatidylserine (PS).
- Amino acids that boost brain neurotransmitters, such as L-5 hydroxytryptophan (5HTP, a natural precursor of serotonin), tyrosine (precursor of serotonin), theanine and S-adenosylmethionine.

All these nutrients are vital in allowing the body to manufacture the levels of catecholamines it needs. This helps explain why nutrient supplementation is often so successful; you are in effect allowing the body to work properly for possibly the first time, and to increase production of catecholamines naturally.

A number of studies show that supplementing ADHD children with nutrients can bring a significant alleviation of ADHD symptoms, allowing them to lead a normal and productive life. So the question should be raised as to why nutritional therapy has been so badly neglected in the treatment of ADHD. Instead of being an alternative option, its far superior safety record and lack of dangerous side-effects should make it the treatment of choice.

Other treatments that have shown to be of benefit to those affected by ADHD include the following:

- Dietary modification.
- Detoxification.
- Correction of intestinal dysbiosis (see page 272).
- Avoidance of artificial sweeteners.

- Avoidance of food additives, such as preservatives, flavourings and colourings (also known as the Feingold diet).
- Cutting down on refined sugars.
- Dealing with food sensitivities/allergies (by cutting out problem foods).
- Homeopathy.
- Herbs (such as passion flower, valerian or lemon balm which all have sedative effects).
- Some children with very large amounts of heavy metals in their bodies have benefited from chelation (see page 276). However, this needs to be carried out under medical supervision and only once other more natural detoxification methods using substances such as MSM-sulphur and glutathionine have been attempted for several months (see Chapter 4).

Preventing autism

Few childhood mental disorders are more emotionally distressing than autism. The combination of socially aloof behaviour, a reduced ability to communicate and an inability to integrate with other family members can push even the strongest child–parent bond to its limits. The effects on the family can be similarly devastating, with siblings getting less attention and the parents' own relationship suffering, resulting in a higher divorce rate. So this distressing disorder is a tragedy not only for the child but also for the whole family.

Until very recently, autism has been uncommon and the previous medical view had been that it was due to a genetic disorder. However, over the past few decades the number of children developing the condition has increased alarmingly. For instance, in the USA, for every one case of autism in 1993, there are now eight. This is powerful evidence that the situation has dramatically worsened.

While genetic makeup is obviously important, the dramatic increase in numbers means that it cannot explain the whole story. More and more scientists now suspect that the growing incidence of this condition is due to a major environmental assault from the increasing load of chemicals we are now pumping into our children in the forms of vaccines, contaminated foods, polluted water and polluted air. The role genetics play is now thought to be closely related to the child's inherited ability to deal with chemicals. Children who are less able to detoxify these chemicals could be more prone to developing autism.

But to find out more about current thinking as to what is behind the autism epidemic, and of course ways in which to deal with and prevent it, we need to know more about what is thought to trigger this disease.

All about autism: In most cases of autism the child develops normally until about two years old and then regresses rapidly. Autism is usually apparent by the age of three. Although symptoms of autism may increase when the child enters adolescence, they often improve in adulthood.

Young children with autism tend to have impaired language development. They may have difficulty expressing their needs verbally (and so use gestures instead of words). They may laugh, cry or show distress for unknown reasons. Some may develop abnormal patterns of speech that lack intonation and expression and may obsessively repeat words or phrases.

In general, autistic children do not express interest in other people and often prefer to be alone. They may resist changes in their

Is autism on the increase?

Any parent of an autistic child would tell you that autism is not something you are likely to miss. Yet many sceptics eager to ignore parents' growing fears that vaccinations trigger autism have been quick to blame the increase in autism on improved diagnosis, rather than an actual rise in the number of sufferers. However, recent facts suggest otherwise. In California, figures taken from the official State statistics produced by the US Department of Education reveal that the number of children with autism increased by 726 per cent over a 10-year period from 1992/3–2001/2. The subsequent detailed 2002 MIND study (Byrd et al) proved that the California increases were not ascribable to better recognition, greater awareness, nor to immigration but to a real increase in number.[294]

routine, repeat actions (such as turning in circles, or flapping their arms over and over), or injure themselves by biting or scratching themselves, or banging their head. The following symptoms of autism occur in various combinations, from mild to severe:

- Appears indifferent to surroundings.
- Appears content to be left alone and happier to play alone.
- Displays lack of interest in toys.
- Displays lack of response to others.
- Does not point out objects of interest.
- Shows marked reduction or increase in activity level.
- Avoids cuddling or touching (indeed touches may be experienced as painful).
- Exhibits frequent behavioural outbursts/tantrums.
- Shows extreme response to sensory stimuli (for instance loud noises, such as from a motorcycle or vacuum cleaner, could be experienced as painful, certain smells may be overwhelmingly unpleasant and bright lights may cause inconsolable crying).
- Shows inappropriate attachment to objects.
- Maintains little or no eye contact.
- Shows over- or undersensitivity to pain.
- Exhibits no fear of danger.
- Exhibits abnormal patterns of play.
- Unresponsive to normal teaching methods and verbal clues (may appear to be deaf despite normal hearing).

The consistency of these symptoms has made autism the most well-validated childhood 'neuropsychiatric' disorder. In addition to the above, many corroborating tests can help to confirm a diagnosis. Unfortunately, not all of these are widely available. A few are used by conventionally trained doctors, some are research tools only and the rest tend to be understood and therefore requested just by doctors specialising in environmental medicine. The following are some of the signs revealed by these tests.

- Most autistic patients show signs of brain dysfunction.
- About half of autistic children have abnormal electro-encephalograms (EEGs), which register electrical activity in the brain.
- Over 25 per cent of autistic children and adolescents have abnormally low levels of the neurotransmitter serotonin in the brain.
- Abnormalities in levels of catecholamines are commonly found.
- The immune system appears to be damaged in many of those affected, with autoimmune disorders a particular problem (antibodies against myelin proteins are frequently found).
- Gut malabsorption problems such as a 'leaky' gut and dysbiosis (a general term for bacterial flora imbalance in the digestive tract) are rife.
- In one study, impaired detoxification of chemicals was found in all of the autistic patients tested. Impaired sulphur metabolism, commonly associated with detoxification disorders, is linked to gut malabsorption problems.
- Food intolerances are frequently present (particularly towards dairy and gluten-containing foods).
- Blood clotting problems have also been reported.

So what could have happened to cause such a significant degree of disturbance in an increasing number of children?

Factors linked to autism

- Genetic predisposition.
- Early exposure to chemicals (such as toxic metals, pesticides, pollutants and medications including anticonvulsants and thalidomide).
- Foods containing gluten (such as wheat, rye, barley and oats) and milk and dairy products. If the gut is 'leaky', more peptides (small protein fragments, see page 273) from inadequately digested foods will escape into the blood, and eventually enter the brain, upsetting normal functioning.
- Vaccination (all types, not just MMR).
- Nutrient deficiencies.

Autism and the environment: The prevailing view is that autism is caused by genetic predisposition together with a series of early environmental shocks to the developing nervous system, mainly from toxic chemicals. The children who develop autism tend to be those who are exposed to higher levels of chemicals (particularly toxic metals such as aluminium and mercury) at certain stages of their development, but are genetically less able to break them down. This could explain why autistic children tend to have a higher body burden of toxic chemicals, in particular toxic metals.[295] Autism could then arise following a final trigger such as an infection, a further vaccination or other factors.

Why do vaccines in the UK still contain mercury preservatives?
In the USA, mercury is being phased out of childhood vaccines because it is known to be neuro-toxic, due to its strong links to autism and because scientists have realised that the amount given in vaccines exceeds Federal safety limits. Despite the growing pile of data linking mercury to autism, several vaccines still use this metal as a preservative (see Appendix C), and the number of vaccines being used on children is continually growing. So is it any wonder that an increasing number of children are becoming autistic?

The links between artificial chemicals and autism are also getting stronger by the day. Indeed, artificial chemicals have even been used to create 'animal models' of autism. They have done this by exposing developing rats to valproic acid – a medicinal drug given to treat epilepsy.[296] These rats then go on to display many of the brain abnormalities associated with autism in humans.

Another group has put forward the hypothesis that autism is more of a metabolic illness than a mental one. The Autism Research Unit of the University of Sunderland has researched more than 1,200 children with autism over 11 years[297] and has evidence that autism is due to natural substances known as peptides. These peptides are tiny fragments of proteins. Autistic patients tend to have higher levels of these substances in the blood. This could be as a result of abnormalities in the gut commonly seen in autistic children. Damage to the gut wall could cause partially digested foods to leak out of the gut and enter the blood, and ultimately the brain. The abnormally high levels of these substances in the brain are thought responsible for triggering the abnormal behaviours characteristic of autism. So what could cause the gut to be damaged in this way?

Again, the same answer crops up – toxic chemicals which can damage the gut, increasing the level of food intolerances and making it more 'leaky' (see Chapter 9). This leads neatly to the ongoing debate on the role of MMR vaccines in triggering autism.

Vaccinations and autism: The link between vaccinations and autism is currently the subject of much controversy. On one hand are the massive vested interests keen to push ahead with an ever-expanding vaccination programme. On the other side are the growing number of families whose children appear to be damaged as a direct result of these vaccines.

Autism and thimerosal

Prompted by growing health fears about vaccine additives, Northeastern University pharmacy professor Richard Deth and colleagues from the University of Nebraska, Tufts, and Johns Hopkins University carried out animal research on the vaccines given to children and have found a link between exposure to certain neurodevelopmental toxins, such as mercury, and an increased possibility of developing neurological disorders such as autism and attention deficit hyperactivity disorder. This work, prompted by the recent increase in the incidence of autism and their previous work in the field, led them to speculate that environmental exposures, including vaccine additives, might contribute to the triggering of this disorder.

Another US-based study found that children who received vaccines containing thimerosal, which is almost 50 per cent mercury, were more than twice as likely to develop autism as children who did not.[298]

Yet, despite these and many other studies which show that symptoms of mercury toxicity in young children are extremely similar to those of autism and ADHD, there is still no research in the pipeline to assess the potential harm children might be experiencing from the highly toxic chemicals used as additives that they are now subjected to as a result of the current childhood vaccination programme.

Dr Andrew Wakefield suspected a connection between vaccination and autism after he saw an increasing number of children with a previously unknown gut disorder (now known as ileocolonic lymphonodular hyperplasia) in a group of children with autism. Of 48 children who had developed autism just after vaccination, 46 exhibited these same bowel abnormalities. In his view, the sheer number of children showing up with this previously extremely uncommon bowel disorder, along with autistic tendencies that started soon after vaccination, was more than chance.[297]

Together with his colleague Paul Shattock, director of the Autism Research Unit at the University of Sunderland, Wakefield postulated that the attenuated (weakened) strain of the measles virus caused a reaction in the gut wall that damaged it and made it more leaky. Wakefield then speculated that the associated deficiencies in vitamin B12, from a reduced ability to absorb this nutrient from food, contributed to the autistic regression seen in those children, since this nutrient is essential for the normal development of the central nervous system.

To sum up, it seems that a number of factors are responsible for triggering the onset of autism. In the case of MMR-triggered autism, the virus in this vaccine could be the final straw that triggers autism in a child whose body has already been damaged by previous exposure to chemicals in vaccines and the environment.

I have a personal view regarding this current controversy. I have already described my second son's close call following his first MMR vaccination. At one year of age, he developed a high temperature and green offensive diarrhoea. From a happy little boy he withdrew into his shell and stopped his baby banter, showing early warning signs of autism. Fortunately, since starting him on nutrients, he improves all the time and is a normal, happy six-year-old.

What to do? The parents of autistic children are in the front line of the battle. They must cope with this condition every day. Owing to the number of factors leading to the development of autism, it should not come as any surprise that the treatments involve several different strands. In addition to reducing the overall exposure to chemicals (see Chapter 3), it is important to lower existing mercury levels in the body by using substances that specifically bind to heavy metals (see box). Both of these actions lead to health benefits.[299]

Ensuring your child gets the right nutrients is just as important as ensuring that their exposure to chemicals is minimised, as about half the children with autism show marked improvements when nutritional supplements are given. These include vitamins A, B3, B6, B12 and folic acid, calcium, magnesium (particularly helpful), zinc and omega-3 oils such as fish oils. Other beneficial nutrients are MSM (a form of sulphur to boost the detoxification

---

Toxic metal chelation

A chelation detox is the opposite of supplementation. Chelation attempts to remove toxic metals that have accumulated over the years, especially in nerve and brain tissue. Chelation can be accomplished with nutrients and/or drugs. The safest way to shift mercury from your or your child's system is to start taking the amino acid NAC (N-acetyl L-cysteine) and glutathione (the body's natural chelator) right away as these feed the body's natural chelating system. Glutathione (and its precursor NAC) binds mercury in the blood and it is then removed by the kidneys. MSM-sulphur is also very beneficial as it enhances the body's natural stores of glutathione and safely carries mercury out of the kidneys. The nutrient ALA (alpha lipoic acid), a powerful antioxidant (which has in the past been classified as a vitamin), also contains sulphur molecules and therefore can bind and remove mercury from your tissues. These natural substances are usually highly effective at removing mercury from the tissues.

Finally, the man-made water-soluble chelators, known as DMSA (DL-2,3,-dimercapto-succinic acid) and DMPS (2,3-dimercapto-1-propane-sulphonic acid) are used to lower levels of mercury, but they can have marked side-effects if the mercury is displaced too quickly and so should only be administered under medical supervision. Moreover, most practitioners practised in using DMPS and DMSA are US based.

Chelation methods appear to have marked benefits in the majority of children affected by autism. These benefits are boosted by taking soluble fibre supplements.[299]

(The nutrients can be found in Appendix B, page 287.)

process) and digestive enzymes – the latter helping to reduce symptoms in over half the children affected.

Dietary restrictions – including removal of milk and other casein dairy products, wheat and other gluten sources, sugar, chocolate, preservatives and food colourings – are essential in getting maximum benefit out of the other treatments. Reducing the intake of the foods that autistic patients find more difficult to digest tends to be among the most beneficial treatments for autism. While these diets do not cure autism, they can make the symptoms more manageable. However, bear in mind that if you exclude certain food groups from the diet, there is an increased risk of nutritional imbalance, so it is best to do this under medical supervision. This will also help ensure that the child gets adequate essential nutrients from supplements.

Gastrointestinal improvements are also assisted by tackling the fungal infections such as *Candida albicans*, which are increasingly common in autism. Here probiotics (beneficial bacteria) and a good nutritional supplementation programme come into their own in correcting dysbiosis and decreasing gut permeability. On the whole, with the exception of antifungal medications such as nystatin, prescription medications appear to offer only very limited benefits in autism.

Minimise dyslexia and other learning disorders

Many years ago, dyslexia was regarded as a condition inherited from your parents with symptoms varying from one generation to another. However, times have changed and with them the number of people affected by dyslexia. Alarmingly, between 1976 and 1993 there was a threefold increase in the prevalence of dyslexia, forcing a change in previous thinking on the causes of this condition.

Many scientists now think that this increase in numbers is due to a significant rise in neuro-toxic chemicals in our environment. These chemicals are known to damage the immature nervous system of infants, leading to abnormal development and result-ing in a raft of behavioural and learning difficulties in childhood.

While this problem cannot usually be totally reversed once it occurs, much can be done to reduce many of the symptoms as well as preventing deterioration. This can be achieved by a combination of a good detox programme (see Chapter 4), together with a number of nutritional supplements that help to support and enhance functioning in existing brain cells. This will enable children with dyslexia to maximise and enhance their existing skills. To understand how this works, we first need to know more about this complex disorder.

What is dyslexia? It is now estimated that 10 per cent of the population of the USA and UK suffer some degree of dyslexia and that 4 per cent are severely affected. Dyslexia is found in families across the full range of socio-economic backgrounds. In practice, the word dyslexia tends to be used as an umbrella term for a number of related disorders of common origins, which occur more frequently in dyslexics, such as:

- Dyslexia (a reduced ability or inability to read or spell).
- Dyspraxia (problems with learning, planning and executing sequences of co-ordinated movements, for example eating with a spoon, riding a bike or speaking clearly).
- Dyscalculia (problems with numbers).
- Dysgraphia (problems with handwriting).

Dyslexia literally means the inability to master the written word. It is usually described as 'word blindness'. A dyslexic brain has problems in seeing, understanding or recognising some words. The result is that some dyslexics are unable to read well, to write fluently or to spell adequately, despite strenuous efforts by both teacher and learner.

Dyslexia symptoms are found in similar disorders, such as ADHD. Interestingly, this could be more than just coincidence, as these conditions share many other features such as abnormal levels of certain neurotransmitters, such as catecholamines, abnormal energy metabolism in the brain, differences in the sizes of structures in the brain, brain symmetry in areas where it should be asymmetrical and also the reverse of this.[300] So what is thought to cause this problem?

The environment and dyslexia: Although there is a powerful genetic predisposition to dyslexia, the increase in the numbers of those with dyslexia symptoms is probably due to the huge amount of toxic chemicals in the environment, which are known to damage the developing nervous system. This form of damage results in abnormal connections forming between different parts of the brain, underdevelopment or overdevelopment in parts of the brain, and an imbalance in the brain's ability to produce neurotransmitters. The upshot of this is that the damaged brain cannot process information as it was designed to do – resulting in reading and learning problems.

It is difficult to point at any particular chemical, but many are known to be strongly linked to dyslexia. For instance, toxic metals are well known to destroy nerves. There is a close correlation between the level of mercury that children are exposed to in the womb, and the degree of language and memory deficits that result. In other words, the higher the level of mercury the greater the degree of dyslexia.[301] Other metals such as cadmium, lead and aluminium also tend to be found in much higher levels in dyslexic children.[302]

Other environmental contaminants such as PCBs (found in high levels in fish and animal products) are known to produce features common to dyslexia, such as abnormal levels of brain

People with dyslexia tend to have problems with a number of the following:

- Learning to speak.
- Organising written and spoken language.
- Learning letters and their sounds.
- Memorising number facts.
- Spelling.
- Reading.
- Learning a foreign language.
- Arithmetic.

catecholamines and an altered brain shape and symmetry. Organochlorine pesticides such as DDT can also affect energy metabolism in the brain, another feature commonly found in dyslexics.

While some of this damage is permanent, looking on the positive side it is possible to improve the situation in a developing child by lowering future exposure to nerve-killing chemicals while simultaneously lowering the existing levels of chemicals in the body. This will help prevent future damage while also allowing the brain to adapt as much as it can in order to restore some of the damage done (the growing brain can be remarkably adaptive). In addition to a good detox programme (see Chapter 4) which includes toxin-binding soluble fibre and essential nutrients, chelation therapy (under medical supervision) is thought to significantly benefit the 1–2 per cent of preschool children whose blood lead levels are too high, by reducing their degree of reading disability in later childhood.[303]

Nutritional support: Many children with dyslexia are known to be deficient in nutrients such as magnesium, zinc, and particularly omega-3 and omega-6 oils.[304] As these nutrients are essential for the brain to work properly, it comes as little surprise that they can bring great improvements in dyslexia, dyspraxia and all the other learning disorders, when given as part of a balanced supplement programme.

Amino acids that help boost normal functioning of brain neurotransmitters, such as L-5 hydroxytryptophan (5HTP) and tyrosine have also been shown to help alleviate symptoms in many dyslexics.

Adjusting the diet to one low in refined sugar is also thought to help. This is because a diet high in refined sugar tends to cause more erratic eye movements in dyslexics, whilst a diet low in refined sugars helps to normalise the eye movements.[305]

Finally, since many children with ADHD also have symptoms of dyslexia, treatments will fortunately help in both areas.

Common Toxic Chemicals

We are exposed to vast numbers of chemicals in a huge amount of everyday products. Although it would be impractical to go through all of them individually, I have picked out some of the most common chemicals, just to highlight some of the places in which they can now be found.

The more you appreciate how widely these chemicals are used, and their individual longevity, the more clearly you will understand why we are now so contaminated with them.

A.1 Organochlorines (and other organohalides)

What are they? Naturally toxic elements such as chlorine, fluorine and bromine, and the synthetic chemicals made with them, such as organochlorines and other organohalogens.

Examples: Chlorine, fluorine and bromine salts, organochlorine pesticides such as DDT, chlordecone, aldrin, dieldrin, endrin, toxaphene, heptachlor, lindane family, HCB (hexachlorobenzene); organochlorine pollutants such as dioxins, PCBs (polychlorinated biphenyls); organobromine fire-retardants such as the PBBs (polybrominated biphenyls – used mainly in the USA) and PBDEs (polybrominated diphenyl ethers – used mainly in northern Europe).

Background information: The halogen salts of chlorine, fluorine and bromine are naturally extremely toxic, and are widely used as pesticides in their own right. Synthetic chemicals made with these elements are also extremely toxic. Although most developed countires have banned or restricted many types of pesticides using either the salt alone or more commonly the synthetic compound containing the salt, such as many types of organochlorines, owing to their previous extensive use and their long-lasting effects, their production is thought to have resulted in the permanent pollution of the entire planet.

Moreover, these pesticides continue to be produced and used in developing countries, largely because of their relatively low cost, even though many of their dangers are well known. As contaminants, they accumulate up the food chain, and because of their high fat solubility and stability they tend to concentrate in fatty tissues.

Intended uses: Water disinfectant, fluorination of water supplies, 'cleaning' substances, general pesticides (herbicides, insecticides and fungicides); wood preservatives and treatment for termite protection; anti-malaria spray; electrical conductors, fire-retardants; paints and dyes; medicines.

Where they are found: In most cleaning products, in swimming pool chlorination chemicals, in food, as deliberately applied pesticide residues; as environmental contaminants in carnivorous fish, fatty meats, dairy products, human tissue, soil, water and air adjacent to pollution sources; as contaminants in combusted leaded petrol; as contaminants in pesticides; as fire-retardants on fabrics, clothes, curtains, furniture coverings and wood; in electrical sealants, small capacitors, old refrigeration units, starter motors for fluorescent light switches; in carpets, carbonless duplicating paper, surface coatings, inks, and adhesives; in medicines such as nit shampoo and treatments for head and crab lice.

Estimated health risk: Extremely powerful, owing to their omnipresence, their extreme stability, our relative inability to expel them and their widespread toxicity to the body's hormonal systems.

A.2 Organophosphates

What are they? Synthetically manufactured chemicals.

Examples: Organophosphate insecticides.

Background information: Organophosphates were originally created in 1845. Later they were developed as a nerve gas and used in the Second World War. Since then, they have been used extensively in many different areas of manufacturing, food production and even medicine. They are now some of the commonest pesticides detected on our foods.

Intended uses: Nerve gas in human warfare; pesticides for crops; sheep dips, cattle treatments, flea treatments for pets; wood infestation treatments; animal growth-promoters; medicines, particularly treatment for lice, crabs and nits; widespread industrial uses such as petrol additives, stabilisers in lubricating and hydraulic oils, synthetic additives, rubber additives and flame-retardants.

Where they are found: In food as pesticide residues, particularly on soft fruit, vegetables and grain products; as pesticides used in agriculture; in household and garden pesticides such as fly spray; in pet treatments; on treated wood; as medicines; in car oil, petrol fumes and rubber.

Estimated health risk: High. Although the toxicity of organophosphates varies, they are some of the most powerful pesticides in current usage, damaging a wide number of different body systems.

A.3 Carbamates

What are they? Synthetically manufactured chemicals.

Examples: Carbamate insecticides, dithiocarbamate fungicides, ETU (ethylenetiourea).

Background information: Action thought to be similar to that of organophosphates, but generally considered to be less toxic. Some effects last for a shorter period than those of organophosphates, but other toxic actions can last for much longer periods and result in permanent organ damage, for instance some carbonates are known to damage the brain.

Intended uses: In pesticides such as insecticide, herbicide, fungicide and anti-microbials; preventing potatoes from sprouting; ridding livestock and chickens of parasites; in flea treatments for pets; in forestry and wood infestation treatments; as animal growth-promoters; in manufacturing synthetic rubber; in other synthetics; as metal chelating agents. Carbamates have been used as growth-promoters in battery farm situations because of their ability to slow down the overall metabolic rate. They are used in medicine for their anti-thyroid hormone actions.

Where they are found: In a wide range of foods and drinks, including potatoes, soya beans, citrus fruits, peanuts, tomatoes, beer and wine; in cigarettes and cigars; in cotton; in household and garden pesticides, including pet treatments, fly sprays and mothballs; in treated wood; in water as contaminants; in medicines (see page 284).

Estimated health risk: Moderate to high. They particularly target our energy metabolism.

A.4 Toxic metals

What are they? Naturally occurring toxic metals.

Examples: Cadmium, lead, mercury, methyl mercury and tributyl tin (TBSPT).

Background information: These toxic substances mainly occur naturally. However, owing to their extensive industrial use, we are now being exposed to them in levels many times greater than are usually found in nature.

Intended uses: Industrial uses include pesticide formulations, electroplating, nickel plating, for soldering, in alloys, in photo-electric cells and in storage batteries. Released in mining practices. Household uses include plumbing, building materials, cable covering and paints; also used in medicine (as disinfectants and in vaccines), in dentistry (as 'silver' amalgam fillings actually contain more mercury than silver), as petrol additives and in insecticides.

Where they are found: As contaminants in drinking water and in food grown near road sides. Found as human contaminants and in effluent in heavily polluted areas; used in amalgam fillings, vaccinations (usually mercury and aluminium), crystal glass, petrol, batteries, roofing.

Estimated health risk: High. Their extreme nerve-damaging actions, combined with a powerful tendency to accumulate and persist in the body for years, or decades, after the initial exposure, makes them very important as health-damaging substances.

A.5 Solvents

What are they? Synthetically manufactured chemicals.

Examples: Organic solvents (styrene and polystyrene), chlorinated solvents (trichloroethylene), industrial solvents.

Background information: These chemicals are very widely used in a whole range of products. Certain liquid solvents, such as styrene, can be converted into polystyrene.

Intended uses: Solvents are used extensively throughout industry to dissolve or dilute oils and fats; as a petrol additive; as a major component of packaging and household materials; a major substance used in the dry-cleaning industry; used in manufacturing synthetic rubbers, latex and resins.

Where they are found: As synthetic fragrances in toiletries, detergents, skincare products, perfumes and aftershaves; in synthetic rubbers; as a heat seal coating on metal foils (on yoghurt and cream containers, for example); as polystyrene cups, plates and packaging; as a solvent for paints, in turpentine substitute, in shoe creams, floor waxes or dyes; in household pesticides and medicines; as an environmental contaminant found in water, in the urban atmosphere and in wildlife; in foods packaged in polystyrene; as a human contaminant; in glass fibre, petrol vapour and exhaust fumes.

Estimated health risk: Moderate. Although many of these chemicals can be broken down by the body, they pose a significant threat to health, particularly to brain and nerve tissues, because of their very extensive presence in the environment.

A.6 Plastics and plasticisers

What are they? Synthetically manufactured chemicals.

Examples: Common plastic additives known as phthalates and the substance known as Bisphenol A.

Background information: The main function of phthalates is to give flexibility to plastic. Since plastics are so widely used, phthalates are now said to be the most abundant industrial contaminant in the environment. Bisphenol was originally created in the 1930s to mimic oestrogen, but is now extremely commonly used as a plastic in food packaging. For example, it is used in the lining of metallic food containers.

Intended uses: Phthalates are used as an additive in PVC and in virtually all other types of plastics; as a pesticide dilutant; as surface active agents (cleaning compounds commonly derived from petroleum); in industry they are widely used in rubber and plastic manufacturing, as industrial cleaning agents, lubricants and corrosion inhibitors.

Where they are found: In plastic wrappings for food, in food containers, in plastic bottles for baby milk, in the lining of cardboard and aluminium food containers, in the lining of metal food cans; in food and water as contaminants; in some types of fish; in fatty foods such as eggs, dairy and breast milk; as human tissue contaminants; in household pesticides and insect repellants; in cosmetics, perfumes, shampoo, hair products and nail polish; in inks, synthetic leather, vinyl floors, carpet backing, water pipes, adhesives and waterproofing; in medical devices such as catheter bags and blood storage bags; in all kinds of tubing; in dental sealant and dental impression material; in detergents and paints.

Estimated health risk: Moderate. Although these can mostly be metabolised in the body, their extensive presence ensures that they are a constant source of metabolic and hormonal disruption in our bodies.

Appendix B
Nutrients, Supplements and Popular Herbals

Note: SONA = suggested optimal nutrient allowance – for long-term use.

B.1 Vitamins

B.1.1 Vitamin A and carotenes

Functions: Carotenes are converted in the body to vitamin A, which is essential for good eyesight and night vision, for bone formation and normal body growth, especially skin and teeth, and assists pregnancy and lactation. Carotenes and vitamin A act as antioxidants, detoxifiers, protect against cancer, heart disease and other diseases. Enhances immune system.

Deficiency signs: Poor night vision, mouth ulcers, dry skin, increased susceptibility to colds and other infections.

How much? Adult RDA 600 mcgRE (2,000 IUs).

SONA: 2,000 mcgRE (6,600 IUs).

   (RE = retinol equivalent. 1 mcgRE = 3.3 IUs)

Food sources: Meat, milk and milk products, fat spreads, cereal products, eggs, fish, dark green, dark yellow and orange vegetables, carrots, sweet potatoes, coloured fruits, peaches, oranges and apples.

Toxicity: Plant-based carotenes are non-toxic, even when consumed in large amounts over long periods of time, except that harmless temporary yellowing of skin may occur. Vitamin A found in animal food is toxic only in prolonged excessive intake and can cause birth defects. If trying to conceive do not exceed 3,000 mcgRE (10,000 IUs) or 3,000–30,000 mcg beta carotene per day, long term.

Comment: Commonly found chemicals, such as PCBs, solvents, insecticides and drugs, can dramatically drain body stores of this essential nutrient, by increasing its usage and excretion. Consequently 20 per cent of those with chemical sensitivities tend to have deficient blood levels of vitamin A. Many medical conditions show improvements following vitamin A supplementation. These conditions include allergies, skin/gum/mouth complaints, asthma, visual problems and an increased vulnerability to infections.

B.1.2 Vitamin B1 (Thiamin)

Functions: Normal functioning of all body cells, especially nerves. Improves reaction time and hand–eye coordination. Aids metabolism of carbohydrates, protein and fats for energy. Vital detoxifier.

Deficiency signs: Poor concentration and memory, irritability, muscle aches and pains, fast heartbeat, tingling fingers and hands.

How much? Adult RDA 0.8–1 mg.

SONA: 3–9 mg.

Food sources: Potatoes, wheatgerm, nutritional yeast, cooked beans and peas, spring greens, raisins, oranges, nuts, whole grains, milk and milk products.

Toxicity: No known toxic levels.

Comment: Up to 30 per cent of people sensitive to chemicals are deficient in vitamin B1. Substances that increase the body's need for this nutrient include alcohol, coffee, tea, diuretics, antacids, excessive refined sugar intake, tobacco, most chemicals and raw fish. Also increased need in hypothyroidism and stress. Vitamin B1 appears to be particularly useful in the treatment of alcoholism, muscle disorders, indigestion, mental illness, diabetes, depression, fatigue, excessive chemical toxicity and failure to detoxify chemicals.

B.1.3 Vitamin B2 (Riboflavin)

Functions: Metabolism of carbohydrates, protein and fats for energy. Important for normal growth and development, detoxifying, hormonal production and regulation, formation of red blood cells, and healthy eyes, hair and nails.

Deficiency signs: Sore tongue, weak nails, cracked lips, burning light-sensitive eyes, low energy levels.

How much? Adult RDA 1.1–1.3 mg.

SONA: 1.8–2.5 mg.

Food sources: Milk and milk products, dark green leafy vegetables, avocado, wheatgerm, whole grains, meat, eggs.

Toxicity: No known toxic levels.

Comment: Up to 30 per cent of people sensitive to chemicals are deficient in this nutrient. Substances that increase the body's need for vitamin B2 are alcohol, tobacco, coffee, excessive refined sugar, toxic synthetic chemicals and medications such as the oral contraceptive pill and antibiotics. Vitamin B2 appears to help in cases of acne, alcoholism, cracked lips, mouth sores, red and sore eyes, light sensitivity and stress.

B.1.4 Vitamin B3 (Niacin)

Functions: Metabolism of carbohydrates, protein and fats for energy. Aids in synthesis of fats and certain hormones, formation of red blood cells and detoxification. Required for the maintenance of all body cells.

Deficiency signs: Poor energy levels, memory problems and other mental disorders such as depression, tiredness and irritability. Bleeding, tender gums and skin disorders such as acne, eczema and dermatitis.

How much? Adult RDA 13–17 mg.

SONA: 25–30 mg.

Food sources: Beef, poultry, other meats, cooked dried beans and peas, nuts, whole wheat and grains, potatoes, nutritional yeast, fish.

Toxicity: None known below 3,000 mg.

Comment: As with most of the other B vitamins, up to 30 per cent of those sensitive to chemicals are deficient in vitamin B3. Substances which increase needs of this nutrient include drugs, alcohol, synthetic chemicals and tea and coffee.

B.1.5 Vitamin B5 (Pantothenic acid)

Functions: Vital for energy production, muscle metabolism, making hormones, and for healthy brain functioning by creating brain neurotransmitters and boosting fat metabolism. Helps maintain skin, hair and nails.

Deficiency signs: Muscle cramps and pains, low energy levels, apathy, poor concentration, teeth grinding and nausea.

How much? Adult RDA 3–7 mg.

SONA: 25 mg.

Food sources: Beef, pork, chicken, legumes, soya beans, avocados, mushrooms, green vegetables, bananas, oranges, whole grains, wheatgerm.

Toxicity: None seen in doses up to 100 times the RDA.

Comment: Pantothenic acid is easily available in a wide variety of foods. Significant amounts are lost in refining of grains. Although most people tend not to be measurably deficient in this nutrient, many people with chemical sensitivities often show positive responses following supplementation, suggesting that their total body levels and reserves must have been low.

B.1.6 Vitamin B6 (Pyridoxine)

Functions: Metabolism of carbohydrates, protein and fats for energy. Involved in production of red blood cells and many enzymes. Aids in formation and maintenance of the nervous system and immune system, regulation of mental processes and mood. Vital in chemical detoxification.

Deficiency signs: Tingling in hands, depression, anxiety, muscle cramps and tremors, low energy levels, dry skin, poor ability to detoxify chemicals.

How much? Adult RDA 1.2–1.4 mg.

SONA: 5–25 mg.

Food sources: Cooked dried beans and peas, nutritional yeast, beef liver, wheatgerm, nuts, bananas, avocados, leafy greens, cabbage, cauliflower, potatoes, whole grains, dried fruit, fish, venison.

Toxicity: Toxic to the nervous system when taken in supplements in doses above 1,000 mg.

Comment: Approximately 60 per cent of people with chemical sensitivities are deficient in vitamin B6. High degrees of vitamin B6 deficiencies are also seen in older people or people taking prescription medications such as the contraceptive pill. Unfortunately, in addition to being one of the most important nutrients with respect to our entire metabolism and detoxification system, it appears to be one of the most vulnerable to deficiency owing to increased usage and problems with absorption. Supplementation is essential in most cases to ensure sufficient levels are received. As with all of the B vitamins, vitamin B6 works better if given as part of a general B vitamin complex.

B.1.7 'Vitamin' B7 (Biotin)

Functions: Metabolism of carbohydrates, protein and fats for energy.

Deficiency signs: Anorexia, depression, fatigue, muscle pain and weakness, anaemia, alopecia.

How much? Adult RDA 10–200 mcg.

SONA: 50–200 mcg.

Food sources: Oatmeal, nutritional yeast, legumes, soya beans, mushrooms, bananas, nuts, whole grains, egg, milk.

Toxicity: No known toxic levels.

Comment: Despite not being a true B vitamin, biotin is included for completeness in this category as it works with other B vitamins, and therefore is best supplemented as part of a B vitamin complex. Because it is used to break down alcohol, chemicals and certain drugs, exposure to these substances can result in biotin deficiency. Supplementation can help improve the above conditions.

B.1.8 Vitamin B12 (Cyanocobalamin)

Functions: Metabolism of carbohydrates, protein and fats for energy. Formation and maintenance of the nervous system. Essential for detoxifying chemicals and for replacement and maintenance of all body cells.

Deficiency signs: Low energy levels, anxiety, mouth sensitivity to heat or cold, irritability, eczema or dermatitis, sore muscles, pale complexion, hair loss.

How much? Adult RDA 1.5 mcg.

SONA: 2–3 mcg.

Food sources: Liver, oysters, kidney, fish (all types), mussels, nutritional yeast, fortified foods and soya milk.

Toxicity: No known toxic levels.

Comment: 15 per cent of people with chemical sensitivities are deficient in vitamin B12. Smoking and alcohol rapidly use up this nutrient, increasing the risk of deficiency. Other similar 'anti-vitamin B12' substances include coffee, laxatives and prescription medications. Liver diseases and bowel absorption problems increase the need for B12. Supplementation of this nutrient is beneficial in many conditions, but particularly helpful in alcoholism, and in those with detoxification problems.

B.1.9 Folate (Folic acid)

Functions: Synthesis of DNA. Essential for normal growth and maintenance of all cells. Involved in the production of neuro-transmitters that regulate mood, sleep and appetite. Important in the creation of new foetal and maternal tissue during pregnancy. Prevents heart disease by reducing homocysteine levels in blood.

Deficiency signs: Stomach pains, eczema, premature greying, cracked lips, poor appetite, poor energy, anaemia, depression.

How much? Adult RDA 200 mcg.

SONA: 400–1,000 mcg.

Food sources: Dark green leafy vegetables, nutritional yeast, beans, avocados, wheatgerm, various fruits like banana and orange, whole grains, walnuts, peanuts.

Toxicity: No known toxic effects, but large doses (4 mg) could mask a B12 deficiency, causing nerve problems to progress unde-tected to an irreversible stage.

Comment: Up to 15 per cent of those sensitive to chemicals are also deficient in folic acid. Deficiency is also found in those with a greater exposure to chemicals, as this increases the demand for this nutrient.

B.1.10 Vitamin C (Ascorbic acid)
Functions: Formation and maintenance of collagen, which strengthens connective tissues and encourages healing. Promotes healthy teeth, gums and bones. Antioxidant. Strengthens immunity. Detoxifies chemicals. Helps boost energy production.
Deficiency signs: Poor general immunity, increased colds, low energy levels, muscle pain, bleeding or tender gums, easy bruising, nose bleeds, slow wound healing.
How much? Adult RDA 40 mg.
SONA: 400–1,000 mg.
Food sources: Fresh fruits and vegetables, green pepper, broccoli, citrus fruits, tomatoes, guava, strawberries, blackcurrants.
Toxicity: May cause bowel looseness in excess, but this is not thought to be a sign of toxicity as it quickly stops when dose is lowered.
Comment: Up to 50 per cent of those sensitive to chemicals may be deficient in or have an abnormally high need for vitamin C. This is because of the increased level of chemical-induced free radicals. This nutrient appears to be very useful in rapidly calming down pollutant- or stress-induced reactions.

B.1.11 Vitamin D
Functions: Regulates absorption and use of calcium and phosphorus. Helps the formation of bones and teeth. Aids in maintenance of healthy nerve and muscle system.
Deficiency signs: Tooth decay, muscle cramps, joint pain or stiffness, hair loss, immune system problems.
How much? Adult RDA 200–600 IUs.
SONA: 400–800 IUs.
Food sources: Sunlight (20 minutes of direct sunshine, three times per week, is enough for our vitamin D needs), butter, cheese, milk, egg, fish, fortified foods and beverages.
Toxicity: Upper recommended limit 2,000 IUs.

Comment: While 15 per cent of people with chemical sensitivities appear to be deficient in this nutrient, another 15 per cent appear to have excess vitamin D. This nutrient has been found to help cases of acne, allergies, colds, tooth decay, lack of sunlight, rickets, diabetes, bone, skin and joint diseases.

B.1.12 Vitamin E (Tocopherol)

Functions: Antioxidant. Protects body cells and tissues from damage; regulates use and storage of vitamin A. Enhances detoxification. Prevents premature ageing, cancer and heart disease. May alleviate symptoms of premenstrual syndrome (PMS). Vital in detoxifying chemicals and tackling tissue-damaging, pollutant-induced free radicals.

Deficiency signs: Exhaustion post-exercise, poor wound healing, infertility, reduced sex drive, varicose veins.

How much? Adult RDA 15 IUs.

SONA: 400–800 IUs.

Food sources: Unrefined vegetable oils, seeds, nuts, wheatgerm, spinach, peaches, avocados, broccoli, dried prunes, whole wheat.

Toxicity: Relatively non-toxic below 1,200 IUs. However, if you have high blood pressure, rheumatic heart disease or are taking blood-thinning (anticoagulant) medications or digitalis, start with 100 IUs and consult your doctor since vitamin E possesses a blood-thinning effect, usually highly beneficial, but together with powerful anticoagulant medication could cause an excess of this effect.

Comment: The rising levels of pollutants has meant that the level of vitamin E we now need to deal with toxins appears to have risen above that which we can reasonably get from our food. To ensure that you get enough, it is best to use supplements. The better supplement form of vitamin E is D-alpha tocopherol and not the synthetic dl-alpha tocopherol. High-temperature cooking, such as frying, can increase the body's need for this nutrient even further, as can prescription medications, such as the contraceptive pill, and excessive intake of refined or processed fats and oils.

B.1.13 Co-enzyme Q10

Functions: Antioxidant. Important in energy metabolism, improves heart function, lowers blood pressure, increases exercise tolerance, improves immunity.

Deficiency signs: Low energy levels, heart disease, low exercise tolerance, poor immunity.

How much? No adult RDA.

SONA: None, but useful levels range from 10–90 mg a day.

Food sources: Fish (mackerel, sardines), soya oil, sesame seeds, walnuts, spinach.

Toxicity: None known.

Comment: The best supplements provide this nutrient in a lipid base, as this enhances absorption.

B.2 Minerals

B.2.1 Magnesium

Functions: Metabolism of carbohydrates, protein and fats for energy. Synthesis of genetic material. Functions in muscle relaxation and contraction, calms down an overactive immune system, improves nerve transmission, prevents tooth decay and heart problems, strengthens bones and teeth, promotes healthy limb and heart muscles.

Deficiency signs: Muscle weakness or tremor and spasm, insomnia, high blood pressure, irregular heartbeat, constipation, fits or convulsions, hyperactivity, depression, poor energy levels, confusion, lack of appetite, calcium deposited in body in form of kidney stones or in other soft tissues.

How much? Adult RDA 300 mg.

SONA: 375–500 mg.

Food sources: Wheatgerm, all nuts and seeds, tofu, broccoli, spinach, Swiss chard, soya beans, tomato purée, all pulses (peas, beans and lentils), brewer's yeast, sweet potato, squash, avocados, bananas, dark green leafy vegetables, low-fat yoghurt, milk.

Toxicity: Kidneys are efficient at excreting excess magnesium.

Comment: This mineral, often referred to as the relaxing mineral, appears to be one of the most important minerals required for all chemical detoxification. It is also essential for alcohol breakdown. However, this increased need, compounded by lower levels in food owing to processing and modern farming methods, has resulted in a very large percentage of people having sub-optimal or deficient levels of magnesium. Supplementation is often highly effective in treating high blood pressure, high cholesterol, depression, anxiety attacks, heart failure, heart attacks, kidney stones, childhood behavioural disorders, overweight, tooth decay and failure to detoxify chemicals. Since most vitamins and mineral multis contain very small amounts of magnesium, in most cases individual supplementation of this nutrient is required.

B.2.2 Zinc

Functions: Essential component in numerous metabolic and detoxing enzymes in the body and for healthy prostate gland function. Detoxifier. Essential for metabolism of carbohydrates, protein and fats for energy. Allows the proper functioning of insulin, maintenance of genetic code, aids wound and burn healing. Needed for healthy teeth and assists bone and hair growth.
Deficiency signs: Low energy, low fertility. White marks on more than two fingernails, poor immune system, frequent infections, stretch marks, acne or greasy skin, depression, loss of appetite.
How much? Adult RDA 15 mg.
SONA: 15–20 mg.
Food sources: Oysters, beef, wheatgerm, nuts, including walnuts and almonds, seeds, including pumpkin and sunflower seeds, fish, beans, mushrooms, whole grain products.
Toxicity: Relatively non-toxic. Larger doses might inhibit copper absorption and reduce iron absorption and cause illness, and 2 g or more would start to cause symptoms of gastric irritation, vomiting, reduced growth and stiffness.
Comment: This mineral is often found lacking in many people, particularly those sensitive to chemicals. As low levels are associated with many of the twenty-first century health problems, supplementation has helped treat many conditions, such as prostate diseases, wound healing, acne, alcoholism, failure of detoxification and lowered immunity.

B.2.3 Selenium

Functions: Antioxidant, protects against cancer and heart disease. Important for normal development of foetus during pregnancy. Protects against increased chemically triggered free radicals, reduces inflammation, stimulates the immune system to fight infections, required for male fertility and for metabolism.

Deficiency signs: Premature ageing, family history of cancer, frequent infections, high blood pressure and cataracts.

How much? Adult RDA 70 mcg.

SONA: 100 mcg.

Food sources: Brazil nuts, kidney, fish, seafoods, dried beans and other pulses, wholemeal bread, liver, all plant foods grown in selenium-rich soil.

Toxicity: Can be toxic if consumed in amounts greater than 600–750 mcg.

Comment: Modern farming techniques and food processing lower levels of this mineral in foods. It appears to be beneficial in cases of toxic metal poisoning and chemical sensitivity.

B.2.4 Iron

Functions: Manufacture of haemoglobin, transportation of oxygen in blood to all the body cells. Strengthens the immune system. Improves athletic performance. Component of a large number of enzymes. Vital for energy production.

Deficiency signs: Low energy, breathlessness, anaemia, pale skin, fatigue, loss of appetite, nausea, sensitivity to cold, underactive immune system.

How much? Adult RDA 10–14 mg.

SONA: 15 mg.

Food sources: Dark green leafy vegetables, pulses, nuts and seeds, blackstrap molasses, sea vegetables, dried fruits, whole and enriched grains.

Toxicity: If excess iron is accumulated this might catalyse the formation of free radicals, and thus increase the risk of cancer and heart disease.

Comment: Iron deficiency is thought to be one of the commonest nutrient deficiencies in the world. Almost half the women and 20 per cent of the men in developing countries suffer from some degree of iron deficiency. Substances that lower iron levels include tea, spinach, fizzy drinks, food additives, antacids and a high zinc intake. Iron can also be beneficial in people with fatigue but who test with apparently normal blood levels of iron, so a trial supplementation of iron could be of value.

B.2.5 Potassium
Functions: Helps maintain normal balance and distribution of fluids throughout the body. Regulates nerve transmission and many cell membrane functions. Controls normal blood pressure, proper calcium balance and heartbeat.

Deficiency signs: Rapid irregular heartbeat, muscle weakness, pins and needles, irritability, vomiting, diarrhoea, low blood pressure, confusion.

How much? Adult RDA 2,000 mg.

SONA: 2,000 mg.

Food sources: Fruits, vegetables, grains, potatoes, avocados, bananas, oranges, cooked dried beans and peas, dried fruits.

Toxicity: Uncommon to reach levels high enough to cause problems.

Comment: Many substances lower the body's levels of potassium, such as salt, alcohol, sugar, diuretics, laxatives and corticosteroids, as does stress.

B.2.6 Calcium
Functions: Main function is development and maintenance of healthy bones and teeth. Aids in blood clotting. Essential in production and activity of numerous enzymes and hormones that regulate digestion, energy and fat metabolism, and in nerve transmission.

Deficiency signs: Muscle cramps or tremors, high blood pressure, joint pain or arthritis, insomnia and nervousness, tooth decay.

How much? Adult RDA 800 mg.

SONA: 800–1,000 mg.

Food sources: Dairy products, fish, eggs, oysters, dark green leafy vegetables, broccoli, cooked dried beans, soya products including milk, nuts, seeds, dried fruits, sea vegetables, calcium-fortified foods such as tofu and orange juice.

Toxicity: Excessive intake might increase risk for calcium deposition into soft tissues, reduce zinc and iron absorption, impair vitamin K metabolism.

Comment: Should not need separate calcium supplement over and above that present in a multivitamin and mineral tablet if you are taking additional magnesium, as this will improve the levels of calcium your body absorbs.

B.2.7 Chromium

Functions: Main value appears to be as a component of glucose tolerance factor, which maintains normal blood sugar levels by increasing and regulating insulin effectiveness. Stimulates synthesis of protein.

Deficiency signs: Addiction to sweet foods, excessive or cold sweats, dizziness or irritability after six hours without food, need for frequent meals, cold hands, need for excessive sleep or drowsiness in the day, excessive thirst.

How much? No adult RDA.

SONA: 100 mcg.

Food sources: Mushrooms, nuts, oysters, beef, nutritional yeast, wholegrain breads, spices and herbs.

Toxicity: Excess intake can inhibit, instead of enhance, the effectiveness of insulin.

Comment: Cases of mild diabetes can respond to chromium supplements.

B.3 Essential fatty acids

B.3.1 Omega-3 (Linolenic acid)

Functions: Important for normal functioning of all body tissues; helps prevent atherosclerosis, reduce incidence of heart disease, depression and stroke, and bring relief from the symptoms associated with ulcerative colitis, menstrual pain and joint pain. Also plays major role in detoxifying chemicals and increasing energy levels, reducing inflammation in the body and in keeping skin supple.

Deficiency signs: Depression, fatigue, low energy, dry, itchy skin, brittle hair and nails, inability to concentrate, joint pain, constipation and frequent colds.

How much? No adult RDA, but the US National Institutes of Health recommend that people consume at least 2 per cent of their total daily calories as omega-3 oils. To meet this recommendation, a person consuming 2,000 calories per day should eat at least 4 g of omega-3 oils. For instance, two tablespoons of flax seeds contain 3.5 g of omega-3 oils. Fish oil contains a more concentrated form of omega-3, but tends to be highly polluted with environmental toxins and heavy metals. There are some much safer fish oil products on the market, such as Dr Sear's OmegaRx Ultra-Refined fish oil, which have had these chemicals actively removed by a distillation process. Four one-gram capsules of this oil contain 2.4 g of omega-3.

Food sources: Found widely in nuts, seeds, vegetables, beans and fruits; vegetable oils such as rapeseed, flax seed, soya bean, walnut and wheatgerm; salmon, halibut, sardines, albacore, trout and herring. Other foods that contain omega-3 include prawns, clams, light chunk tuna, catfish, cod and spinach.

Toxicity: All fats can increase free-radical production, so it's best to ensure you are taking a supplement that contains good levels of vitamin E.

Comment: Recent statistics indicate that nearly 99 per cent of people in the USA do not eat enough omega-3, whilst 60 per cent of Americans are frankly deficient in omega-3, and about 20 per cent have so little that test methods cannot even detect any in their blood. However, the symptoms of omega-3 deficiency are very vague, and can often be attributed to some other health conditions or nutrient deficiencies. Consequently, few people realise that they are not consuming enough omega-3 oils. One of the reasons so few people are getting these oils is because their use is minimised in processed foods as their tendency to go rancid quickly means a shorter shelf life. Omega-3 may play a role in the prevention and/or treatment of the following health conditions: Alzheimer's disease, asthma, attention deficit hyperactivity disorder (ADHD), bipolar disorder, cancer, cardiovascular disease, depression, diabetes, eczema, high blood pressure, Huntington's disease, lupus, migraine headaches, multiple sclerosis, obesity, osteoarthritis, osteoporosis, psoriasis, rheumatoid arthritis. When purchasing an omega-3 supplement, remember that these oils are highly sensitive to damage from heat, light and oxygen. Choose a certified organic or chemical-free product that has been kept refrigerated and is packaged in a dark brown or green glass jar, and be sure to store the product in your refrigerator or freezer.

B.3.2 Omega-6 (Linoleic acid)

Functions: Important for normal functioning of all body tissues; may prevent atherosclerosis, reduce incidence of heart disease and stroke, and bring relief from the symptoms associated with ulcerative colitis, menstrual pain and joint pain.

Deficiency signs: Excessive thirst, frequent urination, rough, dry skin and hair, increased frequency of colds. May follow antibiotic use.

How much? No adult RDA, but omega-6 should make up 3–5 per cent of total daily calorific intake. To meet this recommendation, a person consuming 2,000 calories per day should eat at least 6–10 g of omega-6 oils.

Food sources: Nuts and seeds, especially sunflower seeds; vegetable oils such as blackcurrant, borage, evening primrose, hemp, corn, safflower, sunflower, soya bean and cottonseed.

Toxicity: All fats and oils increase free-radical production.

Comment: Normally most people tend to get sufficient levels of omega-6 in their diet, so supplementation is not as important as omega-3 oils. Indeed, it appears to be more important that the ratio of omega-6 to omega-3 oils is balanced, at around 2:1, as too much omega-6 can upset the system. Since Western diets tend to have a ratio of omega-6 to omega-3 oils of as much as 20:1, in most cases people need only supplement omega-3 oils to get the balance right.

B.4 Amino acids

B.4.1 Glutathione

Functions: This powerful antioxidant helps detoxify the liver of poisonous chemicals, especially alcohol and mercury. In addition to being a neurotransmitter, it promotes healthy immune function, and is crucial in protecting cells against free-radical damage. It also helps protect the stomach lining against stomach acid.

Deficiency signs: Lowered immunity and reduced ability to detoxify chemicals, premature ageing.

How much? No adult RDA.

Supplementary ranges: 200–3,000 mg a day.

Food sources: Fresh fruit and vegetables, especially asparagus and avocados, and fresh meats.

Toxicity: Do not take in very high doses (greater than 7 g per day). Patients with cystinuria (excessive cysteine excretion) should not take it. People with liver or kidney disease should seek their doctor's approval before taking amino acid supplements.

Comment: Glutathione is one of the body's most important and powerful antioxidants. It is a composition of three amino acids (cysteine, glutamic acid and glycine) and protects against damage caused by exposure to pesticides, plastics, smoke, nitrates and drugs. It also helps prevent ageing, cancer, cataracts, Parkinson's disease, rheumatoid arthritis, schizophrenia, heavy metal poisoning (arsenic, lead, mercury) and ulcers caused by medications such as NSAIDS (non-steroidal anti-inflammatory drugs), and helps safeguard fertility.

B.4.2 MSM-sulphur

Functions: MSM stands for methylsulphonylmethane. This is an organic sulphur compound that exists to some extent in all living things and is a basic nutrient required for the proper functioning of the body. As a dietary supplement, MSM is strongly recommended for neutralising and eliminating toxins, particularly toxic metals such as mercury. It also can help alleviate conditions of environmental and food allergies, gives pain relief from inflammatory disorders, such as arthritis and sore muscles, and has been used to treat gastointestinal ailments, emphysema, diabetes (sulphur is a component of insulin), sunburn and infection. It is known as the 'beauty mineral' because it fortifies the skin cells, preventing wrinkling, and strengthens the hair and nails.

Deficiency signs: Slow wound healing, scar tissue, brittle hair and/or nails, gastointestinal problems, arthritis, acne, allergies and immune system disorders, and depression, among others.

How much? 1,500 mg a day.

Supplementary ranges: 500–6000 mg.

Food sources: MSM-sulphur is a natural form of sulphur found in many foods, including meat, seafood, milk, fruit, cabbage, broccoli, wheatgerm, eggs, lentils and asparagus. However, processing, storage and cooking of foods destroys essential MSM-sulphur.

Toxicity: It is thought that you cannot overdose with MSM, since the body will use what it needs then flushes out the rest without harm. An unwanted side effect is wind, which can be avoided by initially taking low levels of this nutrient then building levels up slowly over days/weeks. It is important for people who react to sulphites in wine or other products to avoid using MSM-sulphur. People with a particular inability to detoxify, such as those with inflammatory bowel disease, chemical sensitivities and autism, may possibly also react to it, so this supplement should be taken cautiously a few weeks after the other supplements have been started. Any reaction would therefore be readily identified and the MSM-sulphur easily stopped.

Comment: Most people are deficient in this nutrient, so supplementation is usually greatly beneficial. Its abilities to mobilise and remove mercury from the kidneys safely makes it an essential supplement for all those who have, or have ever had, mercury amalgam fillings, or mercury from vaccinations. All my family take this supplement regularly.

B.5 Fibre

B.5.1 Soluble fibre

Functions: Soluble fibre is vital for enhancing bowel function and providing a food source for gut bacteria to produce essential vitamins and suppress harmful gut micro-organisms. It is also used to lower levels of body cholesterol, by binding to it on its passage through the gut. As it removes these cholesterols it also removes many of the body's most persistent pollutants found in the cholesterol, thereby making it one of the most important substances available in promoting detoxification of both toxic metals and synthetic chemicals, particularly organochlorines.

How much? No adult RDA, but a UK Department of Health committee recommends 18–32 g of fibre per day (from foods and supplements), without specifying the proportion of soluble or insoluble fibre.

Food sources: Oats, barley, pulses (peas, beans and lentils), citrus fruit, apples, brown rice, apricots, plums, broccoli, carrots, peas, potatoes, squash.

Toxicity: Fibre supplements are generally well tolerated. However, allergy to psyllium husks has been reported. Rare cases of intestinal obstruction have occurred in individuals consuming high amounts of fibre supplements in a dry, un-hydrated form without also taking adequate fluids, or with pre-existing gastrointestinal problems. High fibre intake, more than 40 g a day, may reduce the absorption of essential minerals including zinc, calcium and iron, and certain prescription medications.

Comment: Since addition of fibre to the diet may initially result in gas, diarrhoea or constipation, increase slowly over a period of days to minimise this side-effect. Always drink a minimum of eight glasses of water a day to prevent constipation. In the lower intestine, soluble fibre is broken down by bacteria, so unlike insoluble fibre it doesn't help keep you regular. However, soluble fibre has also been linked to reduced risk of some cancers, including colon cancer and cancer of the larynx. It also plays a role in improving weight control, preventing cardiovascular disease, lowering blood pressure and blood cholesterol, improving sugar metabolism, enhancing gastrointestinal health, and promoting healthy gut microflora.

B.5.2 Insoluble fibre

Functions: To enhance bowel regularity. By speeding up the passage of waste products through the bowel it reduces the time toxic waste products are present in the body.

How much? No adult RDA, but a UK Department of Health committee recommends 18–32 g of fibre per day, without specifying the proportion of soluble or insoluble fibre.

Food sources: Wholegrain varieties of starchy foods, such as wholemeal bread, wholegrain breakfast cereals, brown rice, wholegrain pasta and pulses, fruit and vegetables are particularly good sources of insoluble fibre.

Toxicity: A relatively safe substance. However, some studies have shown wheat bran to be an irritant at high levels, and when supplemented in high amounts in the absence of soluble fibre, can actually increase cholesterol levels.

Comment: This type of fibre, also known as roughage, is the kind most people associate with fibre. It's important in preventing constipation and associated problems such as haemorrhoids.

B.6 Popular herbals

B.6.1 Echinacea angustifolia (Purple cone flower)

Main uses: Echinacea is used for its many immune system-enhancing properties. It decreases inflammatory allergic reactions to mild food allergies, has antiviral, antifungal, antibacterial and anti-inflammatory properties, and enhances white-cell stimulation and production.

Toxicity: None known.

Comment: This popular herbal has been used by the Native American Indians for hundreds of years and is thought to help those with the following conditions: AIDS, bronchitis, Crohn's disease, cystitis, herpes simplex, irritable bowel syndrome, mastitis, ear infections, ulcerative colitis, infections such as colds, skin problems such as recurrent boils and acne, and tonsillitis. Reduces recurrence rate of vaginal candidiasis (thrush) when used in conjunction with econazole nitrate cream applied locally.

B.6.2 Milk thistle (Silybum marianum)

Main uses: This commonly used and powerful antioxidant and detoxifier can boost the liver's ability to break down chemicals. It also helps prevent tumours from occurring, fights existing cervical cancer cells and reduces liver inflammation.

Toxicity: Very low. Although not a toxicity as such, owing to its ability to increase bile flow, stools may be looser.

Comment: Milk thistle helps those with cholecystitis, hepatitis, psoriasis, psoriatic arthritis, cirrhosis, cholangitis and fatty infiltration of the liver. It also helps prevent kidney damage from the anti-cancer drug cisplatin without decreasing its anti-tumour effectiveness, and helps prevent liver damage from paracetamol, alcohol, halothane and phenothiazines.

B.6.3 Garlic (Allium sativum)

Main uses: It enhances various immune functions. Garlic has been shown to modify, both directly and indirectly, the function of immune cells that play a leading role in promoting good health and preventing infections and cancer. It helps protect against heart disease, lowers blood pressure and blood cholesterol, is a digestive stimulant and diuretic, and helps thin the blood, preventing excessive blood clotting.

Toxicity: Should not be used in allergic contact dermatitis, in those with goitres, and those with increased white cells in the blood (leukocytosis). Also should not be used in organ transplants and pemphigus. Care should be taken in those on warfarin or other blood-thinning drugs, as garlic can increase their anti-coagulant action. If consuming high doses of garlic, do not take ginkgo biloba or high-dose vitamin E.

Comment: Garlic has been cultivated in the Middle East as a culinary spice and medicinal herb for more than 5,000 years and is an important part of traditional Chinese medicine. Garlic is mentioned in the Bible and the Talmud. Hippocrates, Galen, Pliny the Elder and Dioscorides all mention the use of garlic for its many health benefits. Its use in China was first mentioned in AD 510. It is now thought to benefit the following conditions: AIDS, asthma, atherosclerosis, candidiasis, fatigue, diabetes, high blood pressure, high cholesterol, bacterial, viral and fungal infections and parasitic infestations, cancer, cardiovascular diseases, flatulence, and inflammatory and respiratory conditions. Fresh garlic is the best form.

B.6.4 Ginger (Zingiber officinale)

Main uses: Improves motion sickness, eases nausea symptoms and is used as a digestive aid. Helps prevent deep vein thrombosis in the legs and excessive clotting, lowers cholesterol levels, helps prevent atherosclerosis and strengthens heart muscle.

Toxicity: People with gallstones should not take ginger without consulting a doctor, but otherwise very low toxicity.

Comment: Can cause sensation of heat and burning within the stomach so patients with 'sensitive' stomachs may not always tolerate ginger. Ginger has been used in the treatment of atherosclerosis, bronchitis, congestive heart failure, constipation, high blood pressure, memory loss, migraine, headache, psoriatic arthritis, cardiac diseases, colds, chemotherapy-induced vomiting, menstrual cramps, motion sickness, drug-induced nausea, post-operative nausea, gut cramps due to undigested foods, gas and bloating.

B.6.5 Ginkgo biloba

Main uses: This popular antioxidant improves memory in Alzheimer's patients, enhances blood flow, helps prevent blood clots, reduces brain swelling, improves energy levels, aids brain functioning, helps protect against radiation damage, protects transplanted kidneys against damage from drugs (ciclosporin) used in transplantation patients.

Toxicity: Allergic skin reaction, headaches, gut upsets (rare). Should not be taken with other blood-thinning drugs or high doses of garlic or vitamin E. Aspirin and ginkgo taken concurrently may produce spontaneous bleeding due to reduced platelet clotting activity. Should not be used in amenorrhoea (failure to menstruate), menorrhagia (heavy menstrual bleeding). Since ginkgo increases blood supply to the brain, caution is to be taken in high-risk stroke patients.

Comment: Has been used to counteract the effects of ageing and treat the following conditions: Alzheimer's disease, chronic fatigue syndrome, congestive heart failure, depression, eczema, high blood pressure, hypothyroidism, impotence, visual loss from macular degeneration, memory loss, multiple sclerosis, schizophrenia, bed-wetting, tinnitus, varicose veins, dizziness, dementia, coronary ischaemia, chemical toxicity, diabetic retinopathy, senility.

B.6.6 Ginseng (Chinese ginseng, Korean ginseng)

Main uses: Improves fatigue, enhances physical performance, reduces stress, enhances natural immunity, helps improve diabetic control and prevents excessive blood clotting.

Toxicity: Although side-effects are rare, they include menstrual abnormalities, breast tenderness, high blood pressure and insomnia. Ginseng is not recommended for those with acute illnesses, such as colds or flu, or for those with bronchitis, excessive menstrual bleeding, those on warfarin (as it increases the anticoagulant effect), those with hypertension or who suffer from low blood sugar. It is also not advised in pregnancy or for children, and should not be taken with stimulants including high caffeine intake.

Comment: It is also used to prevent ageing effects, improve concentration and treat congestive heart failure, diabetes mellitus, memory loss, sexual dysfunction, including impotence, insomnia and stress.

B.6.7 St John's wort (Hypericum perforatum)

Main uses: It can be taken in capsule form or applied to the skin to treat wounds, inflammation, muscle aches and first-degree burns. Taken orally it helps treat depression, premenstrual syndrome and seasonal affective disorder (SAD). St John's wort also has immune-enhancing effects, and is used as an antibacterial, anti-inflammatory, and antiviral, and has astringent actions. It also protects the liver from damage, raises the level of melatonin, and has a sedative effect.

Toxicity: It can cause photosensitivity (skin and eyes become sensitive to light), especially in fair-skinned people. It may also cause allergic reactions. It is not recommended for severe or chronic depression. It should not be taken with antidepressants or alcohol and should be avoided in pregnancy.

Comment: St John's wort has also been used to treat AIDS, anorexia nervosa, manic depression, haemorrhoids, herpes simplex type 1 and 2, incontinence, insomnia, migraine, headaches, ear infections, circulatory disorders, facial neuralgia after dental extractions and toothache.

B.6.8 Saw palmetto (Serenoa repens)

Main uses: Its uses are based on its anti-oestrogenic, hormone-balancing actions. It is used to treat benign enlarged prostate and improve overall prostate health, enhance sexual vigour and breast size, and as a diuretic.

Toxicity: Although rare, this includes gut disturbances and headaches, and large amounts can cause diarrhoea.

Comment: This herbal has also been used to treat impotence, chronic emaciating diseases where there is weight loss, weakness, debility and tissue wasting, painful urination, low libido, and bladder stones.

Appendix C
Vaccines and their Chemical Ingredients

This is a list of some of the more commonly used types of vaccines on the market taken from the 1997 Physicians' Desk Reference. This list of ingredients and companies is correct to the best of my knowledge. However, since companies are constantly merging and certain ingredients are in the process of being phased out, some of these details may change.

Name: Acel-Immune DTaP
Headline components: Diphtheria and Tetanus Toxoids and Acellular Pertussis (whooping cough) Vaccine
Produced by: Lederle Laboratories
Ingredients include: Thimerosal (mercury), aluminium hydroxide, aluminium phosphate, formaldehyde, polysorbate 80, gelatin (animal parts/bovine)
Note: This vaccine is commonly known as the 'triple' DTP vaccine and has been given to babies in the UK for many years in the first few months of life. However, by the time of publication of this book, this vaccine is due to have been replaced in the UK by a '5 in 1' vaccine, to be produced by the company Aventis Pasteur. This '5 in 1' jab is due to contain the antigens for diphtheria, tetanus, whooping cough, polio and Hib meningitis (DTaP/IPV/Hib). Despite the absence of thimerosal, these vaccines are likely to contain a number of other chemical toxic metal additives such as aluminium; however, information about

this vaccine and its chemical ingredients was not available at the time of writing from this company's website.

Name: Act HIB
Headline components: Haemophilus Influenzae Type B (Hib) Tetanus Toxoid Conjugate
Produced by: Connaught Laboratories/Aventis Pasteur SA
Ingredients include: Thimerosal (mercury), ammonium sulphate, formalin, sucrose
Medium: Semi-synthetic

Name: Attenuvax
Headline components: Measles Virus Vaccine Live
Produced by: Merck & Co, Inc.
Ingredients include: Neomycin, sorbitol, hydrolised gelatine
Medium: Chick embryo

Name: DPT
Headline components: Diphtheria and Tetanus Toxoids and Pertussis (whooping cough) Vaccine Adsorbed
Produced by: SmithKline Beecham Pharmaceuticals
Ingredients include: Thimerosal, aluminium phosphate, formaldehyde, ammonium sulphate, washed sheep red blood cells, glycerol, sodium chloride
Medium: Porcine (pig) pancreatic hydrolysate of casein

Name: Energix-B
Headline components: Hepatitis B
Produced by: SmithKline Beecham Pharmaceuticals
Ingredients include: Thimerosal, aluminium hydroxide
Medium: Yeast (possibly 5% residual)

Name: Havrix
Headline components: Hepatitis A
Produced by: SmithKline Beecham Pharmaceuticals
Ingredients include: Aluminium hydroxide, formalin, phenoxyethanol (antifreeze), polysorbate 20, residual MRC5

proteins (from medium), medium human diploid cells (originating from human aborted foetal tissue)

Name: Biavax
Headline components: Rubella and Mumps Virus Vaccine Live
Produced by: Merck & Co, Inc.
Ingredients include: Neomycin, sorbitol, hydrolised gelatine
Medium: Human diploid cells (originating from human aborted foetal tissue)

Name: HibTiter
Headline components: Haemophilus Influenzae Type B (Hib)
Produced by: Lederle Laboratories
Ingredients include: Thimerosal (mercury), polyribosylribitol, ammonium sulphate
Medium: Chemically defined, yeast based

Name: Fluvirin
Headline components: Influenza Virus Vaccine
Produced by: Medeva Pharmaceuticals/Evans Vaccines Limited UK
Ingredients include: Thimerosal (mercury), embryonic fluid (chicken egg), neomycin, polymyxin, betapropiolactone
Medium: Embryonic fluid (chicken egg)

Name: FluShield
Headline components: Influenza Virus Vaccine, Trivalent, Types A&B
Produced by: Wyeth–Ayerst
Ingredients include: Thimerosal (mercury), gentamicin sulphate, formaldehyde, polysorbate 80, tri(n)butylphosphate
Medium: Chick embryos

Name: IPOL
Headline components: Inactivated Polio Vaccine
Produced by: Connaught Laboratories
Ingredients include: 3 types of polio virus, formaldehyde,

phenoxyethanol (antifreeze), neomycin, streptomycin, polymyxin B
Medium: VERO cells, a continuous line of monkey kidney cells

Name: MMR
Headline components: Measles Mumps Rubella Live Virus Vaccine
Produced by: Merck & Co., Inc.
Ingredients include: Sorbitol, neomycin, hydrolysed gelatine
Mediums: M&M - chick embryo, Rubella - human diploid cells (originating from human aborted foetal tissue)

Name: M-R-Vax
Headline components: Measles and Rubella Virus Vaccine Live
Produced by: Merck & Co., Inc.
Ingredients include: Neomycin, sorbitol, hydrolysed gelatine
Mediums: M – chick embryo, R – human diploid cells (originating from human aborted foetal tissue)

Name: Menomune
Headline components: Meningococcal Polysaccharide Vaccine (meningitis)
Produced by: Connaught Laboratories
Ingredients include: Thimerosal (mercury), lactose
Medium: Freeze-dried polysaccharide antigens from Neisseria Meningitidis

Name: Meruvax II
Headline components: Rubella Virus Vaccine Live
Produced by: Merck & Co., Inc.
Ingredients include: Neomycin, sorbitol, hydrolysed gelatine
Medium: Human diploid cells (originating from human aborted foetal tissue)

Name: Mumpsvax
Headline components: Mumps Virus Vaccine Live
Produced by: Merck & Co., Inc.
Ingredients include: Neomycin, sorbitol, hydrolysed gelatine

Medium: Human diploid cells (originating from human aborted foetal tissue)

Name: Orimune
Headline components: Poliovirus Vaccine Live Oral Trivalent
Produced by: Lederle Laboratories
Ingredients include: 3 types of attenuated polioviruses, strepto-mycin, neomycin, calf serum, sorbitol
Medium: Monkey kidney cell culture

Name: Pneumovax
Headline components: Pneumococcal Vaccine Polyvalent
Produced by: Merck & Co., Inc.
Ingredients include: Phenol and capsular polysaccharides from the 23 most prevalent pneumococcal types

Name: Imovax
Headline components: Rabies Vaccine Adsorbed
Produced by: Connaught Laboratories
Ingredients include: neomycin sulphate, human albumin, phenol red indicator
Medium: Human diploid cells (originating from human aborted foetal tissue)

Name: Rabies Vaccine Adsorbed
Headline components: Rabies
Produced by: SmithKline Beecham Pharmaceuticals
Ingredients include: ethylmercurithiosalicylate (thimerosal/ mercury), aluminium phosphate, betapropiolactone, sodium phenol red
Medium: Foetal rhesus monkey lung cells

Name: Recombivax
Headline components: Hepatitis B Vaccine Recombinant
Produced by: Merck & Co., Inc.
Ingredients include: Thimerosal (mercury), aluminium hydroxide
Medium: Yeast (residual < 1% yeast protein)

Name: RotaShield
Headline components: Rotavirus Vaccine, Live, Oral, Tetravalent
Produced by: Wyeth–Ayerst Laboratories
Ingredients include: Monosodium glutamate (MSG), 1 rhesus monkey rotavirus, 3 rhesus-human reassortant viruses, sucrose, potassium monophosphate, potassium diphosphate, foetal bovine serum, neomycin sulphate, amphotericin B
Medium: Foetal rhesus diploid cell line

Name: Varivax
Headline components: Varicella Virus Vaccine Live
Produced by: Merck & Co., Inc.
Ingredients include: Produced using sucrose, phosphate, monosodium glutamate, processed gelatine
Medium: Human diploid cells (originating from human aborted foetal tissue)

Profiles of the above chemical additives

Aluminum: A toxic metal known to be toxic to nerves, lungs, etc. (see Appendix A: Common Toxic Chemicals).
Ammonium Sulphate: A toxin thought to damage the liver, gut, lungs and nerves.
Amphotericin B: A drug used to treat fungus infections. Side-effects include blood clots, blood defects, kidney problems, nausea and fever. When used on the skin, allergic reactions can occur.
Beta-Propiolactone: Recognised carcinogen (cancer-triggering chemical), and thought to poison the gut, liver, lung, nerve and skin. On at least five federal regulatory lists, it is ranked as one of the most hazardous compounds (worst 10%) to humans.
Formaldehyde: Recognised carcinogen (cancer-triggering chemical), thought to poison or damage the gut, liver, immune system, nervous system, fertility, lungs and skin. On at least eight federal regulatory lists: ranked as one of the most hazardous compounds (worst 10%) to ecosystems and human health.
Gentamicin Sulfate: An antibiotic.

Hydrolysed Gelatine: Obtained from selected pieces of calf and cattle skins, cattle bones and porkskin.

Neomycin: An antibiotic.

Phenol: Thought to poison the cardiovascular system, developing foetuses and children, gut, liver, kidney, nervous system, lungs and skin.

Phenoxyethanol: Thought to damage child development and fertility. It is commonly used as antifreeze.

Polymyxin: An antibiotic.

Polyribosylribitol: A component of the Hib bacterium.

Polysorbate: Thought to poison the skin and parts of the nervous system.

Sorbitol: Thought to damage the gut and the liver.

Streptomycin: An antibiotic.

Sucrose: Refined sugar.

Thimerosal: The mercury in thimerosal is known to damage many body systems, such as the nervous system, with developing foetuses and children being particularly vulnerable (see Appendix A: Common Toxic Chemicals).

Tri(n)butylphosphate: Kidney and nervous system poison.

Appendix D
Useful Contacts

Visit Dr Paula Baillie-Hamilton's website at
www.slimmingsystems.com

Environmental Medicine
To see a local specialist in environmental medicine, contact one
of the following organisations or individuals:

American Academy of Environmental Medicine
7701 East Kellogg, Suite 625, Wichita, KS 67207, USA
Tel: +1 316 684 5500
Fax: +1 316 684 5709
Website: www.aaem.com

Australasian College of Nutritional and Environmental Medicine
13 Hilton Street, Beaumaris, Victoria 3193, Australia
Tel: +61 3 9589 6088
Fax: +61 3 9589 5158

Australian Society for Environmental Medicine Inc.
2/11 Howell Close, Doncaster East, Victoria 3109, Australia
Tel: +61 3 9842 1886
Fax: +61 3 9841 4336

British Society for Allergy, Environmental and Nutritional
Medicine (BSAENM)
PO Box 7, Knighton, LD7 1WT
Tel: +44 (0) 1547 550378
Fax: +44 (0) 1547 550339
Website: www.jnem.demon.co.uk

Dr Damian Downing
Biolab Medical Unit, 9 Weymouth Street, London W1W 6DB
Appointments: 0845 166 2058/+44 (0) 1904 691591
Website: www.naltd.co.uk
Dr Downing, a specialist in environmental and nutritional medicine, also travels to several clinics around the UK.

Professor Kim Jobst
Herefordshire, United Kingdom
Tel: +44 (0) 1432 761340
Consultant physician and medical homeopath, with a special interest in healthcare and integrative medicine.

Dr John Mansfield
Burghwood Clinic, 34 Brighton Road, Banstead, Surrey SM7 1BS
Appointments: +44 (0) 1737 361177
Website: www.burghwoodclinic.co.uk
A specialist in environmental and nutritional medicine and vaccination issues.

Dr Sarah Myhill
Upper Weston, Llangunllo, Knighton, Powys LD7 1SL
Appointments: +44 (0) 1547 550331
Website: www.drmyhill.co.uk
A specialist in environmental and nutritional medicine, Dr Myhill also has a very good website.

Professor William Rea
Environmental Health Centre Dallas, 8345 Walnut Hill Lane, Suite 220, Dallas, Texas 75231, USA
Tel: +1 214 368 4132
Website: www.ehcd.com

Useful Companies
BioCare
BioCare Ltd, Lakeside, 180 Lifford Lane, Kings Norton, Birmingham B30 3NU
Tel: +44 (0) 121 433 3727

Website: www.biocare.co.uk
A mail-order company that also sells its products in selected
health food shops.

Biolab
Biolab Medical Unit, The Stone House, 9 Weymouth Street,
London W1W 6DB
Tel: +44 (0) 207 636 5959/5905
Website: www.biolab.co.uk
An excellent company that performs a wide range of tests for
doctors specialising in environmental and nutritional medicine.
It tests for toxic chemicals and nutritional status amongst other
factors. It also provides a referral list of medical doctors specialising in nutritional and environmental medicine and allergy
treatment. All doctors on this list are familiar with Biolab investigations and welcome patients who may benefit from their
laboratory tests. All samples have to be referred by medical
doctors.

Higher Nature
Higher Nature Limited, Burwash Common, East Sussex
TN19 7BR
Tel: +44 (0) 1435 882 880
Website: www.higher-nature.co.uk

Holland and Barrett
Tel: 0870 6066605
Website: www.hollandandbarrett.com
Chain of high-street supplement and health-food shops. Phone
for details of nearest branch.

Mynutrition
Tel: +44 (0) 1372 470730
Website: www.mynutrition.co.uk
A mail-order company that sells all the best brands of
supplements on the market. Also a great source for the harder-
to-find amino acids and other supplements.

Solgar Vitamin and Herb
500 Willow Tree Road, Leonia NJ 07605, USA
Tel: +1 877 765 4274
Website: www.solgar.co.uk

Nordic Naturals
One of the exceedingly few companies which make and sell potent, pollution-free fish oils, Nordic Naturals use the latest molecular distillation methods to remove all chemical contaminants. A good one to buy is Omega 3, which is available in soft gel-type oil capsules. You should take the daily dose they recommend, as the concentrated nature of their products means you will probably need to take smaller amounts, compared to those of other companies, to be effective. Nordic Naturals also sell a children's product. Although not widely available in the UK, the products are available from the following UK shop and US websites:

Aromantica
16 St Martin's Walk, Dorking, Surrey RH4 1UT
Tel: +44 (0) 1306 742005
www.nordicnaturals.com
www.natuarlgreens.com

Organic Living
To dig deeper into organic issues, check out the following contacts:

Association for Environmentally-Conscious Building
PO Box 32, Llandysul, SA44 5ZA
Tel/Fax: +44 (0) 1559 370 908
Website: www.aecb.net
They advise on natural and organic materials in new buildings, extensions, etc.

Building Investigations Ltd (Environmental House Doctor)
The Cartshed, Church Lane, Osmington, Dorset DT3 6EW
Tel: +44 (0) 1305 837223
Website: www.building-investigations.co.uk
Tests your home for toxic chemicals.

Construction Resources
16 Great Guildford Street, London SE1 0HS
Tel: +44 (0) 207 450 2211
Fax: +44 (0) 207 450 2212
Website: www.ecoconstruct.com
Ecological builders' merchant and building centre who also
provide useful advice.

GeneWatch UK
The Mill House, Manchester Road, Tideswell, Buxton,
Derbyshire SK17 8LN
Tel: +44 (0) 1298 871898
Website: www.genewatch.org

The Healthy House
The Old Co-Op, Lower Street, Ruscombe, Stroud,
Gloucestershire GL6 6BU
Tel: +44 (0) 1453 752216
Website: www.healthy-house.co.uk/chemical.htm
A very good site to source less polluted non-food products, from
organic carpets to organic mattresses.

Henry Doubleday Research Association (HDRA)
Ryton Organic Gardens, Coventry CV8 3LG
Tel: +44 (0) 24 7630 3517
Fax: +44 (0) 24 7663 9229
Website: www.hydra.org.uk
For gardening products and information.

International Federation of Organic Agriculture Movements
(IFOAM)
Okazentrum Imsbach, D-66636, Tholey-Theley, Germany
Tel: +49 6853 5190
Website: www.ifoam.org
IFOAM's website has comprehensive links to organic organisa-
tions around the world.

The Soil Association
Bristol House, 40–56 Victoria Street, Bristol BS1 6BY
Tel: +44 (0) 117 929 0661
Fax: +44 (0) 117 925 2504
Website: www.soilassociation.org
Another very helpful website. This organisation regulates organic farming in the UK.

The range of organic products on the market is currently increasing at a tremendous pace. To find out how to source these products, there are many books available that contain this information for an ever-expanding number of countries. In addition, the Internet is a very good source of information.

Chemical Information Websites

Fluoride Action Network
PO Box 5111, Burlington VT 05402, USA
Tel: +1 802 355 0999 or +1 315 379 9200
Website: www.fluoridealert.org
An international coalition working to end water fluoridation and alert the public to fluoride's health and environmental risks.

Pesticide Action Network UK (formerly the Pesticides Trust)
Eurolink Centre, 49 Effra Road, London SW2 1BZ
Tel: +44 (0) 20 7274 8895
Website: www.pan-uk.org
For information on the effects of pesticides as well as finding alternatives.

Silent Spring Institute
Newton Office, 29 Crafts Street, Newton, MA 02458, USA
Tel: +1 617 332 4288
Website: www.silentspring.org
This is a non-profit scientific research organisation dedicated to identifying the links between the environment and women's health, especially breast cancer.

Organisations Specialising in Specific Health Problems

Immune system disorders
Action Against Allergy
PO Box 278, Twickenham TW1 4QQ
Tel: +44 (0) 20 8892 2711
Website: www.actionagainstallergy.co.uk
This charity helps those suffering from any kind of allergy. Its aim is to advance understanding, awareness and recognition of allergic medical conditions and allergy-related illness, including the role toxic chemicals play in allergies, and the actions needed for research, diagnosis and treatment. It also provides a database of specialist doctors, allergy specialists and dietitians.

The Food Allergy and Anaphylaxis Network
11781 Lee Jackson Hwy, Suite 160, Fairfax, VA 22033–3309, USA
Tel: 0 800 929 4040
Website: www.foodallergy.org
Deals with most aspects of food allergies, including dietary information.

Nervous system disorders
Mental Health Foundation
7th Floor, 83 Victoria Street, London SW1H 0HW
Tel: +44 (0) 20 7802 0300
Website: www.mentalhealth.org.uk
A leading charity concerned with both mental health and learning disabilities, the organisation plays a vital role in pioneering new approaches to treatment and care.

The National Multiple Sclerosis Society
733 Third Avenue, New York, NY 10017, USA
Website: www.nationalmssociety.org
The stated mission of the National Multiple Sclerosis Society is to end the devastating effects of MS.

The World Parkinson Disease Association
via Zuretti, 35, 20125 Milano, Italy
Tel: +39 02 66713111
Website: www.wpda.org
The website contains information about research and treatments
for Parkinson's disease.

Gut Health
Irritable Bowel Syndrome Network
IBS Network, Northern General Hospital, Sheffield S5 7AU
Tel: +44 (0) 114 261 1531
Website: www.ibsnetwork.org.uk
The IBS Network is a UK national charity offering advice, infor-
mation and support.

Mind Body Digestive Center
80 Central Park West, New York, NY, USA
Tel: +1 212 712 0494
Website: www.mindbodydigestive.com
An interesting website which looks at various treatments for irri-
table bowel syndrome and other digestive disorders.

Hormonal Health
Diabetes.com
Website: www.alternativediabetes.com
Excellent website exploring complementary ways of dealing with
diabetes.

Foresight
Association for the Promotion of Pre-conceptual Care
28 The Paddock, Godalming, Surrey GU7 1XD
Tel: +44 (0) 1483 427839
Website: www.foresight-preconception.org.uk
Excellent site for enhancing fertility and increasing your chances
of giving birth to a healthy baby.

Thyroid-Info
Website: www.thyroid-info.com
Interesting commercial website promoting alternative treatments for thyroid disease.

Circulatory System
Holistic Online
Website: http://holisticonline.com
This website provides a great resource for information on many complementary and alternative ways to improve cardiovascular health.

Cancer
Breast Cancer (see Silent Spring Institute, page 324)

Bristol Cancer Help Centre
Grove House, Cornwallis Grove, Clifton, Bristol BS8 4PG
The national-rate telephone helpline number for people with cancer and their supporters:
Tel: 0845 123 23 10
Website: www.bristolcancerhelp.org
The Bristol Cancer Help Centre is the leading UK charity specialising in the Bristol Approach to cancer care, for people with cancer and those close to them. The Bristol Approach works alongside medical treatment, offering a unique combination of physical, emotional and spiritual support, using complementary therapies and self-help techniques.

International Health News Database
Website: www.yourhealthbase.com/prostatecancer.html
A website that deals with various health issues, including a good section on prostate cancer, as well as other forms of cancer.

The Prostate Health Directory
Website: www.prostatehealthdirectory.com
A website which gives a number of organisations dealing with prostate cancer.

Chemical Sensitivities
Breakspear Hospital
Hertfordshire House, Wood Lane, Hemel Hempstead, Herts
HP2 4FD
Tel: +44 (0) 1442-261333
Website: www.breakspearmedical.com
Breakspear Hospital is a privately owned day patient unit, dedicated to the treatment of environmental illness. It also offers chelation therapy.

The Chronic Syndrome Support Association Inc.
801 Riverside Drive, Lumberton, NC 28358–4625, USA
Website: www.cssa-inc.org
Contains information for people with chemical sensitivities, ME, inflammatory health problems, etc.

Environmental Health Centre Dallas
8345 Walnut Hill Lane, Suite 220, Dallas, Texas 75231, USA
Tel: +1 214 368 4132
Website: www.ehcd.com
A complete testing and outpatient treatment medical facility for chemically sensitive adults and children. Their clinic includes sauna, massage, exercise, oral and intravenous nutrition, oxygen therapy, skin testing for antigens, laboratory tests for evaluation of immune parameters, vitamin, mineral and amino acids, and lipids.

Multiple Chemical Sensitivities International
MCS International, PO Box 431, Southport, Merseyside PR8 1WX
Tel: +44 (0) 1704 547418
Website: www.mcsinternational.org
MCS International is a charity for multiple chemical sensitivity sufferers offering support, a helpline and self-help ideas.

Musculo-skeletal problems
Action for M.E.
PO Box 1302, Wells, Somerset BA5 1YE
Tel: +44 (0) 1749 670799
Website: www.afme.org.uk

Action for M.E. is a national charity campaigning to improve the lives of people with ME in the UK.

The Arthritis Research Campaign (arc)
PO Box 177, Chesterfield, Derbyshire S41 7TQ
Tel: 0870 850 5000 or +44 (0) 1246 558033
Website: www.arc.org.uk
The Arthritis Research Campaign promotes medical research into the causes and treatment of arthritic conditions. It also works to provide information to people affected by arthritis.

The 25% ME Group
Website: www.btinternet.com/%7Esevereme.group/
This UK site offers information and support for severely affected ME sufferers.

Childhood Diseases
Action against Autism
Eastwood Business Centre, Greenhill Avenue, Glasgow G46 6QZ
Tel: +44 (0) 141 638 6131

Autism Research Unit
School of Health, Natural and Social Sciences, University of Sunderland, Sunderland SR1 3SD
Tel: +44 (0) 191 510 8922
Fax: +44 (0) 191 567 0420
Email: autism.unit@sunderland.ac.uk
Website: http://osiris.sunderland.ac.uk/autism/
This centre is an excellent source of information about autism, what it is caused by and ways in which to prevent and treat it. An essential site to visit for any parent or carer of a child with autism.

Autism Society of America
7910 Woodmont Avenue, Suite 300, Bethesda, Maryland 20814–3067, USA
Tel: +1 301 657 0881
Website: www.autism-society.org
Good site for information about autism.

Dyslexia Research Trust
Website: www.dyslexic.org.uk/index.html
An Oxford-based charity that funds cutting-edge interdisciplinary research into dyslexia and other related conditions in addition to supporting clinics for the assessment and treatment of people with dyslexic problems. Their vision is to alleviate the struggles and misery of the nearly 10 million people in Britain who suffer from dyslexia and other related conditions, such as specific language difficulties, developmental coordination disorder (DCD-dyspraxia), attention deficit hyperactivity disorder (ADHD) and Aspberger's and autistic spectrum disorders.

The Hyperactive Children's Support Group (HACSG)
71 Whyke Lane, Chichester, West Sussex PO19 2LD
Tel: +44 (0) 1903 725 182
Website: www.hacsg.org.uk
A UK-based charity offering help and support to hyperactive children and their families, plus advice and support on treating your child without reverting to drugs.

Justice Awareness and Basic Support (JABS)
1 Gawsworth Road, Golborne, Warrington WA3 3RF
Tel: +44 (0) 1942 713565
Website: www.jabs.org.uk
JABS is a self-help group that neither recommends nor advises against vaccinations but aims to promote understanding about immunisations and offer basic support to any parent whose child has a health problem after vaccination.

Stimulants Are Not The Answer (SANTA)
Website: www.santa.inuk.com/frame.htm
SANTA is a website endorsed by professionals, including some of the world's leading experts, wishing to restore balance to the debate on attention deficit hyperactivity disorder (ADHD). One of its aims is to make information on ADHD available via the Internet.

Vaccination.co.uk
Website: www.vaccination.co.uk
A website on vaccinations presented by Dr Richard Lanigan, a member of the International Chiropractic Association. Its aim is to provide information about the risks attached to diseases and vaccines, and to be useful to people in their decision-making process.

Alternative and Complementary Treatments and Information

British Acupuncture Council
63 Jeddo Road, London W12 9HQ
Tel: +44 (0) 20 8735 0400
Website: www.acupuncture.org
Publishes a full list of qualified practitioners and general information on acupuncture.

British Complementary Medicine Society
BCMA, PO Box 5122, Bournemouth BH8 0WG
Tel: 0845 345 5977
Website: www.bcma.co.uk
Provides a list of qualified practitioners.

British Holistic Medical Association
59 Lansdown Place, Hove, East Sussex BN3 1FL
Tel: +44 (0) 1273 725951
Website: www.bhma.org
Publishes *Holistic Health*, which is available to members.

British Homeopathic Association and Faculty of Homeopathy
15 Clerkenwell Close, London EC1R 0AA
Tel: +44 (0) 20 7566 7800
Website: www.trusthomeopathy.org
Can provide a national list of medical doctors qualified in homeopathy along with an information pack on homeopathy.

British Medical Acupuncture Society
12 Marbury House, Higher Whitley, Warrington WA4 4QW
Tel: +44 (0) 1925 730727
Website: www.medical-acupuncture.co.uk
Provides a list of practitioners who are also medical doctors, and gives patient information.

British Reflexology Association
Monks Orchard, Whitbourne, Worcester WR6 5RB
Tel: +44 (0) 1886 821207
Website: www.britreflex.co.uk
Publishes a general information sheet on reflexology and a list of registered practitioners.

Institute for Complementary Medicine
PO Box 194, London SE16 7QZ
Tel: +44 (0) 20 7237 5165
Website: www.icmedicine.co.uk
Publishes a register of complementary practitioners.

International Federation of Aromatherapists
182 Chiswick High Road, London W4 1TH
Tel: +44 (0) 20 8742 2605
Website: www.ifaroma.org
Provides information on aromatherapy along with a code of ethics and practice.

National Institute of Medical Herbalists
56 Longbrook Street, Exeter EX4 6AH
Tel: +44 (0) 1392 426022
Website: www.nimh.org.uk
Provides general information on herbal medicine along with a full list of herbal practitioners.

Appendix E
Glossary of Terms

Addison's disease A disease marked by the atrophy or destruction of the adrenal cortex. Most cases of Addison's disease appear to involve an autoimmune process.

Adjuvants Materials added to a mixture to enhance the activity or performance of the rest.

Adrenaline (epinephrine) One of the most important slimming and energy-giving hormones we possess. It plays an important role in burning up excess fat and carbohydrates, and is very easily damaged by toxic chemicals.

Allergy An abnormally heightened immune system reaction an individual displays to a foreign substance.

Amino acids These are the basic building blocks from which proteins are made.

Angioedema Swelling similar to urticaria (hives), but beneath the skin instead of on the surface. Angioedema is characterised by deep swelling around the eyes and lips and sometimes of the hands and feet.

Antagonist A thing or a person who suffers opposition.

Antioxidants Substances that are able to effectively neutralise harmful free radicals. Examples include vitamin A and beta carotene, vitamins C and E, zinc, selenium, co-enzyme Q10 and the amino acid glutathione.

Arginine An essential amino acid which supports many health systems, such as the immune system, protein metabolism, hormonal functioning and growth.

Asthma A form of breathing disorder associated with airway obstruction. It is marked by recurrent attacks of shortness of breath, with wheezing due to spasmodic constriction of the main airways.

Attention deficit hyperactivity disorder (ADHD) A behaviour disorder originating in childhood in which the essential features are signs of developmentally inappropriate inattention, impulsivity and hyperactivity.

Autism A disorder beginning in childhood marked by the presence of abnormal or impaired development in social interaction and communication, and a markedly restricted repertoire of activity and interest.

Autoimmune diseases Diseases characterised by the production of antibodies that react against the body's own tissues.

Autoimmune haemolytic anaemia Anaemia triggered by the increased destruction of red blood cells caused by abnormal antibodies.

Candidiasis (Candida albicans) A disease caused by a species of the yeast-like fungus candida, usually *C. albicans*. Candidiasis can affect the skin, nails and mucous membranes throughout the body including the mouth (thrush), oesophagus, vagina (yeast infection), intestines and lungs.

Carbamates A class of very widely used pesticides, used primarily as fungicides. They are employed on a vast scale in agriculture and commonly used in veterinary practice, in medicine and as wood preservatives.

Carnitine An amino acid that transports fatty acids into muscle cells for use as energy fuel.

Chelation The solubilisation of a metal salt by forming a chemical complex.

Chelation therapy The removal from the body of toxic metals that have accumulated over the years, especially in nerve and brain tissue. A chelation detox, which requires medical supervision, uses substances known as DMSA/DMPS to bind to toxic metals.

Chronic fatigue syndrome (CFS) A condition characterised by persistent or recurrent fatigue, diffuse musculo-skeletal pain and sleep disturbances of six months' duration or longer.

Coeliac disease A digestive disease that damages the small intestine and inteferes with absorption of nutrients from foods.

Co-enzyme Q10 This is a substance that acts as an antioxidant and is an important molecule involved in the production of energy. Although the body can make this substance, the amount it produces is thought insufficient for the best of health, and therefore extra amounts need to be obtained from foods or supplements.

Colitis Inflammation of the colon.

Connective tissue disorders A group of disorders characterised by abnormalities in one or more of the types of connective tissue, such as collagen, elastin or the mucopolysaccharides, that effectively hold the body together.

Corticosteroids A group of anti-inflammatory drugs, commonly known as steroids, similar to the natural corticosteroid hormones produced by the adrenal glands.

Detoxification The removal of toxic substances from the body by the body's waste disposal systems.

Diabetes Impaired ability to control blood sugar levels.

DMPS Aslo known as the sodium salt of 2,3-dimercapto-1-propane sulphonic acid, this is a drug developed in 1958. It is rich in sulphur and used as a chelating agent for toxic metals, such as mercury. Due to its ability to rapidly mobilise mercury from the body's tissues, it should only be used under the supervision of a licensed practitioner as people who have high blood burdens of mercury may have potentially harmful effects if this substance is used inappropriately.

DMSA Also known as meso 2,3 dimercaptosuccinic acid, this is a drug approved by the FDA for removing lead from the brains of children who are lead poisoned. It can also remove other toxic and non-toxic metals from tissues but should only be used under the supervision of a licensed practitioner. It is rich in sulphur, a substance that acts like a magnet for metals, bonding with them and flushing them out of the body via the urine and faeces.

Dysbiosis An imbalance between the 'good' and 'harmful' bacteria in the gut which could predispose to the disease.

Dyslexia Impaired ability to understand written and printed words or phrases, despite normal vision.

Eczema An itchy, lumpy skin condition characterised by thickening of the skin, redness, small vesicles (fluid-filled spots), crusting, weeping sores and scratching.

Enteritis Inflammation of the intestines, especially the small intestine.

Flavonoids A group of chemical compounds naturally found in certain fruit, vegetables, teas, wines, nuts, seeds and roots; they possess powerful antioxidant actions.

Free radicals Highly damaging particles that are produced in cells in the normal process of energy creation. They are potentially harmful as they can damage and age all the tissues. Certain factors increase their production such as pesticides, smoking, exhaust fumes, pollution, infections, burnt foods, fried foods and sunburn.

Fungicide A chemical that destroys fungi.

Gastritis Inflammation of the lining of the stomach.

Glutathione An antioxidant containing the amino acid cysteine which is produced by the body and needed for cellular production of energy, proper immune function and detoxification.

Good pasture's syndrome An autoimmune disease in which the antibodies are directed against the lungs and kidneys. It causes lung problems, frequently presenting with coughing of blood, and kidney problems including kidney failure.

Growth promoter A chemical or substance that encourages growth in animals.

Hashimoto's thyroiditis (Graves' disease) A slowly developing, persistent inflammation of the thyroid gland that frequently results in hypothyroidism, a condition of decreased function of the thyroid gland.

Hay fever A seasonal type of allergy to tree and grass pollen, otherwise known as seasonal allergic rhinitis, marked by red, itchy and 'weeping' eyes and runny or congested nose.

Herbicide A chemical that is toxic to plants and commonly used as a weedkiller.

Homocysteine An amino acid that occurs naturally in the body. High levels are a risk factor for coronary artery disease as homocysteine helps 'bad' cholesterol (LDL) build fatty plaques in the coronary arteries.

Hormones Natural substances that act as internal messengers in the body. They are released from one part of the body and then carried around in the body fluids to another part, which they then stimulate.

Hypertension Persistently high blood pressure. Currently accepted threshold levels are 140 mmHg systolic and 90 mmHg diastolic pressure.

Idiopathic thrombocytopenic purpura A blood disorder characterised by an abnormal decrease in the number of blood platelets, which results in internal bleeding. It is normally an autoimmune disorder involving the creation of antibodies against blood platelets.

Inflammatory bowel disease (IBD) Diseases that cause irritation and ulcers in the intestinal tract. Crohn's disease and ulcerative colitis are the most common inflammatory bowel diseases.

Insecticide A substance used to kill insects.

Insulin A hormone, the main role of which is to regulate blood sugar levels. It also has a role in controlling fat metabolism.

Irritable bowel syndrome (IBS) This condition includes a group of gastrointestinal symptoms for which a cause is not known. It is characterised by a combination of abdominal pain and altered bowel function.

Isoflavones A type of flavonoid (see above). These compounds, commonly found in soya products, are known antioxidants and thought to have benefits against cancer and heart disease.

L-5 hydroxytryptophan (5-HT) A neurotransmitter (see below) made of proteins, created in the central nervous system and involved in appetite, mood and the regulation of normal body temperature.

Leukoplakia A white spot or plaque in the mouth, thought to be a pre-cancerous condition and often tobacco-induced.

Metabolic rate The rate at which energy is released in the body as a result of all the individual chemical reactions taking place.

Metabolism All the chemical reactions that occur within a living organism in order to maintain life.

Metabolite Something essential for metabolism or a product of metabolism, including intermediate or waste products.

Methionine An amino acid that contains sulphur and plays an essential role in the detoxification of synthetic chemicals. It is also a natural chelating agent for toxic metals and helps prevent disorders of the skin, nails and hair. Levels are frequently deficient in people with multiple chemical sensitivities.

Mineral An inorganic substance that occurs naturally and is needed by the human body in small quantities for good health.

MSM-sulphur MSM stands for methylsulphonylmethane. MSM is an organic sulphur compound that exists to some extent in all living things. MSM is a basic nutrient required for the proper functioning of the body, including the safe detoxification and removal of toxic metals such as mercury.

Multiple chemical sensitivity A disorder characterised by immediate recurrent symptoms in one or more of the major organ systems in response to demonstrable exposure to many chemical compounds at doses below those established in the general population to cause harmful effects.

Multiple sclerosis A nerve disorder mainly affecting young adults and characterised by destruction of myelin (fatty sheath surrounding nerve fibres) in the brain and spinal cord.

Myasthenia gravis A lifelong condition in which the body's immune system fights its own body. This causes problems with the nerve connections to the muscles, resulting in muscle weakness.

N-acetylcysteine (NAC) An amino acid which acts as an antioxidant and may keep cancer cells from developing or reduce the severity of existing cancer. It also helps the body synthesise glutathione, an important antioxidant, and helps protect the liver from the adverse effects of exposure to toxic chemicals.

Neurotransmitter A chemical messenger (e.g. dopamine or serotonin) used to transmit or prevent messages being relayed through nerves, between nerves in the central nervous system and other types of cells.

Nutrient A substance that provides nourishment essential for the maintenance of life and growth.

Oestrogens A group of female hormones that promotes the development of female sexual characteristics.

Oilgomeric proanthocyanidins A type of flavonoid (see above) which contains antioxidant properties. They are commonly found in grapes, pine bark and cranberries.

Omega-3 oils The omega-3s are one of two families of essential fatty acids which are necessary for growth and development and cannot be made by the body. Omega-3s are the building blocks of eicosanoids, hormone-like compounds that regulate blood pressure, clotting and other bodily functions. Our bodies function best when there is a balance between the levels of omega-3s and -6s in our diet.

Omega-6 oils The omega-6s are one of two families of essential fatty acids which are necessary for growth and development and cannot be made by the body. Omega-6s tend to be found in most people's diets, whilst levels of omega-3s tend to be deficient. As it is the balance of omega-6s to omega-3s which is important, omega-6 supplements are probably not necessary in the majority of people.

Organic The term organic has two popular definitions that can result in a certain amount of confusion. In the first, organic means natural plants and animals, or made from natural substances, or allowed to grow naturally.

The second popular definition describes food legally certified as being free from artificial pesticides, antibiotics, hormones and other additives; that is meat, eggs, vegetables and fruit produced without the use of synthetic chemicals. These two meanings are ambiguous, allowing manufacturers to say that shampoos, cosmetics and other products are made from organic ingredients when they simply contain plant extracts that have been grown in a conventional way.

Organic chemicals Substances derived from living organisms, containing carbon.

Organic solvents A solvent is a liquid that dissolves other substances. The solvent is the component of a solution that is present in greater amount. Organic solvents include substances such as benzene, tetrachloroethylene and turpentine. They are usually flammable materials and may pose certain physical and chemical hazards.

Organochlorines A number of organic chemicals that contain chlorine. These types of compounds do not occur naturally. Owing to our inability to remove them from our bodies, and their longevity, they tend to be extremely persistent in the body as well as toxic. This varied group includes the chemicals DDT, PCBs and lindane.

Organohalogens A number of artificial and highly toxic compounds that include the organochlorines, pesticides, PCBs and the PBB fire-retardants. They are particularly persistent and toxic as these substances tend not to be found in nature. Because of their complex molecular shape, the body's waste disposal systems can find it very difficult to get rid of them.

Organophosphates Synthetic organic compounds containing phosphorus, which include highly toxic pesticides and nerve gases.

Parkinson's disease A progressive, degenerative brain disease characterised by a tremor that is most marked at rest, a tendency to fall backwards, stiff rigid limbs, stooped posture, slowness of voluntary movements, and a mask-like facial expression.

PBBs (polybrominated biphenyls) Organohalogen compounds that contain bromine. These substances are not usually found in nature and include a number of highly stable compounds that are particularly heat resistant – and because of these qualities they are commonly used as fire-retardants. However, owing to our relative inability to remove them from our bodies, levels of these chemicals tend to accumulate in the tissues throughout our lives.

PCBs (polychlorinated biphenyls) Although the manufacture of this type of organochlorine is now banned, these very stable organochlorines are still found in our environment as they are extremely persistent. They are no less persistent in our bodies.

Pemphigoid Pemphigoid is a chronic blistering disease which tends to occur on mucous membranes, such as in the mouth, and less frequently the skin, and with a tendency to scarring.

Pemphigus vulgaris This very rare condition is one of a group of chronic relapsing autoimmune diseases causing blistering of the skin and mucous membranes.

Pentachlorophenol A highly toxic chemical used as a herbicide and fungicide. Formerly an extremely commonly used substance in wood preservative for fences and power line poles and around the home as a pesticide and herbicide, its use has now been restricted due to its known toxicities.

Pernicious anaemia Condition caused by vitamin B12 deficiency and characterised by anaemia and nerve abnormalities.

Pesticide A general term used for substances that destroy insects or other organisms harmful to cultivated plants or to animals and humans, including insecticides, herbicides and fungicides.

Phosphatidylserine A natural nutrient found as part of the cell membrane. It is most commonly found in nerve cells, comprising about 7 to 10 per cent of its lipid content. The phosphatidylserine currently available over the counter is normally derived from soya.

Plasticisers Chemicals added to plastics (synthetic resins) to produce or promote flexibility and to reduce brittleness.

Pollutants Substances that pollute or contaminate the environment, especially harmful chemical or waste material discharged into the atmosphere and water, including gases, particulate matter, pesticides, radioactive isotopes, sewage, organic chemicals and phosphates, solid wastes and many others.

Polydermatomyositis An autoimmune disease which targets muscles.

Primary biliary cirrhosis An inflammation (irritation and swelling) of the bile ducts of the liver resulting in narrowing and obstruction of the flow of bile. This obstruction damages liver cells.

Primary myxoedema Underactive thyroid causing hypothyroidism, marked by dry skin and swellings around the lips and nose as well as mental deterioration.

Rheumatoid arthritis A chronic autoimmune disease characterised by painful and stiff joints on both sides of the body and marked deformities.

S-adenosylmethionine An important compound in the human body which participates in over 40 essential biochemical reactions, particularly those involving detoxification and mood regulation: preventing depression, reducing inflammation, improving antioxidant reactions and joint health.

Scleroderma A chronic disorder marked by hardening and thickening of the skin. It can be localised or can affect the whole body.

Serotonin A neurotransmitter that has many actions, including blood vessel constriction and appetite and sleep control.

Sjögren's syndrome A chronic inflammatory autoimmune disorder characterised by dry eyes, dry mouth, arthritis and other autoimmune disorders.

Slimming Systems ™ A set of highly evolved body functions that work together to control body weight to bring about weight loss.

Stroke A sudden loss of brain function due to a blockage in, or a bleed from, a blood vessel in the brain.

Supplement A substance taken to remedy the deficiencies in a person's diet.

Sympathetic nervous system (SNS) A specialised part of the body's nervous system that plays a key role in controlling our body weight.

Synthetic chemical A substance made by chemical synthesis, especially to imitate a natural product. These substances do not exist in nature.

Systemic lupus erythematosus (SLE) An autoimmune disorder characterised by periodic episodes of inflammation of joints, tendons and other connective tissues and organs.

Testosterone A hormone that promotes the development of male sexual characteristics. It is very vulnerable to chemical damage.

Threonine An essential amino acid and an important constituent of collagen and elastin (the 'glue' holding tissues together). Helps the gut function more smoothly.

Thrombosis Formation or presence of clot within a blood vessel. This blockage can prevent the normal flow of blood within the blood vessel.

Thyroid hormones A group of hormones that regulate growth and development by altering the body's metabolic rate.

Thyrotoxicosis (Graves' disease) An overactive thyroid gland, in which the level of thyroid hormone is elevated, triggering characteristic symptoms such as weight loss, overactivity and intolerance to heat.

Tyrosine An amino acid created in the body and used as a building block for several important brain chemicals, such as adrenaline, noradrenaline and dopamine, all of which work to regulate mood and weight. Some people whose diets lack certain nutrients (such as vitamin B6) or who have multiple chemical sensitivities often have problems in making this important amino acid. It is available as a supplement.

Ulcerative colitis A disease that causes irritation and ulcers in the lining of the large intestine and rectum. Also known as inflammatory bowel disease.

Vitamin Any of a group of organic compounds that are essential for normal growth and nutrition. They are required in small quantities in a person's diet because they cannot be created by the body.

VOCs (volatile organic chemicals) Organic compounds that evaporate readily at normal pressures and temperatures. Organic chemicals are widely used as ingredients in household products. Paints, varnishes and waxes all contain organic solvents, as do many cleaning, disinfecting and cosmetic products, wood preservatives, air fresheners, dry-cleaned clothes, aerosol sprays, degreasing and hobby products. Fuels are made up of organic chemicals. All of these products can release organic compounds when you are using them, and to some degree when they are stored.

Wegener's granulomatosis An autoimmune disorder mainly affecting the lungs and kidneys.

Xenobiotics Foreign or unnatural compounds or chemicals that mimic natural substances but do not exist in nature.

Xenoestrogen An artificial chemical that mimics the actions of natural oestrogens (female hormones).

Appendix F
Recommended Reading

Beaumont, P, *Pesticides, Policies and People: A Guide to the Issues*, The Pesticides Trust, London, 1993.

Caton, H, Buttram, H and Downing, D, *The Fertility Plan: A Holistic Program for Conceiving a Healthy Baby*, Simon and Schuster, New York, 2000.

Clarke, A, *Living Organic: Easy Steps to an Organic Family Lifestyle*, Time-Life Books, London, 2001.

Erasmus, U, *Fats that Heal, Fats that Kill*, Alive Books, Burnaby, 1987/1993.

Heaton, S, *Organic Farming, Food Quality and Human Health*, Soil Association, Bristol, 2001.

Holford, P, *The Optimum Nutrition Bible*, Piatkus, London, 1998.

McTaggart, L, ed., *The Medical Desk Reference*, What Doctors Don't Tell You Publications Ltd., London, 2000.

McTaggart, L, *The Vaccination Bible*, What Doctor's Don't Tell You Publications Ltd., London, 2000.

Rea, W, *Chemical Sensitivity: Volume 1*, Lewis Publishers, Boca Raton, 1992.

Rea, W, *Chemical Sensitivity: Volume 2*, CRC Press, Boca Raton, 1993.

Rea, W, *Chemical Sensitivity: Volume 3*, Lewis Publishers, Boca Raton, 1995.

Rea, W, *Chemical Sensitivity: Volume 4*, CRC Press, Boca Raton, 1996.

Teitelbaum, J, *From Fatigued to Fantastic!: A Proven Program to Regain Vibrant Health*, Avery Publishing Group, Inc., New York, 2001.

Cancer and Natural Medicine, New York, 2001.

Appendix G
References

1. Baillie-Hamilton P. Chemical toxins: a hypothesis to explain the global obesity epidemic. *J Altern Complement Med* 2002;**8**(2):185–92.
2. Miller CS. The compelling anomaly of chemical intolerance. *Ann N Y Acad Sci* 2001;**933**:1–23.
3. Cheraskin EJ. Antioxidants in health and disease. *Journal of the Optometric Association* 1996;**67**(1):50–57.
4. Rea W. Nutritional Replacement. *Chemical Sensitivity*. Boca Raton, Florida: Lewis Publishers, 1996: 2541–2684.
5. Vidal J. Scientists suspect health threat from GM maize. *The Guardian* 2004 Friday February 27.
6. Bjorntorp P. Endocrine abnormalities of obesity. *Metabolism* 1995;**44**(9 Suppl 3):21–3.
7. Tapiero H BG, Tew KD. Estrogens and environmental estrogens. *Biomed Pharmacother.* 2002;**56**(1):36–44.
8. Robert Repetto SB. Pesticides and the Immune System: The Public Health Risks. The World Resources Institute, 1996.
9. Dewailly EAP, Bruneau S, Gingras S, Belles-Isles M, Roy R. Susceptibility to infections and immune status in Inuit infants exposed to organochlorines. *Environ Health Perspect* 2000;**108**(3):205–11.
10. King LE FP. Zinc deficiency in mice alters myelopoiesis and hematopoiesis. *Journal of Nutrition* 2002;**132**(11):3301–7.
11. Alexander J. Immunoenhancement via enteral nutrition. *Arch Surg* 1993;**128**(11):1242–5.
12. Yates C. Parameters for the treatment of urticaria and angioedema. *J Am Acad Nurse Pract* 2002;**14**(11):478–83.
13. Sly R. Changing prevalence of allergic rhinitis and asthma. *Ann Allergy Asthma Immunol* 1999;**82**(3):248–52.
14. Seaton A GD, Brown K. Increase in asthma: a more toxic environment or a more susceptible population? *Thorax* 1994;**49**(2):171–4.
15. Drouet M LSJ, Bonneau JC, Sabbah A. Mercury – is it a respiratory tract allergen? *Allerg Immunol (Paris).* 1990;**22**(3):84–8.
16. Hoppin JA UD, London SJ, Alavanja MC, Sandler DP. Chemical predictors of wheeze among farmer pesticide applicators in the Agricultural Health Study. *Am J Respir Crit Care Med* 2002;**165**(5):683–9.

17. Peden D. Pollutants and asthma: role of air toxics. *Environ Health Perspect* 2002;**110**(Suppl 4):565–8.

18. Thickett KM MJ, Gerber JM, Sadhra S, Burge PS. Occupational asthma caused by chloramines in indoor swimming-pool air. *Eur Respir J* 2002;**19**(5):827–32.

19. Seaton A DG. Diet, infection and wheezy illness: lessons from adults. *Pediatr Allergy Immunol* 2000;**11**(Suppl 13):37–40.

20. Dominguez LJ BM, Di Lorenzo G, Drago A, Scola S, Morici G, Caruso C. Bronchial reactivity and intracellular magnesium: a possible mechanism for the bronchodilating effects of magnesium in asthma. *Clin Sci (Lond)* 1998;**95**(2):137–42.

21. Cipolla C OT, Orciari P, Lugo G, D'Antuono G. Magnesium pidolate in the treatment of seasonal allergic rhinitis. Preliminary data. *Magnes Res* 1990;**3**(2):109–12.

22. McKeever TM LS, Smith C, Hubbard R. The importance of prenatal exposures on the development of allergic disease: a birth cohort study using the West Midlands General Practice Database. *Am J Respir Crit Care Med* 2002;**166**(6):827–32.

23. Reichrtova E CP, Prachar V, Palkovicova L, Veningerova M. Cord serum immunoglobulin E related to the environmental contamination of human placentas with organochlorine compounds. *Environ Health Perspect* 1999;**107**(11):895–9.

24. Schoenthaler SJ BI, Young K, Nichols D, Jansenns S. The effect of vitamin-mineral supplementation on the intelligence of American schoolchildren: a randomized, double-blind placebo-controlled trial. *J Altern Complement Med* 2000;**6**(1):19–29.

25. Schoenthaler SJ BI. The effect of vitamin-mineral supplementation on juvenile delinquency among American schoolchildren: a randomized, double-blind placebo-controlled trial. *J Altern Complement Med* 2000;**6**(1):7–17.

26. Hebert LE BL, Scherr PA, Evans DA. Annual incidence of Alzheimer disease in the United States projected to the years 2000 through 2050. *Alzheimer Dis Assoc Disord* 2001;**15**(4):169–73.

27. Berrino F. Western diet and Alzheimer's disease. *Epidemiol Prev* 2002;**26**(3):107–15.

28. Nishiwaki Y MK, Ogawa Y, Asukai N, Minami M, Omae K. Effects of sarin on the nervous system in rescue team staff members and police officers 3 years after the Tokyo subway sarin attack. *Environ Health Perspect* 2001;**109**(11):1169–73.

29. Rosenstock L KM, Daniell WE, McConnell R, Claypoole K. Chronic central nervous system effects of acute organophosphate pesticide intoxication. The Pesticide Health Effects Study Group. *Lancet* 1991;**338**(8761):223–7.

30. Karczmar A. Invited review: Anticholinesterases: dramatic aspects of their use and misuse. *Neurochem Int* 1998;**32**(5–6):401–11.

31. Kukull WA BJ. Dementia epidemiology. *Med Clin North Am* 2002;**86**(3):573–90.

32. Baker EL FR, White RA, Harley JP, Niles CA, Dinse GE, Berkey CS. Occupational lead neurotoxicity: a behavioural and electrophysiological evaluation. Study design and year one results. *Br J Ind Med* 1984;**41**(3):352–61.

33. Ryglewicz D RM, Kunicki PK, Bednarska-Makaruk M, Graban A, Lojkowska W, Wehr H. Plasma antioxidant activity and vascular dementia. *J Neurol Sci* 2002;**203–204**:195–7.

34. Miller A. The methionine-homocysteine cycle and its effects on cognitive diseases. *Altern Med Rev* 2003;**8**(1):7–19.

35. Ananth J GA. Drug-induced mood disorders. *Int Pharmacopsychiatry* 1980;**15**(1):59–73.

36. Whitlock FA EL. Drugs and depression. *Drugs* 1978;**15**(1):53–71.

37. Baldi I FL, Mohammed-Brahim B, Fabrigoule C, Dartigues JF, Schwall S, Drevet JP, Salamon R, Brochard P. Neuropsychologic effects of long-term exposure to pesticides: results from the French Phytoner study. *Environ Health Perspect* 2001;**109**(8):839–44.

38. Parron T HA, Villanueva E. Increased risk of suicide with exposure to pesticides in an intensive agricultural area. A 12-year retrospective study. *Forensic Sci Int* 1996;**79**(1):53–63.

39. Rehner TA KJ, Trump R, Smith C, Reid D. Depression among victims of south Mississippi's methyl parathion disaster. *Health Soc Work* 2000;**25**(1):33–40.

40. Gottwald B TI, Kupfer J, Ganss C, Eis D, Schill WB, Gieler U. 'Amalgam disease' – poisoning, allergy, or psychic disorder? *Int J Hyg Environ Health* 2001;**204**(4):223–9.

41. Lindh U HR, Danersund A, Eriksson S, Lindvall A. Removal of dental amalgam and other metal alloys supported by antioxidant therapy alleviates symptoms and improves quality of life in patients with amalgam-associated ill health. *Neuroendocrinol Lett* 2002;**23**(5–6):459–82.

42. Baker EL FR, White RF, Harley JP. The role of occupational lead exposure in the genesis of psychiatric and behavioral disturbances. *Acta Psychiatr Scand Suppl* 1983;**303**:38–48.

43. Morrow LA SL, Bagovich GR, Condray R, Scott A. Neuropsychological assessment, depression, and past exposure to organic solvents. *Appl Neuropsychol* 2001;**8**(2):65–73.

44. Snyder JW PR, Stubbins JF, Garrettson LK. Acute manic psychosis following the dermal application of N,N-diethyl-m-toluamide (DEET) in an adult. *J Toxicol Clin Toxicol* 1986;**24**(5):429–39.

45. Jorm AF KA, Jacomb PA, Rodgers B, Pollitt P, Christensen H, Henderson S. Helpfulness of interventions for mental disorders: beliefs of health professionals compared with the general public. *Br J Psychiatry* 1997;**171**:233–7.

46. Wynn V. Vitamins and oral contraceptive use. *Lancet* 1975;**1**(7906):561–4.

47. Kaplan BJ SJ, Ferre RC, Gorman CP, McMullen DM, Crawford SG. Effective mood stabilization with a chelated mineral supplement: an open-label trial in bipolar disorder. *J Clin Psychiatry* 2001;**62**(12):936–44.

48. Rodriguez Jimenez J RJ, Gonzalez MJ. Indicators of anxiety and depression in subjects with different kinds of diet: vegetarians and omnivores. *Bol Asoc Med P R* 1998;**90**(4–6):58–68.

49. Riise T MB, Kyvik KR. Organic solvents and the risk of multiple sclerosis. *Epidemiology* 2002;**13**(6):718–20.

50. Ingalls T. Clustering of multiple sclerosis in Galion, Ohio, 1982–1985. *Am J Forensic Med Pathol* 1989;**10**(3):213–5.

51. Ingalls T. Endemic clustering of multiple sclerosis in time and place, 1934–1984. Confirmation of a hypothesis. *Am J Forensic Med Pathol* 1986; 7(1):3–8.

52. Gout O. Vaccinations and multiple sclerosis. *Neurol Sci* 2001;**22**(2):151–4.

53. Siblerud R. A comparison of mental health of multiple sclerosis patients with silver/mercury dental fillings and those with fillings removed. *Psychol Rep* 1992;**70**(3 Pt 2):1139–51.

54. Blisard KS KM, McFeeley PJ, Smialek JE. The investigation of alleged insecticide toxicity: a case involving chlordane exposure, multiple sclerosis, and peripheral neuropathy. *J Forensic Sci* 1986;**31**(4):1499–504.

55. Besler HT CS, Okcu Z. Serum levels of antioxidant vitamins and lipid peroxidation in multiple sclerosis. *Nutr Neurosci* 2002;**5**(3):215–20.

56. Yasui M OK. Experimental and clinical studies on dysregulation of magnesium metabolism and the aetiopathogenesis of multiple sclerosis. *Magnes Res* 1992;**5**(4):295–302.

57. Frequin ST WR, Braam M, Barkhof F, Hommes OR. Decreased vitamin B12 and folate levels in cerebrospinal fluid and serum of multiple sclerosis patients after high-dose intravenous methylprednisolone. *J Neurol Sci* 1993;**240**(5): 305–8.

58. Wade DT YC, Chaudhuri KR, Davidson DL. A randomised placebo controlled exploratory study of vitamin B-12, lofepramine, and L-phenylalanine (the 'Cari Loder regime') in the treatment of multiple sclerosis. *J Neurol Neurosurg Psychiatry* 2002;**73**(3):246–9.

59. Johnson S. The possible role of gradual accumulation of copper, cadmium, lead and iron and gradual depletion of zinc, magnesium, selenium, vitamins B2, B6, D, and E and essential fatty acids in multiple sclerosis. *Med Hypotheses* 2000;**55**(3):239–41.

60. Thiruchelvam M RE, Goodman BM, Baggs RB, Cory-Slechta DA. Developmental exposure to the pesticides paraquat and maneb and the Parkinson's disease phenotype. *Neurotoxicology* 2002;**23**(4–5):621–33.

61. Derex L T, P. Reversible parkinsonism, hypophosphoremia, and hypocalcemia under vitamin D therapy. *Mov Disord* 1997;**12**(4):612–3.

62. Grundy J MS, Bateman B, Dean T, Arshad SH. Rising prevalence of allergy to peanut in children: Data from 2 sequential cohorts. *J Allergy Clin Immunol* 2002;**110**(5):784–9.

63. Ascher H KI, Kristiansson B. Increasing incidence of coeliac disease in Sweden. *Arch Dis Child* 1991;**66**(5):608–11.

64. Ring J BK, Behrendt H. Adverse reactions to foods. *J Chromatogr B Biomed Sci Appl* 2001;**756**(1–2):3–10.

65. Dotterud. Role of food in atopic eczema. *Tidsskr Nor Laegeforen* 1996;**116**(28):3335–40.

66. Bahna. Cow's milk allergy versus cow's milk intolerance. *Ann Allergy Asthma Immunol* 2002;**89**(6 Suppl 1):56–60.

67. Finamore A RM, Merendino N, Nobili F, Vignolini F, Mengheri E. Zinc deficiency suppresses the development of oral tolerance in rats. *J Nutr* 2003;**133**(1):191–8.

68. Ojuawo A LK, Milla PJ. Serum zinc, selenium and copper concentration in children with allergic colitis. *East Afr Med J* 1996;**73**(4):236–8.

69. Chandra RK. Food allergy and nutrition in early life: implications for later health. *Proc Nutr Soc* 2000;**59**(2):273–7.

70. Cathcart RF. The vitamin C treatment of allergy and the normally unprimed state of antibodies. *Med Hypotheses* 1986;**21**(3):307–21.

71. Hijazi N AB, Seaton A. Diet and childhood asthma in a society in transition: a study in urban and rural Saudi Arabia. *Thorax* 2000;**55**(9):775–9.

72. Yamashiro Y OY, Yabuta K. The regulation of intestinal hypersensitivity reactions to ovalbumin by omega-3 fatty acid enriched diet: studies of IEL and LPL in mucosal damage. *Acta Paediatr Jpn* 1994;**36**(5):550–6.

73. Henriksen C EM, Halvorsen R, Botten G. Nutrient intake among two-year-old children on cows' milk-restricted diets. *Acta Paediatr* 2000;**89**(3):272–8.

74. Christie L HR, Parker JG, Burks W. Food allergies in children affect nutrient intake and growth. *J Am Diet Assoc* 2002;**102**(11):1648–51.

75. Hovdenak N HE, Aksnes L, Fluge G, Erichsen MM, Eide J. High prevalence of asymptomatic coeliac disease in Norway: a study of blood donors. *Eur J Gastroenterol Hepatol* 1999;**11**(2):185–7.

76. Armitage E DH, Wilson DC, Ghosh S. Increasing incidence of both juvenile-onset Crohn's disease and ulcerative colitis in Scotland. *Eur J Gastroenterol Hepatol* 2001;**13**(12):1439–47.

77. Colombel JF G-RC. Etiology of Crohn's disease. Current data. *Presse Med* 1994;**23**(12):558–60.

78. Guo X WW, Ko JK, Cho CH. Involvement of neutrophils and free radicals in the potentiating effects of passive cigarette smoking on inflammatory bowel disease in rats. *Gastroenterology* 1999;**117**(4):884–92.

79. Murphy MJ CE, Parsons V. Resuscitation. *A case of poisoning with mercuric chloride.* 1979;**7**(1):35–44.

80. Powell JJ AC, Harvey RS, Mason IM, Kendall MD, Sankey EA, Dhillon AP, Thompson RP. Characterisation of inorganic microparticles in pigment cells of human gut associated lymphoid tissue. *Gut* 1996;**38**(3):390–5.

81. Fogarty U PD, Good P, Ensley S, Seawright A, Noonan J. A cluster of equine granulomatous enteritis cases: the link with aluminium. *Vet Hum Toxicol* 1998;**40**(5):297–305.

82. Demling. Crohn's disease caused by antibiotics? A medical hypothesis based on epidemiologic data. *Fortschr Med* 1994;**112**(14):195–6.

83. Krzystyniak K TH, Fournier M. Approaches to the evaluation of chemical-induced immunotoxicity. *Environ Health Perspect* 1995;**103 Suppl** 9:17–22.

84. Gupta RK SG. Adjuvants for human vaccines – current status, problems and future prospects. *Vaccine* 1995;**13**(14):1263–76.

85. Afzal MA MP. Vaccines, Crohn's disease and autism. *Mol Psychiatry* 2002;7 **Suppl 2**:S49–50.

86. Lomer MC TR, Powell JJ. Fine and ultrafine particles of the diet: influence on the mucosal immune response and association with Crohn's disease. *Proc Nutr Soc* 2002;**61**(1):123–30.

87. Mahmud N WD. The urban diet and Crohn's disease: is there a relationship? *Eur J Gastroenterol Hepatol* 2001;**13**(2):93–5.

88. Smith CJ LS, Doolittle DJ. An international literature survey of 'IARC Group I carcinogens' reported in mainstream cigarette smoke. *Food Chem Toxicol* 1997;**35**(10–11):1107–30.

89. Saito YA SP, Locke GR 3rd. The epidemiology of irritable bowel syndrome in North America: a systematic review. *Am J Gastroenterol* 2002;**97**(8):1910–5.

90. Van den Driessche M V-WG. Functional foods in pediatrics. *Acta Gastroenterol Belg.* 2002;**65**(1):45–51.

91. Alleva E. Statement from the work session on environmental endocrine-disrupting chemicals: neural, endocrine and behavioural effects. *Toxicology and Industrial Health* 1998;**14**(1–2):1–7.

92. Ruhe RC MR. Use of antioxidant nutrients in the prevention and treatment of type 2 diabetes. *J Am Coll Nutr* 2001;**20**(5 Suppl):363S–369S & discussion 381S–383S.

93. Muir T ZM. Societal costs of exposure to toxic substances: economic and health costs of four case studies that are candidates for environmental causation. *Health Perspect* 2001;**109**(Suppl 6):885–903.

94. Silink M. Childhood diabetes: a global perspective. *Horm Res* 2002;**57**(Suppl 1):1–5.

95. Glynn AW GF, Aune M, Atuma S, Darnerud PO, Bjerselius R, Vainio H, Weiderpass E. Organochlorines in Swedish women: determinants of serum concentrations. *Environ Health Perspect* 2003;**111**(3):349–55.

96. Tiemann U KU. Influence of organochlorine pesticides on ATPase activities of microsomal fractions of bovine oviductal and endometrial cells. *Toxicol Lett* 1999;**104**(1–2):75–81.

97. Lissner L AR, Muller DC, Shimokata H. Body weight variability in men: metabolic rate, health and longevity. *Int J Obes* 1990;**14**(4):373–83.

98. Vena J BP, Becher H, Benn T, Bueno-de-Mesquita HB, Coggon D, Colin D, Flesch-Janys D, Green L, Kauppinen T, Littorin M, Lynge E, Mathews JD, Neuberger M, Pearce N, Pesatori AC, Saracci R, Steenland K, M. K. Exposure to dioxin and nonneoplastic mortality in the expanded IARC international

cohort study of phenoxy herbicide and chlorophenol production workers and sprayers. *Environ Health Perspect.* 1998;**106**(Suppl 2):645–53.

99. Shobha TR PO. Glycosuria in organophosphate and carbamate poisoning. *J Assoc Physicians India* 2000;**48**(12):1197–9.

100. Ho E QN, Tsai YH, Lai W, Bray TM. Dietary zinc supplementation inhibits NFkappaB activation and protects against chemically induced diabetes in CD1 mice. *Exp Biol Med (Maywood)* 2001;**226**(2):103–11.

101. Bener A OE, Gillett M, Pasha MA, Bishawi B. Association between blood levels of lead, blood pressure and risk of diabetes and heart disease in workers. *Int Arch Occup Environ Health* 2001;**74**(5):375–8.

102. Gist GL BJ. Benzene – a review of the literature from a health effects perspective. *Toxicol Ind Health* 1997;**13**(6):661–714.

103. Yeh GY ED, Kaptchuk TJ, Phillips RS. Systematic review of herbs and dietary supplements for glycemic control in diabetes. *Diabetes Care.* 2003;**26**(4):1277–94.

104. Borissova AM TT, Kirilov G, Dakovska L, Kovacheva R. The effect of vitamin D3 on insulin secretion and peripheral insulin sensitivity in type 2 diabetic patients. *Int J Clin Pract* 2003;**57**(4):258–61.

105. Evans JL GI. Alpha-lipoic acid: a multifunctional antioxidant that improves insulin sensitivity in patients with type 2 diabetes. *Diabetes Technol Ther.* 2000;**2**(3):401–13.

106. Fox CH MM, Ramsoomair D, Carter CA. Magnesium deficiency in African-Americans: does it contribute to increased cardiovascular risk factors? *J Natl Med Assoc* 2003;**95**(4):257–62.

107. Cam MC BR, McNeill JH. Mechanisms of vanadium action: insulin-mimetic or insulin-enhancing agent? *Can J Physiol Pharmacol* 2000;**78**(10):829–47.

108. Suresh Y DU. Long-chain polyunsaturated fatty acids and chemically induced diabetes mellitus. Effect of omega-3 fatty acids. *Nutrition* 2003;**19**(3): 213–28.

109. Pandey M KA. Hypoglycaemic effect of defatted seeds and water soluble fibre from the seeds of Syzygium cumini (Linn.) skeels in alloxan diabetic rats. *Indian J Exp Biol* 2002;**40**(10):1178–82.

110. Cater NB GA. The effect of dietary intervention on serum lipid levels in type 2 diabetes mellitus. *Curr Diab Rep.* 2002;**2**(3):289–94.

111. Bagchi N BT, Parish RF. Thyroid dysfunction in adults over age 55 years. A study in an urban US community. *Arch Intern Med.* 1990;**150**(4):785–7.

112. Fahey TJ 3rd RT, Delbridge L. Increasing incidence and changing presentation of thyroid cancer over a 30 year period. *Br J Surg* 1995;**82**(4):518–20.

113. Wong GW CP. Increasing incidence of childhood Graves' disease in Hong Kong: a follow-up study. *Clin Endocrinol (Oxf)* 2001;**54**(4):547–50.

114. Ghinea E SL, Oprescu M. Studies on the action of pesticides upon the endocrines using in vitro human thyroid cells culture and in vivo animal models. I. Herbicides – aminotriasole (amitrol) and atrazine. *Endocrinologie.* 1979;**17**(3):185–90.

115. Heeremans A EA, De Wasch KK, Van Peteghem C, De Brabander HF. Elimination profile of methylthiouracil in cows after oral administration. *Analyst* 1988;**123**(12):2629–32.

116. Frakes R. Drinking water guidelines for ethylene thiourea, a metabolite of ethylene bisdithiocarbamate fungicides. *Regul Toxicol Pharmacol* 1988;**8**(2): 207–18.

117. Sala M SJ, Herrero C, To-Figueras J, Grimalt J. Association between serum concentrations of hexachlorobenzene and polychlorobiphenyls with thyroid hormone and liver enzymes in a sample of the general population. *Occup Environ Med* 2001;**58**(3):172–7.

118. Kosuda LL GD, Bigazzi PE. Effects of HgCl2 on the expression of autoimmune responses and disease in diabetes-prone (DP) BB rats. *Autoimmunity* 1997;**26**(3):173–87.

119. Krivosheeva SS PA, Anchikova LI, Dautov FF. Effects of working conditions in the production of synthetic rubber on workers' health. *Gig Sanit* 2001;**3**:47–9.

120. Gaitan E. Endemic goiter in western Colombia. *Ecol Dis* 1983;**2**(4):295–308.

121. Mesaros-Kanjski E KI, Kusic Z, Kaic-Rak A, Dakovic N, Kuser J, Antonic K. Endemic goitre and plasmatic levels of vitamins A and E in the schoolchildren on the island of Krk, Croatia. *Coll Antropol* 1999;**23**(2):729–36.

122. Bouzas EA KP, Mastorakos G, Koutras DA. Antioxidant agents in the treatment of Graves' ophthalmopathy. *Am J Ophthalmol* 2000;**129**(5):618–22.

123. Yamashita H NS, Takatsu K, Koike E, Murakami T, Watanabe S, Uchino S, Yamashita H, Kawamoto H. High prevalence of vitamin D deficiency in Japanese female patients with Graves' disease. *Endocr J* 2001;**48**(1):63–9.

124. Pehowich D. Thyroid hormone status and membrane n-3 fatty acid content influence mitochondrial proton leak. *Biochim Biophys Acta*. 1999;**1411**(1): 192–200.

125. Inhorn M. Global infertility and the globalization of new reproductive technologies: illustrations from Egypt. *Soc Sci Med* 2003;**56**(9):1837–51.

126. Veeramachaneni D. Deteriorating trends in male reproduction: idiopathic or environmental? *Anim Reprod Sci* 2000;**60–61**:121–30.

127. Slutsky M LJ, Levy BS. Azoospermia and oligospermia among a large cohort of DBCP applicators in 12 countries. *Int J Occup Environ Health* 1999;**5**(2): 116–22.

128. Younglai EV FW, Hughes EG, Trim K, Jarrell JF. Levels of environmental contaminants in human follicular fluid, serum, and seminal plasma of couples undergoing in vitro fertilization. *Arch Environ Contam Toxicol* 2002;**43**(1): 121–6.

129. Tielemans E vKR, te Velde ER, Burdorf A, Heederik D. Pesticide exposure and decreased fertilisation rates in vitro. *Lancet* 1999;**354**(9177):484–5.

130. Choy CM LC, Cheung LT, Briton-Jones CM, Cheung LP, Haines CJ. Infertility, blood mercury concentrations and dietary seafood consumption: a case-control study. *BJOG* 2002;**109**(10):1121–5.

131. Gerhard I MB, Waldbrenner A, Runnebaum B. Heavy metals and fertility. *J Toxicol Environ Health A* 1998;**54**(8):593–611.

132. Bukowski J. Review of the epidemiological evidence relating toluene to reproductive outcomes. *Regul Toxicol Pharmacol* 2001;**33**(2):147–56.

133. Axmon A RL, Stromberg U, Hagmar L. Time to pregnancy and infertility among women with a high intake of fish contaminated with persistent organochlorine compounds. *Scand J Work Environ Health* 2000;**26**(3): 199–206.

134. Potashnik G CR, Belmaker I, Levine M. Spermatogenesis and reproductive performance following human accidental exposure to bromine vapor. *Reprod Toxicol* 1992;**6**(2):171–4.

135. Das UB MM, Debnath JM, Ghosh D. Protective effect of ascorbic acid on cyclophosphamide-induced testicular gametogenic and androgenic disorders in male rats. *Asian J Androl* 2002;**4**(3):201–7.

136. Wong WY MH, Thomas CM, Menkveld R, Zielhuis GA, Steegers-Theunissen RP. Effects of folic acid and zinc sulfate on male factor subfertility: a double-blind, randomized, placebo-controlled trial. *Fertil Steril* 2002;**77**(3):491–8.

137. Nikolaev AA LD, Lozhkina LV, Bochanovskii VA, Goncharova LA. Selenium correction of male subfertility. *Urologiia* 1999;**4**:29–32.

138. Bennett M. Vitamin B12 deficiency, infertility and recurrent fetal loss. *J Reprod Med* 2001;**46**(3):209–12.

139. Gonick HC BJ. Is lead exposure the principal cause of essential hypertension? *Med Hypotheses* 2002;**59**(3):239–46.

140. Maschewsky. Do workplace chemicals harm the heart? *Soz Praventivmed* 1993;**38**(2):71–6.

141. Fletcher RH FK. Vitamins for chronic disease prevention in adults: clinical applications. *JAMA* 2002;**287**(23):3127–9.

142. van Guldener C NP, Stehouwer CD. Homocysteine and blood pressure. *Curr Hypertens Rep* 2003;**5**(1):26–31.

143. Carvalho W. Risk factors related with occupational and environmental exposure to organochlorine insecticides in the state of Bahia, Brazil, 1985. *Bol Oficina Sanit Panam* 1991;**111**(6):512–24.

144. Laden F NL, Spiegelman D, Hankinson SE, Willett WC, Ireland K, Wolff MS, Hunter DJ. Predictors of plasma concentrations of DDE and PCBs in a group of U.S. women. *Environ Health Perspect* 1999;**107**(1):75–81.

145. DeVoto E KL, Heeschen W. Some dietary predictors of plasma organochlorine concentrations in an elderly German population. *Arch Environ Health* 1998;**53**(2):147–55.

146. Walsh LP WD, Stocco DM. Dimethoate inhibits steroidogenesis by disrupting transcription of the steroidogenic acute regulatory (StAR) gene. *J Endocrinol* 2000;**167**(2):253–63.

147. Nikiforov B BL, Petrov I. Heavy metal exposure of the population in an area of nonferrous metallurgy – a prerequisite for the development of atherosclerotic diseases. *Probl Khig* 1987;**12**:27–37.

148. Subramanyam G BM, Govindappa S. The role of cadmium in induction of atherosclerosis in rabbits. *Indian Heart J* 1992;**44**(3):177–80.

149. Meltzer HM MH, Alexander J, Bibow K, Ydersbond TA. Does dietary arsenic and mercury affect cutaneous bleeding time and blood lipids in humans? *Biol Trace Elem Res* 1994;**46**(1–2):135–53.

150. Zeighami EA WA, Craun GF. Chlorination, water hardness and serum cholesterol in forty-six Wisconsin communities. *Int J Epidemiol* 1990;**19**(1):49–58.

151. Mukamal K. Alcohol use and prognosis in patients with coronary heart disease. *Prev Cardiol* 2003;**6**(2):93–8.

152. Kumar P PA, Dutta KK. Steroidogenic alterations in testes and sera of rats exposed to trichloroethylene (TCE) by inhalation. *Hum Exp Toxicol* 2000;**19**(2):117–21.

153. Rezaian GR TM, Mozaffari BE, Mosleh AA, Ghalambor MA. The salutary effects of antioxidant vitamins on the plasma lipids of healthy middle aged-to-elderly individuals: a randomized, double-blind, placebo-controlled study. *J Med Liban* 2002;**50**(1–2):10–3.

154. Shidfar F KA, Jallali M, Miri R, Eshraghian M. Comparison of the effects of simultaneous administration of vitamin C and omega-3 fatty acids on lipoproteins, apo A-I, apo B, and malondialdehyde in hyperlipidemic patients. *Int J Vitam Nutr Res* 2003;**73**(3):163–70.

155. Singh RB NN, Kartikey K, Pella D, Kumar A, Niaz MA, Thakur AS. Effect of coenzyme Q10 on risk of atherosclerosis in patients with recent myocardial infarction. *Mol Cell Biochem.* 2003;**246**(1–2):75–82.

156. Ziakka S RG, Kountouris S, Doulgerakis C, Karakasis P, Kourvelou C, Papagalanis N. The effect of vitamin B6 and folate supplements on plasma homocysteine and serum lipids levels in patients on regular hemodialysis. *Int Urol Nephrol.* 2001;**33**(3):559–62.

157. Ardawi MS RA, Qari MH, Dahlawi FM, Al-Raddadi RM. Influence of age, sex, folate and vitamin B12 status on plasma homocysteine in Saudis. *Saudi Med J* 2002;**23**(8):959–68.

158. Lal J VK, Kela AK, Jain SK. Effect of oral magnesium supplementation on the lipid profile and blood glucose of patients with type 2 diabetes mellitus. *J Assoc Physicians India* 2003;**51**:37–42.

159. Chevalier CA LG, Murphy MD, Suneson J, Vanbeber AD, Gorman MA, Cochran C. The effects of zinc supplementation on serum zinc and cholesterol concentrations in hemodialysis patients. *J Ren Nutr.* 2002;**12**(3):183–9.

160. Miyazaki Y KH, Nojiri M, Suzuki S. Relationship of dietary intake of fish and non-fish selenium to serum lipids in Japanese rural coastal community. *J Trace Elem Med Biol.* 2002;**16**(2):83–90.

161. Aguilar MV M-PM, Gonzalez MJ. Effects of arsenic (V)-chromium (III) interaction on plasma glucose and cholesterol levels in growing rats. *Ann Nutr Metab.* 1997;**41**(3):189–95.

162. Caron MF WC. Evaluation of the antihyperlipidemic properties of dietary supplements. *Pharmacotherapy.* 2001;**21**(4):481–7.

163. Saadeh AM FN, al-Ali MK. Cardiac manifestations of acute carbamate and organophosphate poisoning. *Heart* 1997;77(5):461–4.

164. O'Malley MA MS. Subacute poisoning with phosalone, an organophosphate insecticide. *West J Med* 1990;153(6):619–24.

165. Cox A. Ventricular dysrhythmia secondary to select environmental hazards. *AACN Clin Issues Crit Care Nurs* 1992;3(1):233–42.

166. Sauviat MP PN. Cardiotoxicity of lindane, a gamma isomer of hexachlorocyclohexane. *J Soc Biol* 2002;196(4):339–48.

167. Howard MD PC. In vitro effects of chlorpyrifos, parathion, methyl parathion and their oxons on cardiac muscarinic receptor binding in neonatal and adult rats. *Toxicology* 2002;170(1–2):1–10.

168. Wang CH JJ, Yip PK, Chen CL, Hsu LI, Hsueh YM, Chiou HY, Wu MM, Chen CJ. Biological gradient between long-term arsenic exposure and carotid atherosclerosis. *Circulation* 2002;105(15):1804–9.

169. Tollestrup K DJ, Allard J. Mortality in a cohort of orchard workers exposed to lead arsenate pesticide spray. *Arch Environ Health* 1995;50(3):221–9.

170. Lustberg M SE. Blood lead levels and mortality. *Arch Intern Med.* 2002;162(21):2443–9.

171. Bockelmann I PE, McGauran N, Robra BP. Assessing the suitability of cross-sectional and longitudinal cardiac rhythm tests with regard to identifying effects of occupational chronic lead exposure. *J Occup Environ Med* 2002;44(1): 59–65.

172. Guloglu C KI, Erten PG. Acute accidental exposure to chlorine gas in the Southeast of Turkey: a study of 106 cases. *Environ Res* 2002;88(2):89–93.

173. Klasaer AE SA, Blume C, Johnson P, Thompson MW. Marked hypocalcemia and ventricular fibrillation in two pediatric patients exposed to a fluoride-containing wheel cleaner. *Ann Emerg Med* 1996;28(6):713–8.

174. Strubelt O IH, Younes M. The pathophysiological profile of the acute cardiovascular toxicity of sodium fluoride. *Toxicology* 1982;24(3–4):313–23.

175. Cedergren MI SA, Lofman O, Kallen BA. Chlorination byproducts and nitrate in drinking water and risk for congenital cardiac defects. *Environ Res* 2002;89(2):124–30.

176. Hooiveld M HD, Kogevinas M, Boffetta P, Needham LL, Patterson DG Jr, Bueno-de-Mesquita HB. Second follow-up of a Dutch cohort occupationally exposed to phenoxy herbicides, chlorophenols, and contaminants. *Am J Epidemiol* 1998;147(9):891–901.

177. Hay A TJ. Mortality of power workers exposed to phenoxy herbicides and polychlorinated biphenyls in waste transformer oil. *Ann NY Acad Sci* 1997;837:138–56.

178. Flesch-Janys D BJ, Gurn P, Manz A, Nagel S, Waltsgott H, Dwyer JH. Exposure to polychlorinated dioxins and furans (PCDD/F) and mortality in a cohort of workers from a herbicide-producing plant in Hamburg, Federal Republic of Germany. *Am J Epidemiol* 1995;142(11):1165–75.

179. Toren K HS, Westberg H. Health effects of working in pulp and paper mills: exposure, obstructive airways diseases, hypersensitivity reactions, and cardiovascular diseases. *Am J Ind Med* 1996;**29**(2):111–22.

180. Sunyer J BF, Tertre AL, Atkinson R, Ayres JG, Forastiere F, Forsberg B, Vonk JM, Bisanti L, Tenias JM, Medina S, Schwartz J, Katsouyanni K. The association of daily sulfur dioxide air pollution levels with hospital admissions for cardiovascular diseases in Europe (The Aphea-II study). *Eur Heart J* 2003;**24**(8):752–60.

181. Gustavsson P PN, Hallqvist J, Hogstedt C, Lewne M, Reuterwall C, Scheele P. A population-based case-referent study of myocardial infarction and occupational exposure to motor exhaust, other combustion products, organic solvents, lead, and dynamite. Stockholm Heart Epidemiology Program (SHEEP) Study Group. *Epidemiology* 2001;**12**(2):222–8.

182. Morris CD CS. Routine vitamin supplementation to prevent cardiovascular disease: a summary of the evidence for the U.S. Preventive Services Task Force. *Ann Intern Med* 2003;**139**(1):56–70.

183. Haynes WG. Hyperhomocysteinemia, vascular function and atherosclerosis: effects of vitamins. *Cardiovasc Drugs Ther* 2002;**16**(5):391–9.

184. Oster O PW. Selenium and cardiovascular disease. *Biol Trace Elem Res* 1990;**24**(2):91–103.

185. Seelig MS. Interrelationship of magnesium and congestive heart failure. *Wien Med Wochenschr* 2000;**150**(15–16):335–41.

186. Roth A EY, Keren G, Kerbel S, Harsat A, Villa Y, Laniado S, Miller HI. Effect of magnesium on restenosis after percutaneous transluminal coronary angioplasty: a clinical and angiographic evaluation in a randomized patient population. A pilot study. The Ichilov Magnesium. *Eur Heart J* 1994;**15(9):1164–73**(9):15(9):1164–73.

187. Shechter M BMC, Stuehlinger HG, Slany J, Pachinger O, Rabinowitz B. Effects of oral magnesium therapy on exercise tolerance, exercise-induced chest pain, and quality of life in patients with coronary artery disease. *Am J Cardiol* 2003;**91**(5):517–21.

188. Nordoy A MR, Arnesen H, Videbaek J. n-3 polyunsaturated fatty acids and cardiovascular diseases. *Lipids* 2001;**36 Suppl**:S127–9.

189. Berger MM MI. Metabolic and nutritional support in acute cardiac failure. *Curr Opin Clin Nutr Metab Care* 2003;**6**(2):195–201.

190. Lemaitre RN KI, Mozaffarian D, Kuller LH, Tracy RP, Siscovick DS. n-3 Polyunsaturated fatty acids, fatal ischemic heart disease, and nonfatal myocardial infarction in older adults: the Cardiovascular Health Study. *Am J Clin Nutr* 2003;**77**(2):319–25.

191. Mulvad G PH, Hansen JC, Dewailly E, Jul E, Pedersen M, Deguchi Y, Newman WP, Malcom GT, Tracy RE, Middaugh JP, Bjerregaard P. The Inuit diet. Fatty acids and antioxidants, their role in ischemic heart disease, and exposure to organochlorines and heavy metals. An international study. *Arctic Med Res* 1996;**55 Suppl 1**:20–4.

192. Jeejeebhoy F KM, Freeman M, Barr A, McCall M, Kurian R, Mazer D, Errett L. Nutritional supplementation with MyoVive repletes essential cardiac myocyte nutrients and reduces left ventricular size in patients with left ventricular dysfunction. *Am Heart J* 2002;**143**(6):1092–100.

193. Kondo Y MS, Oda H, Nagate T. Taurine reduces atherosclerotic lesion development in apolipoprotein E-deficient mice. *Adv Exp Med Biol* 2000;**483**: 193–202.

194. Marek K Z-NM, Rola E, Wocka-Marek T, Langauer-Lewowicka H, Witecki K. Examination of health effects after exposure to metallic mercury vapors in workers engaged in production of chlorine and acetic aldehyde. I. Evaluation of general health status. *Heavy metals* 1995;**46**(2):101–9.

195. Weihe P DF, White RF, Sorensen N, Budtz-Jorgensen E, Keiding N, Grandjean P. Environmental epidemiology research leads to a decrease of the exposure limit for mercury. *Ugeskr Laeger* 2003;**165**(2)(2):107–11.

196. Kinoshita H HY, Tanaka T, Hori Y, Nakajima M, Fujisawa M, Oseki M. A case of carbamate poisoning in which GCMS was useful to identify causal substance and to decide the appropriate treatment. *Chudoku Kenkyu* 2001;**14**(4):343–6.

197. Agarwal SB. A clinical, biochemical, neurobehavioral, and sociopsychological study of 190 patients admitted to hospital as a result of acute organophosphorus poisoning. *Environ Res* 1993;**62**(1):63–70.

198. Kundiev Y. Actual medical and ergonomic problems in agriculture in the Ukraine. *Int J Occup Med Environ Health* 1994;**7**(1):3–11.

199. Morton WE CE, Maricle RA, Douglas DD, Freed VH. Hypertension in Oregon pesticide-formulating workers. *J Occup Med* 1975;**17**(3):182–5.

200. Morgan DP LL, Saikaly HH. Morbidity and mortality in workers occupationally exposed to pesticides. *Arch Environ Contam Toxicol* 1980;**9**(3):349–82.

201. Anand M GA, Gopal K, Gupta GS, Khanna RN, Ray PK, Chandra SV. Hypertension and myocarditis in rabbits exposed to hexachlorocyclohexane and endosulfan. *Vet Hum Toxicol* 1990;**32**(6):521–3.

202. Anand M AA, Saxena PR. Effect of a neurotic pesticide, endosulfan, on tissue blood flow in cats, including regional cerebral circulation. *Vet Hum Toxicol* 1981;**23**(4):252–8.

203. Kreiss K ZM, Kimbrough RD, Needham LL, Smrek AL, Jones BT. Association of blood pressure and polychlorinated biphenyl levels. *JAMA* 1981;**245**(24): 2505–9.

204. Pesatori AC ZC, Guercilena S, Consonni D, Turrini D, Bertazzi PA. Dioxin exposure and non-malignant health effects: a mortality study. *Occup Environ Med* 1998;**55**(2):126–31.

205. Klatsky AL. Alcohol and cardiovascular diseases: a historical overview. *Ann NY Acad Sci* 2002;**957**:7–15.

206. Kotseva K PT. Study of the cardiovascular effects of occupational exposure to organic solvents. *Int Arch Occup Environ Health* 1998;**71** **Suppl**:S87-91.

207. Taylor. Cardiovascular effects of environmental chemicals. *Otolaryngol Head Neck Surg* 1996;**114**(2):209–11.

208. Laplanche A C-CF, Contassot JC, Lanouziere C. Exposure to vinyl chloride monomer: results of a cohort study after a seven year follow up. The French VCM Group. *Br J Ind Med* 1992;**49**(2):134–7.

209. Das UN. Nutritional factors in the pathobiology of human essential hypertension. *Nutrition* 2001;**17**(4):337–46.

210. Jee SH MEr, Guallar E, Singh VK, Appel LJ, Klag MJ. The effect of magnesium supplementation on blood pressure: a meta-analysis of randomized clinical trials. *Am J Hypertens* 2002;**15**(8):691–6.

211. Touyz RM. Role of magnesium in the pathogenesis of hypertension. *Mol Aspects Med* 2003;**24**(1–3):107–36.

212. Zittermann A. Vitamin D in preventive medicine: are we ignoring the evidence? *Br J Nutr* 2003;**89**(5):552–72.

213. Hill WD HD, Carroll JE, Wakade CG, Howard EF, Chen Q, Cheng C, Martin-Studdard A, Waller JL, Beswick RA. The NF-kappaB inhibitor diethyldithiocarbamate (DDTC) increases brain cell death in a transient middle cerebral artery occlusion model of ischemia. *Brain Res Bull.* 2001;**55**(3): 375–86.

214. Hollis G. Organophosphate poisoning versus brainstem stroke. *Med J Aust* 1999;**170**(12):596–7.

215. Shindell S US. Mortality of workers employed in the manufacture of chlordane: an update. *J Occup Med* 1986;**28**(7):497–501.

216. Kurth T KC, Berger K, Schaeffner ES, Buring JE, Gaziano JM. Smoking and the risk of hemorrhagic stroke in men. *Stroke.* 2003;**34**(5):1151–5.

217. Hong YC LJ, Kim H, Kwon HJ. Air pollution: a new risk factor in ischemic stroke mortality. *Stroke.* 2002;**33**(9):2165–9.

218. Spence J. Nutritional and metabolic aspects of stroke prevention. *Adv Neurol* 2003;**92**:173–8.

219. Muir K. Magnesium in stroke treatment. *Postgrad Med J.*2002;**78**(925):641–5.

220. Muir K. Magnesium for neuroprotection in ischaemic stroke: rationale for use and evidence of effectiveness. *CNS Drugs* 2001;**15**(12):921–30.

221. Bazzano LA HJ, Ogden LG, Loria C, Vupputuri S, Myers L, Whelton PK. Dietary intake of folate and risk of stroke in US men and women: NHANES I Epidemiologic Follow-up Study. National Health and Nutrition Examination Survey. *Stroke.* 2002;**33**(5):1183–8.

222. Kelly PJ SV, Kistler JP, Barron M, Lee H, Mandell R, Furie KL. Low vitamin B6 but not homocyst(e)ine is associated with increased risk of stroke and transient ischemic attack in the era of folic acid grain fortification. *Stroke.* 2003;**34**(6):51–4.

223. Maxwell CJ HD, Ebly EM. Serum folate levels and subsequent adverse cerebrovascular outcomes in elderly persons. *Dement Geriatr Cogn Disord* 2002;**13**(4):225–34.

224. Kim GW LA, Copin J, Watson BD, Chan PH. The cytosolic antioxidant, copper/zinc superoxide dismutase, attenuates blood-brain barrier disruption

and oxidative cellular injury after photothrombotic cortical ischemia in mice. *Neuroscience* 2001;**105**(4):1007–18.

225. Kadoya C DE, Yang GY, Stern JD, Betz AL. Preischemic but not postischemic zinc protoporphyrin treatment reduces infarct size and edema accumulation after temporary focal cerebral ischemia in rats. *Stroke.* 1995;**26**(6):1035–8.

226. Skerrett PJ HC. Consumption of fish and fish oils and decreased risk of stroke. *Prev Cardiol* 2003;**6**(1):38–41.

227. Iso H SS, Umemura U, Kudo M, Koike K, Kitamura A, Imano H, Okamura T, Naito Y, Shimamoto T. Linoleic acid, other fatty acids, and the risk of stroke. *Stroke.* 2002;**33**(8):2086–93.

228. Zajicek G. A new cancer hypothesis. *Med Hypotheses* 1996;**47**(2):111–5.

229. Korach K VD, Sylvia Curtis, Wayne Bocchinfuso. Xenoestrogens and estrogen receptor action. In: John Thomas HC, ed. *Endocrine Toxicology.* second ed. Washington: Taylor and Francis, 1997.

230. Dodds EL, W. Synthetic Oestrogenic agents without the phenanthrene nucleus. *Nature* 1936.

231. Gottlieb MS CJ. Case-control cancer mortality study and chlorination of drinking water in Louisiana. *Environ Health Perspect* 1982;**46**:169–77.

232. Lu-Yao GL GE. Changes in prostate cancer incidence and treatment in USA. *Lancet.* 1994;**343**(8892):251–4.

233. Edwards T. Prostate cancer. What your doctor doesn't tell you, 2002: 1–4.

234. Johansson JE AH, Andersson SO, Bergstrom R, Holmberg L, Krusemo UB. High 10-year survival rate in patients with early, untreated prostatic cancer. *JAMA* 1992;**267**(16):2191–6.

235. Couldwell C. Prostate cancer. *What Doctors Don't Tell You* 1995;**6**(4).

236. Wetherill YB PC, Monk KR, Puga A, Knudsen KE. The xenoestrogen bisphenol A induces inappropriate androgen receptor activation and mitogenesis in prostatic adenocarcinoma cells. *Mol Cancer Ther* 2002;**1**(7):515–24.

237. Huang HY AA, Norkus EP, Hoffman SC, Comstock GW, Helzlsouer KJ. Prospective study of antioxidant micronutrients in the blood and the risk of developing prostate cancer. *Am J Epidemiol.* 2003;**157**(4):335–44.

238. Vogt TM ZR, Graubard BI, Swanson CA, Greenberg RS, Schoenberg JB, Swanson GM, Hayes RB, Mayne ST. Serum selenium and risk of prostate cancer in U.S. blacks and whites. *Int J Cancer* 2003;**103**(5):664–70.

239. Liang JY LY, Zou J, Franklin RB, Costello LC, Feng P. Inhibitory effect of zinc on human prostatic carcinoma cell growth. *Prostate* 1999;**40**(3):200–7.

240. Krishnan AV PD, Feldman D. The role of vitamin D in prostate cancer. *Recent Results Cancer Res* 2003;**164**:205–21.

241. Baris D ZS. Epidemiology of lymphomas. *Curr Opin Oncol* 2000;**12**(5): 383–94.

242. Costantini AS ML, Kriebel D, Ramazzotti V, Rodella S, Scarpi E, Stagnaro E, Tumino R, Fontana A, Masala G, Vigano C, Vindigni C, Crosignani P, Benvenuti A, Vineis P. A multicenter case-control study in Italy on hematolymphopoietic neoplasms and occupation. *Epidemiology* 2001;**12**(1):78–87.

243. van Zaanen HC vdLJ. Thiamine deficiency in hematologic malignant tumors. Cancer 1992;**69**(7):1710–3.

244. Schreurs WH OJ, Egger RJ, Wedel M, Bruning PF. The influence of radiotherapy and chemotherapy on the vitamin status of cancer patients. *Int J Vitam Nutr Res* 1985;**55**(4):425–32.

245. Krishnan AV PD, Feldman D, Zhang SM GE, Hunter DJ, Rimm EB, Ascherio A, Colditz GA, Speizer FE, Willett WC. Vitamin supplement use and the risk of non-Hodgkin's lymphoma among women and men. *Am J Epidemiol* 2001;**153**(11):1056–63.

246. Kreutzer R NR, Lashuay N. Prevalence of people reporting sensitivities to chemicals in a population-based survey. *Am J Epidemiol* 1999;**150**(1):1–12.

247. Miller CS MH. Chemical sensitivity attributed to pesticide exposure versus remodeling. *Arch Environ Health* 1995;**50**(2):119–29.

248. Staudenmayer H. Psychological treatment of psychogenic idiopathic environmental intolerance. *Occup Med.* 2000;**15**(3):627–46.

249. Schumm WR RE, Jurich AP, Bollman SR, Webb FJ, Castelo CS, Stever JC, Sanders D, Bonjour GN, Crow JR, Fink CJ, Lash JF, Brown BF, Hall CA, Owens BL, Krehbiel M, Deng LY, Kaufman M. Self-reported changes in subjective health and anthrax vaccination as reported by over 900 Persian Gulf War era veterans. *Psychol Rep* 2002;**90**(2):639–53.

250. Abdel-Rahman A SA, Abou-Donia MB. Disruption of the blood-brain barrier and neuronal cell death in cingulate cortex, dentate gyrus, thalamus, and hypothalamus in a rat model of Gulf-War syndrome. *Neurobiol Dis* 2002;**10**(3):306–26.

251. Black DW DB, Voelker MD, Clarke WR, Woolson RF, Barrett DH, Schwartz DA. Multiple chemical sensitivity syndrome: symptom prevalence and risk factors in a military population. *Arch Intern Med.* 2000;**160**(8):1169–76.

252. Lohmann K PA, Schwarz E. Multiple chemical sensitivity disorder in patients with neurotoxic illnesses. *Gesundheitswesen* 1996;**58**(6):322–31.

253. Evengard B KN. Chronic fatigue syndrome: probable pathogenesis and possible treatments. *Drugs* 2002;**62**(17):2433–46.

254. Desaiah D. Interaction of chlordecone with biological membranes. *J Toxicol Environ Health A* 1981;**8**(5–6):719–30.

255. Holmuhamedov EL KG, Baimuradov TB. Non-cholinergic toxicity of organophosphates in mammals: interaction of ethaphos with mitochondrial functions. *J Appl Toxicol* 1996;**16**(6):475–81.

256. Arrhenius E RL, Johansson L, Zetterqvist MA. Disturbance of microsomal detoxication mechanisms in liver by chlorophenol pesticides. *Chem Biol Interact* 1977;**18**(1):35–46.

257. Leonard C BC, O'Keane C, Doyle JS. 'Golf ball liver': agent orange hepatitis. *Gut* 1997;**40**(5):687–8.

258. Nohl H dSD, Summer KH. 2,3,7,8, tetrachlorodibenzo-p-dioxin induces oxygen activation associated with cell respiration. *Free Radic Biol Med* 1989;**6**(4):369–74.

259. Lovett GS SA. The analysis of drug action on mitochondrial oxidative phosphorylation. The choice of organic solvent for water-insoluble drugs. *Methods Find Exp Clin Pharmacol.* 1983;**5**(10):695–9.

260. Bereznowski Z. Effect of methyl methacrylate on mitochondrial function and structure. *Int J Biochem* 1994;**26**(9):1119–27.

261. Lardy H RP, Lin CH. Antibiotic inhibitors of mitochondrial ATP synthesis. *Fed Proc* 1975;**34**(8):1707–10.

262. Masubuchi Y YS, Horie T. Diphenylamine as an important structure of non-steroidal anti-inflammatory drugs to uncouple mitochondrial oxidative phosphorylation. *Biochem Pharmacol.* 1999;**58**(5):861–5.

263. Martin RJ RA, Bjorn H. Target sites of anthelmintics. *Parasitology* 1997;**114** (Suppl:S111–24).

264. Starkov AA WK. Structural determinants of fluorochemical-induced mitochondrial dysfunction. *Toxicol Sci.* 2002;**66**(2):244–52.

265. Jacobs G. ME: The latest theories. In: McTaggart L, ed. The Medical Desk Reference. London: What Doctors Don't Tell You Ltd, 2000: 19–21.

266. McCauley LA JS, Barkhuizen A, Shuell T, Tyree WA, Bourdette DN. Chronic fatigue in a population-based study of Gulf War veterans. *Arch Environ Health* 2002;**57**(4):340–8.

267. Tahmaz N SA, Cherrie JW. Chronic fatigue and organophosphate pesticides in sheep farming: a retrospective study amongst people reporting to a UK pharmacovigilance scheme. *Ann Occup Hyg* 2003;**47**(4):261–7.

268. Bell IR BC, Schwartz GE. Illness from low levels of environmental chemicals: relevance to chronic fatigue syndrome and fibromyalgia. *Am J Med* 1998;**105**(3A):74S–82S.

269. Artsimovich NG CV, Kornev AV, Ivanova TM, Chugunov AV, Oprishchenko MA. The chronic fatigue syndrome. *Zh Nevropatol Psikhiatr Im S S Korsakova* 1994;**94**(5):47–50.

270. Logan AC WC. Chronic fatigue syndrome: oxidative stress and dietary modifications. *Altern Med Rev* 2001;**6**(5):450–9.

271. Gray JB MA. Eicosanoids and essential fatty acid modulation in chronic disease and the chronic fatigue syndrome. *Med Hypotheses* 1994;**43**(1):31–42.

272. Thompson AE PJ. Increased prevalence of scleroderma in southwestern Ontario: a cluster analysis. *J Rheumatol* 2002;**29**(9):1867–73.

273. Mayes M. Epidemiologic studies of environmental agents and systemic autoimmune diseases. *Environ Health Perspect.* 1999;**107**(Suppl 5):743–8.

274. Galland L. Magnesium and immune function: an overview. *Magnesium* 1988;**7**(5–6):290–9.

275. Zhang Y GA. Animal models for scleroderma: an update. *Curr Rheumatol Rep* 2002;**4**(2):150–62.

276. Haustein UF ZV. Scleroderma and scleroderma-like diseases caused by environmental pollutants. *Derm Beruf Umwelt* 1986;**34**(3):61–7.

277. D'Cruz D. Autoimmune diseases associated with drugs, chemicals and environmental factors. *Toxicol Lett.* 2000;**112–113**:421–32.

278. Thomas P. Lupus erythematosus. In: McTaggart L, ed. Medical Desk Reference: What Doctors Don't Tell You Ltd, 2000: 27–29.

279. McTaggart L. Arthritis: the price of painkillers. In: McTaggart L, ed. The Medical Desk Reference. London: What Doctors Don't Tell You Ltd, 2000: 299–304.

280. McCarty MF RA. Niacinamide therapy for osteoarthritis – does it inhibit nitric oxide synthase induction by interleukin 1 in chondrocytes? *Med Hypotheses* 1999;**53**(4):350–60.

281. Brown A. Lupus erythematosus and nutrition: a review of the literature. *J Ren Nutr.* 2000;**10**(4):170–83.

282. Patavino T BD. Natural medicine and nutritional therapy as an alternative treatment in systemic lupus erythematosus. *Altern Med Rev* 2001;**6**(5):460–71.

283. Jacobson JL JS. Association of prenatal exposure to an environmental contaminant with intellectual function in childhood. *J Toxicol Clin Toxicol* 2002;**40**(4):467–75.

284. Olshan AF SJ, Bondy ML, Neglia JP, Pollock BH. Maternal vitamin use and reduced risk of neuroblastoma. *Epidemiology* 2002;**13**(5):575-80.

285. Rowland AS LC, Abramowitz AJ. The epidemiology of attention-deficit/hyperactivity disorder (ADHD): a public health view. *Ment Retard Dev Disabil Res Rev* 2002;**8**(3):162–70.

286. Edwards T. Ritalin: A recipe for cancer? *What Doctors Don't Tell You* 2003;**14**(3):1–4.

287. Sowell ER TP, Welcome SE, Henkenius AL, Toga AW, Peterson BS. Cortical abnormalities in children and adolescents with attention-deficit hyperactivity disorder. *Lancet* 2003;**362**(9397):1699–707.

288. Paule MG RA, Ferguson SA, Chelonis JJ, Tannock R, Swanson JM, Castellanos FX. Attention deficit/hyperactivity disorder: characteristics, interventions and models. *Neurotoxicol Teratol* 2000;**22**(5):631–51.

289. Schettler T. Toxic threats to neurologic development of children. *Environ Health Perspect.* 2001;**109**(Suppl 6):813–6.

290. He Y YX, Xu F. Application of Conners Rating Scales in the study of lead exposure and behavioral effects in children. *Zhonghua Yu Fang Yi Xue Za Zhi.* 2000;**34**(5):290–3.

291. Hardell L LG, Van Bavel B. Is DDT exposure during fetal period and breastfeeding associated with neurological impairment? *Environ Res.* 2002;**88**(3):141–4.

292. Kidd P. Attention deficit/hyperactivity disorder (ADHD) in children: rationale for its integrative management. *Altern Med Rev* 2000;**5**(5):402–28.

293. Kozielec T S-HB. Assessment of magnesium levels in children with attention deficit hyperactivity disorder (ADHD). *Magnes Res* 1997;**10**(2):143–8.

294. Institute M.I.N.D. M.I.N.D. Institute study confirms autism increase. Sacramento, California: M.I.N.D. Institute, 2002.

295. Collins V. Scots study on autism poses new question of MMR link. *The Herald* 2002 Jul 22.

296. Ingram JL PS, Tisdale B, Rodier PM. Prenatal exposure of rats to valproic acid reproduces the cerebellar anomalies associated with autism. *Neurotoxicol Teratol* 2000;**22**(3):319–24.

297. Shattock P. Autism. What Doctors Don't Tell You, 2000: 1–4.

298. Geier DA GM. A comparative evaluation of the effects of MMR immunization and mercury doses from thimerosal-containing childhood vaccines on the population prevalence of autism. *Med Sci Monit* 2004;**10**(3):I33–9.

299. Kidd P. Autism, an extreme challenge to integrative medicine. Part 2: medical management. *Altern Med Rev* 2002;**7**(6):472–99.

300. Leonard CM LL, Walsh K, Eckert MA, Mockler JL, Rowe LA, Williams S, DeBose CB. Anatomical risk factors that distinguish dyslexia from SLI predict reading skill in normal children. *J Commun Disord.* 2002;**35**(6):501–31.

301. Rice D BSJ. Critical periods of vulnerability for the developing nervous system: evidence from humans and animal models. *Environ Health Perspect* 2000;**108**(Suppl 3):511–33.

302. Capel ID PM, Dorrell HM, Williams DC, Grant EC. Comparison of concentrations of some trace, bulk, and toxic metals in the hair of normal and dyslexic children. *Clin Chem* 1981;**27**(6):879–81.

303. Glotzer DE FK, Bauchner H. Management of childhood lead poisoning: clinical impact and cost-effectiveness. *Med Decis Making* 1995;**15**(1):13–24.

304. Grant EC HJ, Davies S, Chasty H, Hornsby B, Galbraith J. Zinc deficiency in children with dyslexia: concentrations of zinc and other minerals in sweat and hair. *Br Med J (Clin Res Ed)* 1988;**296**(6622):607–9.

305. Hardman PK CJ, Lieberman AD. The effects of diet and sublingual provocative testing on eye movements with dyslexic individuals. *J Am Optom Assoc.* 1989;**60**(1):10–3.

Index